Recent Advances in
OBSTETRICS AND GYNAECOLOGY

JOHN BONNAR MA MD FRCOG
Professor of Obstetrics and Gynaecology, University of Dublin; Fellow of Trinity College, Dublin; Consultant Obstetrician and Gynaecologist, Rotunda Hospital, Adelaide Hospital and St. James' Hospital, Dublin, Ireland

Recent Advances in
OBSTETRICS AND GYNAECOLOGY

EDITED BY

JOHN BONNAR

NUMBER FOURTEEN

CHURCHILL LIVINGSTONE
EDINBURGH LONDON MELBOURNE AND NEW YORK 1982

CHURCHILL LIVINGSTONE
Medical Division of Longman Group Limited

Distributed in the United States of America by
Churchill Livingstone Inc., 19 West 44th Street, New
York, N.Y. 10036, and by associated companies,
branches and representatives throughout
the world.

First published 1982

ISBN 0 443 02209 7
ISSN 0143 6848

British Library Cataloguing in Publication Data
Recent advances in obstetrics and gynaecology.
   —14
   1. Gynaecology—Periodicals
   2. Obstetrics—Periodicals
   618'.05   RG1

Library of Congress Catalog Card Number 79–40258

Printed in Great Britain at The Pitman Press, Bath

Preface

Recent Advances in Obstetrics and Gynaecology was first published in 1926 by Mr Alex Bourne, the distinguished obstetrician and gynaecologist, of St Mary's Hospital, London. It is my privilege to accept the invitation of the Publishers, Churchill Livingstone to edit the 14th volume of *Recent Advances in Obstetrics and Gynaecology*. In so doing, I am conscious of the international reputation which Recent Advances achieved under the previous editors Sir John Stallworthy of Oxford and Mr Gordon Bourne of London, two renowned obstetricians and gynaecologists and outstanding teachers.

My own background is one of clinical obstetrics and gynaecology first in the teaching hospitals of Glasgow, followed by Oxford and now in Dublin. Throughout I have had a continuing involvement in laboratory research related mainly to the problems of haemorrhage and thrombosis in obstetrics and gynaecology. University departments attract a constant stream of young men and women from home and abroad for specialist training. These doctors seek not only the most up-to-date scientific knowledge but also its application in their individual clinical practice. The 1970s witnessed an explosion of applied technology in obstetrics and gynaecology. The practitioner was bombarded with batteries of hormone assays, advances in ultrasound and the introduction of sophisticated electronic monitoring equipment. Much of this technology was introduced in an uncontrolled way with the assumption that better results would automatically follow. More extensive experience with these often high cost developments has revealed both limitations and unsuspected complications. In the 1980s a more selective approach to the use of technology is already evident partly as a consequence of painstaking research but also as a result of pertinent questions arising from well informed sections of the public. We are now more than ever conscious of the complex interplay of physical, emotional and psychological factors involved in patient care. These changes are reflected in the contributions to this 14th volume of *Recent Advances in Obstetrics and Gynaecology*.

The opening chapters of the fourteenth volume deal with the management of high-risk pregnancy, fetal monitoring in labour and the practice of amniocentesis. These are followed by up-dates on renal disease and diabetes in pregnancy. In Section 2 the care of the low birthweight infant is critically reviewed and new insights into the complex area of mother–infant interaction are presented. The chapters on fertility after childbirth and on trends in perinatal mortality in the developing world will be of special interest to readers in Asia and Africa. In the gynaecology section the chapters on the detection of ovulation for fertility and infertility, the management of dysovulatory infertility, in vitro fertilization and embryo transfer, and sexual dysfunction, contain a wealth of new material which will be of great help, especially to gynaecologists dealing with the infertile couple. The last two chapters provide detailed analyses of hormone therapy after the menopause and the advances in the treatment of carcinoma of the cervix and corpus uteri.

The subjects included in the 14th volume are of major concern to the practising obstetrician and gynaecologist. Specialists of international standing who have a major involvement in research have been invited to write on the individual topics to provide for the clinician a distillation of current research and scientific knowledge and its significance for present clinical practice. For this to be an up-to-date publication the time schedule followed by the contributors has to be strict. I would like to express my thanks to the individual authors who have generously given of their time and knowledge to produce such high quality contributions for this international publication.

Finally, may I thank Churchill Livingstone for their help and efficiency which enabled rapid publication of this volume and may you, the reader, find it of help in keeping abreast of the many developments in our rapidly evolving speciality.

Dublin, 1982   J.B.

Contributors

ALAN D. G. BROWN MB ChB FRCOG
Senior Lecturer in Obstetrics and Gynaecology, University of Manchester; Honorary Consultant, University Hospital of South Manchester, Manchester

JOHN M. DAVISON MSc MB BS MRCOG
Scientific Staff, MRC Human Reproduction Group, Newcastle upon Tyne; Consultant Obstetrician and Gynaecologist, Newcastle Area Health Authority (Teaching)

M. IVO DRURY MD FRCP FRCOG
Physician in Charge, Diabetes/Endocrine Unit, Mater Misericordiae Hospital, Dublin; Consultant Physician, National Maternity Hospital, Dublin; Consultant Endocrinologist, Coombe Lying-in Hospital, Dublin; Diabetologist, Rotunda Hospital, Dublin

ANNA M. FLYNN MRCOG
Senior Research Fellow, Birmingham Maternity Hospital, Birmingham

JOHN T. FRANCE PhD FAACB
Associate Professor in Steroid Biochemistry, Postgraduate School of Obstetrics and Gynaecology, University of Auckland, National Women's Hospital, Auckland, New Zealand

ALFRED WHITE FRANKLIN MB BCh FRCP
Consultant Paediatrician to St Bartholomew's and Queen Charlotte's Maternity Hospitals

SIMON R. HENDERSON MA BM BCh MRCOG FACOG DPhil
Assistant Clinical Professor of Obstetrics, Gynecology and Reproductive Sciences, University of California; Attending Gynecologist and Reproductive Endocrinologist, Microsurgeon and Infertility Specialist, Children's Hospital, San Francisco

PETER W. HOWIE MD FRCOG
Professor of Obstetrics and Gynaecology, University of Dundee, Ninewells Hospital and Medical School, Dundee; Consultant Obstetrician and Gynaecologist, MRC Reproductive Biology Unit, University of Edinburgh Centre for Reproductive Biology, Edinburgh

ADRIAN KATZ MD
Professor of Medicine; Head, Section of Nephrology, University of Chicago Pritzker School of Medicine, Chicago

JOHN KELLY FRCS FRCOG
Consultant Obstetrician and Gynaecologist, Birmingham Maternity Hospital, Birmingham

PER KOLSTAD MD FRCOG
Chief, Department of Gynaecological Oncology, The Norwegian Radium Hospital; Professor of Gynaecology, University of Oslo, Norway

MARSHALL D. LINDHEIMER MD
Professor of Obstetrics and Gynaecology and Medicine, University of Chicago Pritzker School of Medicine, Chicago

A. LUCAS MA MB BChir MRCP
Lecturer in Paediatrics, University of Cambridge; Registrar, The Cambridge Maternity Hospital, Cambridge

ALAN S. McNEILLY PhD
MRC Unit of Reproductive Biology, University of Edinburgh Centre for Reproductive Biology, Edinburgh

JAMES F. PEARSON MD FRCOG
Reader in Obstetrics and Gynaecology, Welsh National School of Medicine, Cardiff

J. W. K. RITCHIE MD MRCOG
Senior Lecturer in Midwifery and Gynaecology, Queen's University, Belfast

CLIFF ROBERTON MA MB FRCP
Consultant Paediatrician to the Cambridge Maternity Hospital and Addenbrooke's Hospital, Cambridge; Associate Lecturer in Paediatrics, University of Cambridge, Cambridge

JOHN M. STRONGE MAO MRCOG
Consultant Obstetrician and Gynaecologist, National Maternity Hospital, Dublin

R. L. TAMBYRAJA PhD FRCSE MRCOG
Associate Professor, Department of Obstetrics and Gynaecology, National University of Singapore, Kandang Kerbau Hospital, Singapore

W. THOMPSON BSc MD FRCOG
Professor of Midwifery and Gynaecology, Queen's University, Belfast

ALAN TROUNSON MSc PhD
Senior Lecturer in Obstetrics and Gynaecology, Monash University, Queen Victoria Medical Centre, Melbourne, Australia

WULF H. UTIAN MB BCh PhD FRCOG FACOG FICS
Director of Obstetrics and Gynecology, Mount Sinai Medical Centre of Cleveland; Associate Professor, Department of Reproductive Biology, Case Western Reserve University, Cleveland, Ohio

CARL WOOD FRCS FRCOG FRACOG
Chairman, Department of Obstetrics and Gynaecology, Monash University, Queen Victoria Medical Centre, Melbourne, Australia

Contents

Section 1   OBSTETRICS

1. Monitoring high-risk pregnancy *James F. Pearson*   3

2. Fetal monitoring in labour *Anna M. Flynn   John Kelly*   25

3. A critical review of amniocentesis in clinical practice *J. W. K. Ritchie   W. Thompson*   47

4. Renal disease in pregnancy *John M. Davison   Adrian Katz   Marshall D. Lindheimer*   71

5. Diabetes mellitus and pregnancy *M. Ivo Drury   John M. Stronge*   95

Section 2   PERINATAL MEDICINE

6. The care of the low birthweight infant *A. Lucas   Cliff Roberton*   115

7. Mother-infant interaction: the bonding of affection *Alfred White Franklin*   161

8. Fertility after childbirth *Peter W. Howie   Alan S. McNeilly*   181

9. Trends in perinatal mortality in the developing world *R. L. TambyRaja*   201

Section 3 GYNAECOLOGY

10. The detection of ovulation for fertility and infertility *John T. France*   215

11. The management of dysovulatory infertility *Simon R. Henderson*   241

12. In vitro fertilisation and embryo transfer *Carl Wood   Alan Trounson*   259

13. Sexual dysfunction in gynaecological and obstetrical practice *Alan D. G. Brown*   283

14. Cost-effectiveness of hormone therapy after the menopause *Wulf H. Utian*   307

15. Advances in the treatment of carcinoma of the cervix and corpus uteri *Per Kolstad*   325

Index   341

SECTION 1

Obstetrics

1. Monitoring high-risk pregnancy

James F. Pearson

The highest risk of perinatal death usually occurs amongst those mothers who suffer from multiple problems of social, biological and pathological origin. The Second Report of the Perinatal Mortality Survey demonstrated the cumulative risks of adverse maternal age, parity, social class, smoking habits, maternal height and complications of pregnancy such as pre-eclampsia (Goldstein, 1969). Furthermore, those women who had the highest cumulative risk were those who were likely to have had the poorest medical care. Indeed, it has been suggested that 'no amount of technical expertise will help a woman who cannot or will not accept it' (Alberman, 1976). It therefore follows that such 'high risk' mothers, who constitute a dense core of obstetric morbidity, must be persuaded to cooperate so that effective monitoring is used for those who most need it.

THE IDENTIFICATION OF THE HIGH RISK PREGNANCY

Clinical techniques

Provided that the pregnant woman presents herself for advice as early as possible, the first and most important step is to obtain a good history. The main purpose of this should be to highlight those factors which may predispose to perinatal death or injury.

Critical review of records at perinatal mortality meetings often reveal important omissions in the history or failure to 'flag' or to emphasise vital items. It follows that perhaps the traditional type of history-taking has many faults and that a more structured and formalised approach might be better. Various schematic approaches have been tried in different institutions. One of the best, in the opinion of the writer, is that which originated in Edinburgh (Boddy et al, 1976) which is described here in some detail. The main characteristics of the scheme may be summarised as follows:

Each patient is formally assessed by noting features of the pregnancy against a check-list of risk factors, and appraising their significance. A pre-planned programme of management automatically follows the identification of risk factors, and assessment is continually updated, thus focusing attention on the problems arising in the individual pregnancy.

A special feature of the system is a risk card which is reproduced in Tables 1.1(a) and (b). One side of the card summarises relevant factors at booking and the reverse side is designed to record adverse factors arising during pregnancy. The use of a formal and objective assessment of risk has certain advantages over traditional methods of management. However, it is acknowledged that such an assessment is not an exact science but a deductive process. The advantages of the system can be categorised as follows:

1. It ensures that all patients receive a comprehensive and identical assessment during pregnancy and therefore encourages a high standard of care.
2. It enables the obstetrician to give advice to the family doctor on clinical problems without the need for a formal referral to hospital.
3. It encourages the use of planned protocols for the management of pregnancy complications and lays the foundations for the subsequent evaluation of different forms of treatment.
4. It provides a mechanism whereby innovations in management may be introduced in an orderly manner thus ensuring that all patients receive the benefit.

Table 1.1a   Front side of the Edinburgh 'risk card'

NAME:	DOCTOR: ....

BOOKING HISTORY
- [ ] Age less than 18 yrs.
- [ ] Age over 38 yrs.
- [ ] Primigravid age 30 yrs or more
- [ ] Parity = / more than 5

LMP DETAILS
- [ ] LMP uncertain ± 2 weeks
- [ ] Pill stopped 1 or 2 periods before LMP
- [ ] Cycle length prior to LMP greater than 30 days
- [ ] IUCD in situ/on Pill after conception
- [ ] Out of wedlock pregnancy
- [ ] Vaginal bleeding since LMP

PAST OBSTETRIC HISTORY
- [ ] SB/NND
- [ ] Small for dates (<10th Centile)
- [ ] Large for dates (>90th Centile)
- [ ] Fetal abnormality ....
- [ ] Antibodies in previous pregnancy
- [ ] Hypertension/Eclampsia
- [ ] Termination of Pregnancy/Spon. Abortion × 2
- [ ] Premature labour (20–37 weeks)
- [ ] Previous Cervical Suture
- [ ] Previous Caesarean Section
- [ ] PPH/MROP
- [ ] Labour of less than 4 hours

MATERNAL HEALTH
- [ ] Chronic Illness/Drugs ....
- [ ] Hypertension/Proteinuria
- [ ] Infertility with Medical Advice
- [ ] Uterine Anomaly including Fibroids
- [ ] Smoking 10/day at Conception
- [ ] Soc. Sec. Benefits
- [ ] Isolated at Home
- [ ] Family History of Diabetes/Fetal Abnormality ....
- [ ] Completed by .... Date ....

BOOKING EXAMINATION
- [ ] BP = / more than 140/90
- [ ] Maternal Weight = / more 85 kg
- [ ] Maternal Weight = / less than 45 kg
- [ ] Maternal Height = / less than 5 ft
- [ ] Cardiac Murmur Detected/Referred
- [ ] Uterus large/small for dates
- [ ] Other Pelvic Mass Detected
- [ ] Blood Group Rh Negative
- [ ] Completed by .... Date ....

5. It provides a practical method of identifying high risk pregnancies for intensive management during labour.

Once the risk card is completed the doctor may then refer to Table 1.2 to identify the clinical problems which are more likely to occur when a particular risk factor has been noted. An appropriate line of action is also suggested in the right hand column.

Having followed the formal booking and screening procedure it is necessary to have a continuing plan of management. The high-risk pregnancy commonly raises problems regarding the adequacy of fetal growth and the state of oxygenation of the

Table 1.1b Reverse side of the Edinburgh 'risk card'

FACTORS ARISING DURING PREGNANCY																
Weeks of Pregnancy																
FM Not felt																
Hb < 10 gm %																
Poor Weight Gain																
Wt. loss																
Proteinuria																
Glycosuria																
Bacilluria																
BP Systolic > 155																
Diastolic > 88																
Rh Ne/Antibodies																
Uterus large for dates																
Uterus small for dates																
No increase in fundus (Zone)																
Excess liquor																
Mal presentation																
ECV Successful																
Unsuccessful																
Head not engaged																
Any bleeding PV																
Premature labour																
Vaginal infection																
Sign when completed																
Insert Date																

Table 1.2 Prenatal assessment and consequences

Prenatal assessment factors	Potential adverse effect on pregnancy	Clinical programme
Age and parity		
Age less than 18 years	Unplanned pregnancy. Poor attendance at clinics. Premature labour.	See health visitor for counselling. Early diagnosis of premature labour and prompt referral.
Age over 38 years	Down's Syndrome. Feto-placental dysfunction	Prenatal counselling. Amniocentesis at 16 weeks. Serial tests of feto-placental function.
Primigravid aged 30 years or more — (Women aged 30 years or more who have previously conceived but aborted before 20 weeks should be included)	Pregnancy hypertension Feto-placental dysfunction	Estimate plasma creatinine and urate at first visit. Serial tests of feto-placental function.
Parity = / more than 5 — (5 or more pregnancies of gestational age over 20 weeks or birth weights of 500 g)	Feto-placental dysfunction Postpartum haemorrhage	Serial tests of feto-placental function. Active management of the third stage of labour.
LMP details		
LMP uncertain ± 2 weeks	Uncertain gestational age	*Clinical assessment* of gestational age including measurement of fundal height
Pill stopped 1 or 2 periods before LMP — oral contraceptives discontinued within 1 or 2 cycles before LMP		*Sonar assessment* of gestational age is indicated in pregnancies at risk from feto-placental dysfunction.
Cycle length prior to LMP greater than 30 days — (refers to menstrual pattern within 3 months of LMP)		
IUCD in situ/or pill after conception (refers to the estimated date of conception)	IUCD in situ-abortion/premature labour	IUCD may be removed during pregnancy; Early diagnosis of premature labour and prompt referral.
Out of wedlock pregnancy — (Unmarried at conception and no prospect of marriage during pregnancy)	Unplanned pregnancy: Poor attendance at clinics	See health visitor for counselling
Vaginal Bleeding since LMP — (refers to bleeding in early pregnancy)	Molar pregnancy	Estimation of urinary HCG; sonar examination
Past obstetric history		
SB/NND — Fetal death in utero after 20 weeks gestation (or birth wt of 500 gm or more) or death in the first 4 weeks after birth	Depends on cause of death — fetal malformation, prematurity, feto-placental dysfunction	Determine cause of death from previous records. Serial tests of feto-placental function may be indicated.

Prenatal assessment factors	Potential adverse effect on pregnancy	Clinical programme
Small for dates (<10th centile) — delivered of an infant whose birth weight, corrected for gestational age, is below the 10th centile	Small for dates infant. Feto-placental dysfunction	Sonar examination in early pregnancy if gestational age in doubt. Serial tests of feto-placental function may be indicated.
Large for dates (>90th centile) — delivered of an infant whose birth weight, corrected for gestational age, is above 90th centile	Gestational diabetes Large fetus, dystocia, birth injury	Glucose Tolerance Test in pregnancy. Intensive care in labour.
Fetal abnormality — (refers to congenital malformations and inherited disorders)	Congenital malformation Inherited disorder	Discuss with Neonatologist before 14 weeks. Genetic counselling and amniocentesis may be indicated.
Antibodies in previous pregnancy — ABO/Rh antibodies in maternal blood or feto-maternal incompatibility	Feto-maternal blood group incompatibility	Serology and Coomb's test in early pregnancy, 20, 32 and 38 weeks
Hypertension/eclampsia — Hypertension is defined as BP 140/90 on two occasions during the prenatal/intrapartum/postnatal period)	Pregnancy hypertension; Renal disease	Estimate plasma creatinine and urate at first visit. Serial tests of feto-placental function may be indicated
Termination of pregnancy/spon. abortion — X2	Cervical incompetence	A cervical suture may be required; Early diagnosis of premature labour and prompt referral. Tests of feto-placental function are indicated if uterine relaxant (Beta mimetic) therapy is anticipated
Premature Labour – (20–37 weeks) Previous cervical suture	Premature labour	
Previous Caesarean section — including hysterotomy	Uterine rupture (usually after 37 weeks)	X-ray pelvimetry may be requested at 36 weeks. Discuss method of delivery with specialist
PPH/MROP — (postpartum haemorrhage/manual removal of placenta)	Recurrent third stage problems; uterine abnormality	Confinement in specialist hospital is advisable
Labour of less than 4 hours	'Born before arrival'; Neonatal asphyxia, hypothermia	Prompt admission to hospital at or before the onset of labour

Maternal health

Chronic Illness/Drugs — including cardiac, renal, collagen, diabetic, epileptic, haematological, gastro-intestinal, nervous disorders)	There may be adverse effects of the disease on pregnancy and pregnancy on the disease	A plan of management to be outlined in collaboration with obstetrician, physician and neonatologist
Hypertension/proteinuria — (BP 140/90 or proteinuria on two or more occasions in the non-pregnant state)	Pregnancy hypertension: Renal disease Feto-placental dysfunction	Estimate plasma creatinine and urate at first visit; Hypotensive drugs may be indicated. Serial tests of feto-placental function

Prenatal assessment factors	Potential adverse effect on pregnancy	Clinical programme
Infertility with medical advice	Anxiety during pregnancy Feto-placental dysfunction	Reassurance by good prenatal care Serial tests of feto-placental function may be indicated
Uterine anomaly including fibroids — (bicornuate, unicornuate uterus and fibroids)	Premature labour; malpresentation Degeneration of a fibroid	Sonar examination. Increased uterine activity controlled by bed rest and Beta-mimetic therapy. Tests of feto-placental function.
Smoking 10/day at conception	Feto-placental dysfunction	Serial tests of feto-placental function after 30 weeks if fundal height in Zone 4
Soc. Sec. Benefits — (the couple qualify for social security benefits)	Poor attendance at clinics Feto-placental dysfunction	Counselling by health visitor
Isolated at home — (applies to rural areas at distance from hospital)	Delivery in transit, neonatal asphyxia, hypothermia	Timely admission to hospital before onset of labour
Family history of diabetes — (Siblings, mother or maternal grandmother)	Gestational diabetes	Glucose tolerance test in pregnancy
Family history of fetal abnormality (Siblings, parents, grandparents)	Fetal malformation	Genetic counselling by 14th week of pregnancy. Amniocentesis at 16 weeks may be indicated
Booking examination		
BP = / more than 140/90	Pregnancy hypertension	Exclude aortic coarctation by clinical examination; phaeochromocytoma by 24 hour urinary VMA excretion; estimate plasma creatinine and urate
Maternal weight = / more than 85 kg	Pregnancy hypertension Gestational diabetes	Plasma urate and creatinine at first visit. Seek dietetic advice. Glucose tolerance test during pregnancy
Maternal weight = / less than 45 kg	Feto-placental dysfunction	Serial tests of feto-placental function may be indicated
Cardiac murmur detected/referred to cardiologist	Asymptomatic heart disease	Refer for cardiological opinion
Uterus large/small for dates	Multiple pregnancy Dates in doubt	Sonar examination
Other pelvic mass detected	Uterine fibroid or ovarian cyst	Sonar examination; bimanual examination under anaesthesia may be necessary
Blood group Rh negative	Rhesus isoimmunization	Blood group, serology and Coomb's test at booking, 20, 32 and 38 weeks

fetus. Some traditional clinical methods can be utilised with advantage. The two indices of maternal weight and uterine size have long been utilised but the value of such measurements will only be appreciated if normality and the degree of variation are defined. The pattern of weight gain and total weight increase during pregnancy vary widely and are related to the patient's initial body weight. Mothers whose initial body weights are outside the range 45 to 85 kg have weight gain characteristics which are significantly different from those of the remainder of the population. To correct for these differences would be difficult and would necessitate the construction of weight gain graphs based on initial body weight. For clinical purposes the authors of this scheme have highlighted only 'static weight' or 'weight loss' after the 20th week of pregnancy as being of practical importance.

Uterine growth in pregnancy
Starting with a reliable menstrual history and early bimanual clinical examination to confirm gestational age, the most commonly used method of assessing fetal growth is based upon serial clinical examination during pregnancy by abdominal palpation, where the observer tries to measure relative growth of the uterus and its contents. The growth-retarded fetus shows poor or static incremental growth and a diminution in the quantity of liquor amnii. There are so many drawbacks to this form of assessment that no obstetrician should ever consider himself to be precise. For instance, the distances between the symphysis pubis, umbilicus and xiphisternum — the tradition-al landmarks — vary widely. Even measurements of the distance of the uterine fundus from the symphysis with a tape or calipers show considerable discrepancies between patients at any given period of gestation (Beazley & Underhill, 1970). To determine that a given fetus is 'small for dates', the duration of gestation must be accurately known. The accurate dating of a pregnancy is often difficult since as many as 30 per cent of women do not remember the date of their last menstrual period (LMP) and even when they do, the menstrual cycle may be irregular, or their LMP may have been a withdrawal bleed following oral contraceptive usage.

Nevertheless, in Sweden, Westin (1977), whilst acknowledging the disadvantages as outlined above, has demonstrated an impressive fall in perinatal mortality following the introduction of his 'gravidogram' in a Stockholm hospital. He also showed convincingly that the serial measurement of the symphysis-fundus distance when plotted on an experimentally derived nomogram (which he called a gravidogram) was superior to both HPL and urinary oestriol in detecting growth retardation. Belizan et al (1978) developed a similar nomogram for use in an Argentinian population. Of 44 neonates who were light for gestational age, 38 had a uterine height below the 10th centile (sensitivity 86 per cent). Of 95 neonates with adequate birth weight, 85 had uterine heights above the 10th centile (specificity 90 per cent).

Quaranta et al (1981) found that 30 out of 41 small-for-dates infants were detected using this technique and suggested that a single measurement was most accurate for detecting low birthweight for gestation at 32 to 33 weeks.

The Edinburgh scheme uses the chart illustrated in Figure 1.1 which was derived from the local population. To surmount the problem of differing maternal abdominal lengths, the distance between the symphysis and xiphisternum is recorded separately. Women with short abdominal lengths (less than 37 cm in their population) tend to have measurements recorded in zone 3 or even in zone 4 and may appear falsely as being small-for-dates.

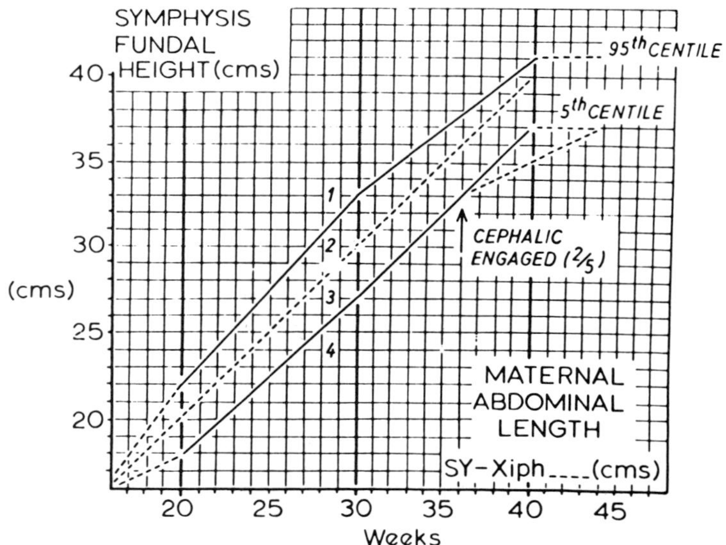

Fig. 1.1 Symphysis-fundus nomogram (from Boddy et al, 1976). The measurement of total abdominal length is measured from the upper border of the symphysis to the xiphisternum. Women with short abdominal lengths (<37 cm) usually have measurements in the lower part of zone 3 but may fall into zone 4 and appear SFD.

Estimation of the duration of pregnancy by measurements of fundal height is only approximate, but uniformity of recording technique allows more confidence to be placed in results from different observers, and simplifies interpretation. From the 20th week of pregnancy the symphysis-fundus length has an almost linear relationship to the weeks of pregnancy (approximately 1 cm per week). This is represented on the graph by the central dotted line. The variation around this is ±3 cm, and for a given gestational age measurements recorded in zones 2 and 3 would be considered normal for the Edinburgh population. Such measurements are useful confirmatory evidence of dates and satisfactory growth, but in the absence of an adequate menstrual history cannot be used to assess gestational age.

Measurements recorded in zones 1 and 4 on the chart identify the large and small uterus and raise several possibilities, all of which are important and justify specialist opinion and sonar examination. For example, the estimated gestational age may be wrong, fetal growth may be inappropriate or the pregnancy may be multiple.

Ultrasonography and the high-risk pregnancy

Routine scanning in early pregnancy
A very good case can be made for routine scanning in early pregnancy: to determine gestational age in the face of poor menstrual data, to spot multiple pregnancies and to identify certain early pregnancy abnormalities. Measurement of the fetal crown-rump length (CRL) in the first trimester (Robinson, 1973) or the biparietal diameter (BPD)

to 24 weeks (Campbell, 1976) are accurate measures of gestational age. An accurate knowledge of gestational age is necessary for the interpretation of serum alpha feto-protein levels and for the timing of diagnostic amniocentesis for fetal chromosome analysis. Because it is difficult to determine that a given fetus is small-for-dates (SFD) later on in pregnancy unless gestational age has first been ascertained, there are great advantages in scanning all patients.

Poor intrauterine fetal growth
Though it has been shown that up to 73 per cent of SFD fetuses can be identified by serial cephalometry (Campbell & Dewhurst, 1971) actual detection rates in routine clinical practice are worse (Neilson & Hood, 1980).

In the SFD baby the organs most affected by undernutrition are the thymus, the spleen and the liver (Gruenwald, 1974). On the other hand the brain is the organ least affected by the process. This brain-sparing effect is likely to be due to the preferential redistribution of blood to the brain (Assali & Brinkman, 1973). Thus the biparietal diameter represents an index of the size of the organ least affected by poor nutrition, a fact which probably explains the poor results of serial cephalometry in the routine management of the high risk pregnancy. It has also been recognised that two distinct types of fetal growth impairment occur: symmetrical and asymmetrical.

Symmetrical growth retardation
These infants do not appear to be wasted at birth. The growth of the BPD shows early departure from the normal curve but continues at a slower than normal rate until delivery. Many of these infants have a poor growth potential despite a satisfactory intrauterine environment. It has been suggested that this is the result of an insult in early pregnancy which may be genetic, as in chromosomal abnormalities, or due to a viral infection during organogenesis. In such cases there is a permanent loss of cells and the fetal brain is not spared (Winick, 1971).

Asymmetrical growth retardation
These infants have a wasted appearance at birth with large heads when compared to the size of the trunk — although it must be pointed out that the head size is somewhat smaller than normal (McLean & Usher, 1970). BPD growth in such cases is usually normal until the third trimester when marked slowing of growth may be observed. These infants have a high incidence of perinatal asphyxia and neonatal hypoglycaemia as one would expect in infants suffering from failing placental exchange which is the cause of this type of growth deficit.

In order better to differentiate between these groups, various ultrasonic measurements of the fetus have been tried. Total intra-uterine volume (Hobbins et al, 1978) depends on the fact that an SFD infant is usually associated with a small placenta and oligohydramnios. But not only may growth retardation co-exist with a normal volume of liquor, polyhydramnios may be present with an SFD fetus which may have an abnormality. The head to abdomen area ratio can identify and categorise the SFD fetus in about 80 per cent of cases (Varma et al, 1979). This measurement is time-consuming and is abnormal in only half the cases before 36 weeks (Wittman et al, 1979).

The development of a rapid ultrasonic screening procedure to identify the SFD fetus is an attractive concept. Based on the Scottish figures for 1977 where it was shown that 45 per cent of intrauterine deaths in growth-retarded fetuses occurred after the 36th week (McIlwaine et al, 1979), Neilson et al (1980) showed that the measurement of the crown-rump length × the cross-sectional area of the trunk gave an index which correctly identified 34 out of 36 SFD fetuses (94 per cent) when scanned between 34 and 36 weeks gestation. One advantage claimed for this measurement is that the entire examination takes only four minutes.

Whilst such a screening procedure is a useful advance, many SFD infants die earlier than the 36th week, and although it is of value to know that an infant is growth-retarded, this knowledge, of itself, does not indicate to the clinician the length of time the fetus will survive undelivered. Other indices of feto-placental function are thus required.

Hormone assays
Although still in widespread use, hormone assays as a means of judging fetal wellbeing have been disappointing.

Two hormonal tests of fetal wellbeing are currently popular: oestriol and human placental lactogen (HPL).

Concentrations of the three principal oestrogens in the maternal urine (oestrone, 17β-oestradiol and oestriol) are markedly raised during pregnancy. The excretion of oestrone is increased a hundredfold and oestriol a thousandfold. The great increase in the excretion of oestriol is due to an enzyme (16α-hydroxylase) present in the fetal adrenal and liver. Thus, measurement of oestriol in urine or plasma is commonly used as an index of feto-placental function. The normal range of values of oestriol is wide, and as there is a diurnal variation, serial measurements are required to determine a trend, although any acute fall of 40 to 50 per cent may be considered abnormal (Hull & Chard, 1976). Furthermore, as the levels of oestriol increase markedly during the last trimester in the normal patient, it is necessary not only to perform serial assays, but also to have a reasonably accurate idea of gestational age for the proper interpretation of this test.

Human placental lactogen (HPL) is a protein hormone produced by the syncytio-trophoblast with many similarities to growth hormone and prolactin. The precise physiological role of HPL remains unclear. It is easy to measure in maternal blood and results can be available within two hours.

HP levels in the mother rise progressively with gestational age, reaching a plateau for the last month. As with oestriol measurements, the normal range is wide and serial sampling is required to determine a trend. It is also necessary to know the gestational age to evaluate the results. Although low levels of HPL have been reported prior to fetal death (Ward et al, 1973), HPL levels sometimes remain within the normal range until after fetal death has occurred (Hull & Chard, 1976).

In practice hormonal tests of placental function have not fulfilled the expectations of their originators, due to the variety of pathophysiology found in pregnancy and the overlap of values found between normal and abnormal pregnancy.

Dynamic tests of fetal wellbeing
The development of dynamic tests of fetal wellbeing has been advantageous. These tests tell us how a baby is behaving 'in utero' and, as such, help the clinician to

distinguish between an 'at risk' but healthy baby from one suffering from oxygen deprivation.

Two main categories of such tests are in general use: fetal movement recording and antenatal cardiotocography. The ultrasonic evaluation of fetal breathing movements as an indicator of fetal vitality is promising, but its value in clinical management has yet to be determined. Fetal breathing and its possible clinical significance was recently reviewed by Wilds (1978), who concluded that the available ultrasonic instrumentation for such recordings has important theoretical and practical drawbacks and that even these technical difficulties seemed less formidable than the biological problems of ascertaining how breathing movements are controlled.

Fetal movement recording

Sadovsky & Yaffe (1973) made the important observation that in cases of placental insufficiency where the fetus died, fetal movements decreased and stopped 12 to 48 hours before the fetal heart ceased to beat. They called this the 'movement alarm signal' and suggested that when this signal became manifest, immediate delivery could save the life of the baby. This observation pointed the way to the development of a dynamic non-invasive test which could help to distinguish an 'at risk' but healthy baby from one about to die. It was hoped that this would be of sufficient predictive value to enable therapeutic action to be undertaken.

In cases where intrauterine fetal death occurs, a 12-hour daily fetal movement count (DFMC) recorded by the mother shows a characteristic pattern. Fetal activity diminishes over the course of several days and movements cease altogether between 12 to 48 hours before the fetal heart stops. The four charts shown in Figure 1.2 illustrate this.

Reinold (1973) used ultrasound to record fetal movements in early pregnancy and found that spontaneous movements were absent, infrequent or sluggish in cases of disturbed fetal wellbeing. The same group of workers later demonstrated that death of the fetus even as early as the third month of pregnancy was preceded by a reduction of fetal activity over several days, fetal movements ceasing shortly before abortion took place.

Maternal observations of fetal movements are subjective with all the disadvantages that this implies, but in an objective study (Sadovsky et al, 1973) about 87 per cent of fetal movements recorded on an electromagnetic device were felt by the mother.

Comparison of subjective and ultrasonic assessments of fetal movements later confirmed a significant positive correlation between the two methods of recording, but the scatter was wide and low subjective movement counts correlated poorly with ultrasonic measurement (Gettinger et al, 1978). In this study there were wide differences in the rapidity, degree and vigour of observed movements. However, a group of workers from the same centre (Hertogs et al, 1979), using more definitive methods, have recently shown that the mother tended to perceive the more major fetal movements; those incorporating movements of all limbs, the trunk and the head. They found that most of their subjects were consistent and accurate in their perception of such large movements and concluded that fetal movement counts kept by mothers would be accurate and that low counts should indicate the need for closer monitoring of the fetus.

A range of fetal activity as measured by the 12-hour DFMC was published by

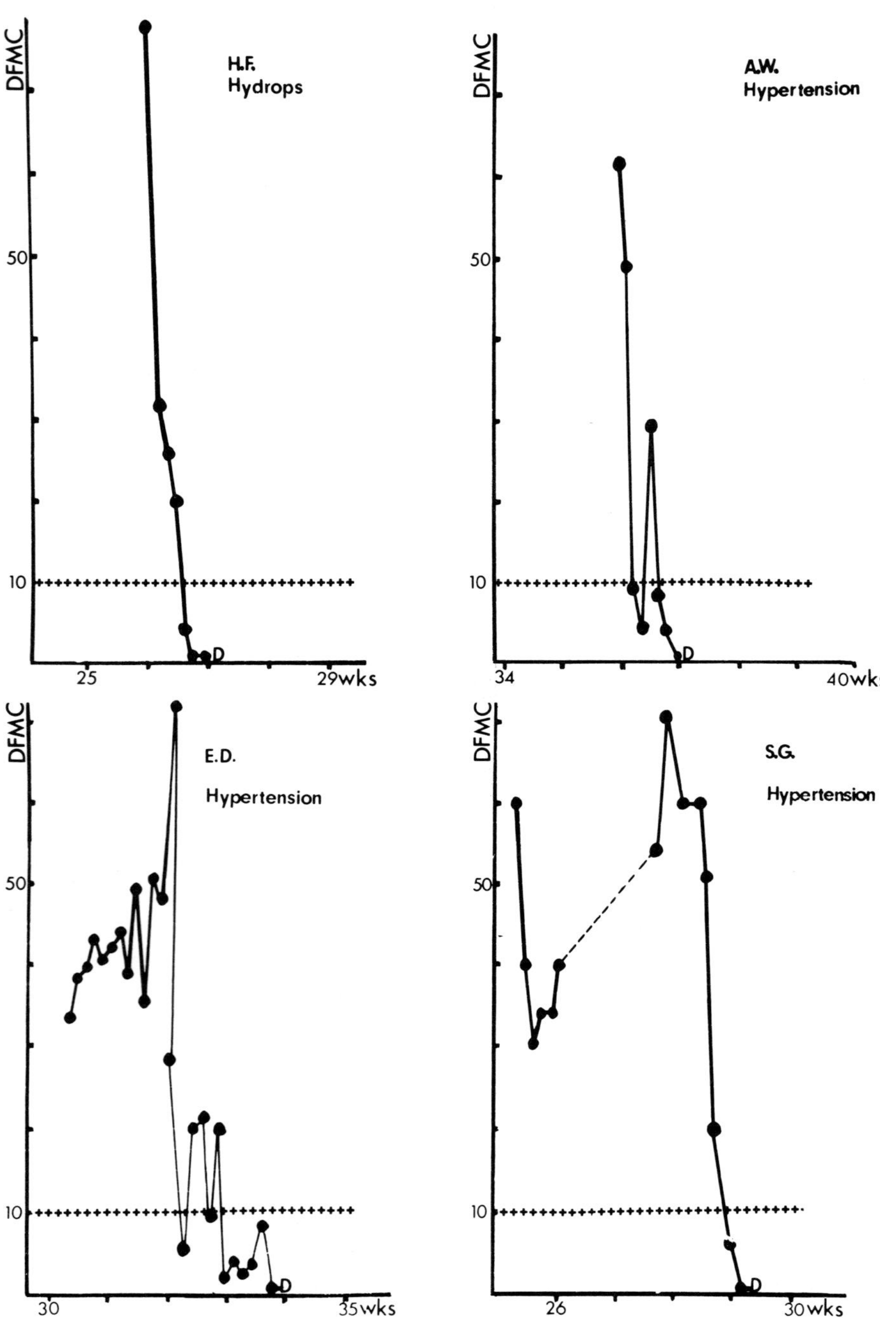

Fig. 1.2   12 hour daily fetal movement counts (DFMC) in four patients who suffered intrauterine fetal death before labour. Time of death is indicated (D). (From Pearson J F & Weaver J B, 1976.)

Pearson & Weaver in 1976 (Fig. 1.3), which showed that the lowest 2.5 per cent of 1654 DFMCs by 61 women who subsequently gave birth to healthy infants fell below 10 movements per 12 hours.

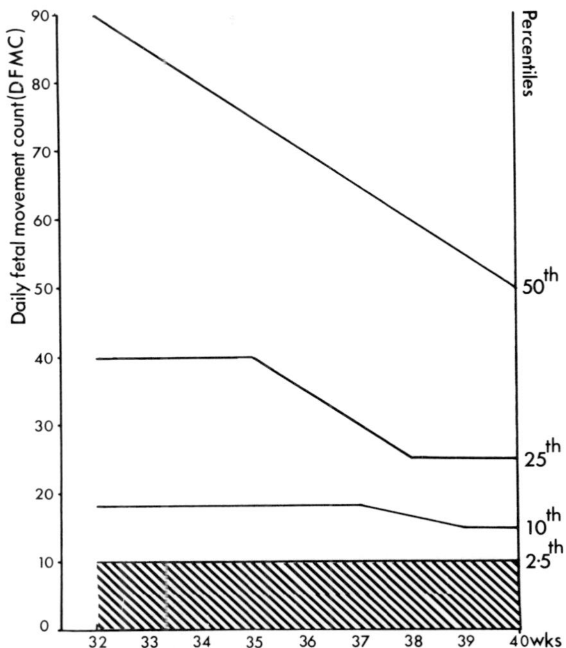

Fig. 1.3   Percentile distribution of 12 hour daily fetal movement counts below 50th percentile in 1654 counts from 61 patients between 32 and 40 weeks of pregnancy. (From Pearson J F & Weaver J B, 1976.)

Generally, fetal movements gradually decreased in number from the 32nd week of pregnancy to term, but the 2.5 per cent line remained constant at 10 movements per 12 hours and this they adopted as the lower limit of normal for clinical purposes. DFMC was also evaluated in a 'high risk' group of patients where the method compared favourably with a commonly used placental function test — the 24-hour urinary excretion of total oestrogen.

Sadovsky et al (1974) compared urinary oestriol findings with the DFMC and found that the DFMC was more reliable in predicting impending fetal death in utero. Spellacy et al (1976), using serum HPL as a yardstick, also advocated the use of maternal movement counts as a useful additional parameter of fetal vitality.

The most convincing evidence of the effectiveness of maternal monitoring of fetal movements came from a well conducted randomised controlled trial involving 2250 mothers, where there were eight intrauterine deaths of infants weighing more than 1500 g without major malformations in the patients not counting movements, and none in those who did (Neldam, 1980).

As has previously been explained, most traditional placental function tests depend for their interpretation upon an accurate knowledge of the duration of pregnancy. Whilst it is possible to determine that the fetus may be suffering from placental insufficiency by clinical and ultrasonic assessment of poor growth rate and by the finding of low values of biochemical placental function tests, the difficulty often facing the obstetrician is to decide whether or not to expedite delivery in the interests of the infant. This is a particularly vexing problem when the infant is very premature. If the fetus is delivered it runs the risk of respiratory distress, but if delivery is deferred to await pulmonary maturity, the price of delay might be intrauterine fetal death. The DFMC offers a solution to this dilemma in that normal activity is almost always associated with the survival of a healthy infant, even in the face of placental insufficiency, thus reassuring the clinician who wishes to defer delivery of the 'at risk' fetus to gain further maturity.

THE CLINICAL APPLICATION OF THE DFMC

A full 12-hour DFMC is costly in terms of the patient's time and therefore it is unrealistic to expect outpatients to do a full DFMC. Suggestions have been made to simplify counting by using shorter periods of time. For instance, Sadovsky (personal communication), in the current Jerusalem protocol suggests that the number of fetal movements are assessed by the patient two to three times during the day for 30 minutes. If movements are less than three per hour the patient should then monitor the movements for six to 12 hours per day. From these observations is calculated a 12-hour 'daily fetal movement count'.

The Cardiff 'Count-to-Ten' system was devised to be as simple as possible (Fig. 1.4). This chart begins at 9 a.m. and continues in half-hourly blocks of time until 9 p.m. The patient decides for herself what constitutes a movement and fills in the half-hour block of time in which the tenth movement falls.

A very active baby should move ten times fairly early on in the day, leaving the mother free to go about her business, but a relatively sluggish infant will take longer to reach ten movements. High levels of fetal activity are not recorded with much accuracy, though this is not important, but as one gets to low levels of activity, accuracy automatically improves. If by 9 p.m. ten movements have not been recorded, the actual number counted are entered in below the thick black line and here the chart is completely accurate (Pearson, 1977). Jarvis & MacDonald (1979) have suggested on the basis of their observations that a 'Count-to-20' system might be an improvement, but the principle remains the same.

THE CLINICAL INTERPRETATION OF THE DFMC

Maternal appreciation of fetal activity is subjective and some women are unaware of many of the movements that the infant makes, whereas other women will count several hundreds of fetal movements during the day. Many women are more aware of movements on retiring to bed at night and when resting during the day. On the other hand, they tend to be less aware of fetal activity when busy with children and housework.

Each infant tends to have its own rhythm of activity and may be inactive for several hours at a time, probably corresponding to periods of intrauterine sleep. Sedatives not only sedate the mother and lessen her awareness but also sedate the fetus, whose activity is correspondingly diminished.

Should a patient report a low DFMC it is important to determine whether or not the fetus is suffering from hypoxia.

Firstly, the general state of the patient and her baby should be clinically assessed. If

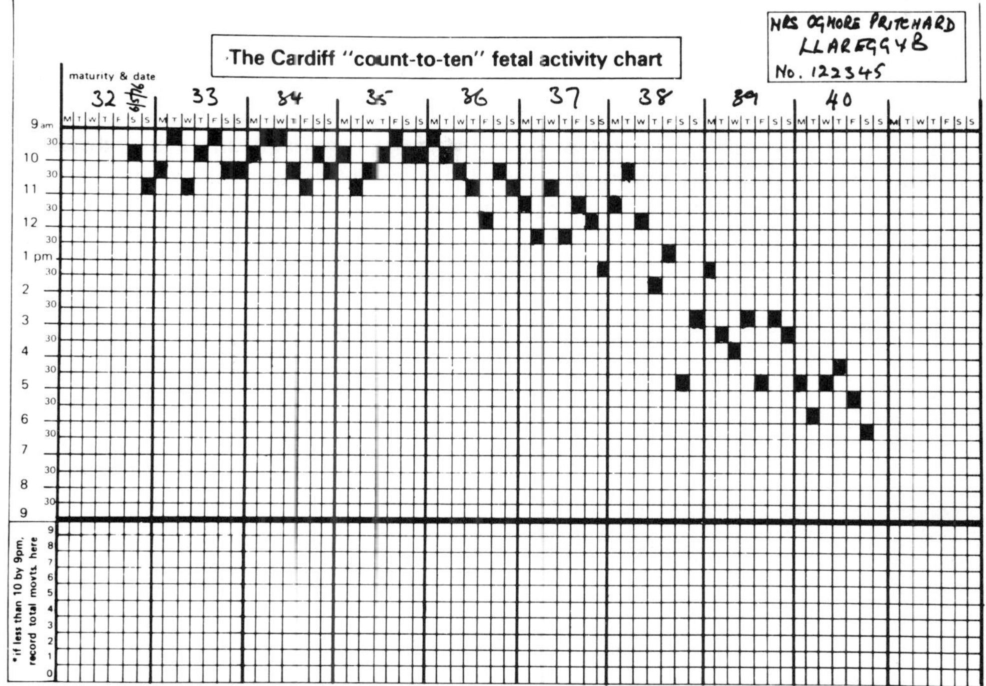

Fig. 1.4 Completed Cardiff 'Count-to-Ten' fetal movement chart.

the baby is clinically small-for-dates then the low DFMC must be taken seriously and the patient needs closer investigation using cardiotocography (CTG). If the infant is well grown, then the elicitation of the 'startle' response by external manipulation of the fetus is all that is required to provoke considerable activity, which is usually clearly visible to the clinician (Rosen et al, 1979). The DFMC cannot always predict fetal demise. One obstetric condition causing sudden death of the fetus which is not preceded by the characteristic slowing of fetal activity is abruptio placentae. Our experience suggests that when this occurs fetal death is immediately preceded by a sudden flurry of movement. Episodes of bleeding sometimes occur in late pregnancy which are not immediately fatal to the fetus, but might represent minor degrees of placental separation. It is therefore good practice to perform antenatal cardiotocography in such cases following each episode of bleeding, because in this situation fetal movement counting is unreliable.

Pregnancy complicated by hydramnios is a special problem because of the coexistence of diminished fetal movements and hydramnios is suggestive of fetal malformation (Sadovsky & Perlman, 1978).

About 5 per cent of women, at either extreme of the IQ scale, are unable to fill in a 'Count-to-Ten' chart. Furthermore, some patients are so determined to have an uneventful pregnancy that they 'forge' a favourable record, while some other patients, hoping to have labour induced, have claimed extremely low counts. External cardiotocography distinguishes the latter group, but the former group is more difficult to evaluate.

Despite these difficulties, the DFMC is a useful non-invasive test of fetal wellbeing by which each pregnant patient can monitor her own fetus. Compared with conventional placental function tests it has been shown to be equally reliable, is inexpensive and it does not require an accurate knowledge of gestational age for its proper interpretation. Most importantly, it helps the obstetrician to identify the 'at risk' but healthy baby. If widely used this test should contribute not only to a lowering of the perinatal mortality rate, but also to a lowering of the rate of induction of labour in women possessing 'at risk' factors, but carrying healthy infants.

Possible future developments

Phased-array ultrasonography provides a means for the continuous observation of moving structures. Using this technique Birnholz et al (1978) identified no less than 11 separate spontaneous fetal movement patterns in clinically normal women examined from the sixth week to term. A trend of increasingly complex movements with advancing gestational age was noted. Discrete movements such as isolated extension of the body, thumb sucking and repetitive chest wall movements could be recognised after 24 weeks. They were also able tentatively to identify a fetal 'startle' response to an externally applied pressure stimulus. Ultimately, holography (Holbrooke et al, 1973), three-dimensional imaging or stereogeometric reconstructions will become available.

Antenatal cardiotocography

The history of this technique dates back to the preliminary observations of Hammacher (1962), although it has been widely used only during the last decade.

There are two main types of test, the oxytocin stress test (OCT) and unstressed cardiotocography. The oxytocin stress test purports to evaluate placental reserve by stressing the fetus by means of oxytocin-induced uterine contractions. This test has certain theoretical and practical disadvantages. It is invasive, it cannot be used safely in cases of antepartum bleeding, particularly when a placenta praevia is suspected and there is a danger of initiating labour. It is also time-consuming, probably unphysiological and may, by causing uterine hypertonus, constitute an iatrogenic hazard to the compromised fetus. Although the American literature has concentrated almost exclusively on this test, it has been little used in Europe and has never been popular in Britain. Even in the USA the trend has now shifted in favour of the non-invasive, safe technique of unstressed cardiotocography. The term unstressed cardiotocography should not be confused with the term non-stress test (NST), which is a test currently popular in the USA. The NST is often used as a screening procedure for large numbers of patients. The rationale of the NST is that the presence of FHR accelerations associated with fetal movements indicates an intact and responsive central nervous system (Paul & Keegan, 1979). Infants showing this response are said to be 'reactive' and those not responding are termed 'non-reactive'. Depression of reactivity occurs in hypoxia, but is also present in fetal sleep, with fetal anomalies and following maternal sedation (Keegan et al, 1979). There is also a high false positive rate for this test. Because of these drawbacks the slightly more demanding but more exact technique of unstressed antenatal cardiotocography is here preferred as a first-line procedure, whereas in the USA a non-reactive NST tends to be regarded as an indication for the performance of an OCT.

The principles of unstressed cardiotocography (CTG)
The ease or otherwise of interpretation of a CTG tracing depends entirely upon the technical quality of the recording. It therefore follows that time, care and expertise need consistently to be expended to achieve this. In the UK most units visited by the writer perform too many CTGs. The result is that those which matter most tend to be swamped by a mélange of short uninterpretable tracings engendered by too heavy a monitoring work load, which, with other conflicting priorities, leads to lack of technical care in the individual case. Kubli et al (1977) make this point emphatically.

From what is already known from FHR monitoring in labour, late and variable decelerations of the FHR in response to uterine contractions are signs of substantial fetal hypoxia. We take the view proposed by Simmonds (1974) that the precise time relationship between the contraction and the deceleration is unimportant. Kubli et al (1977) concur, and Figure 1.5 demonstrates the occurrence of moderate variable deceleration patterns within 30 minutes of fetal death.

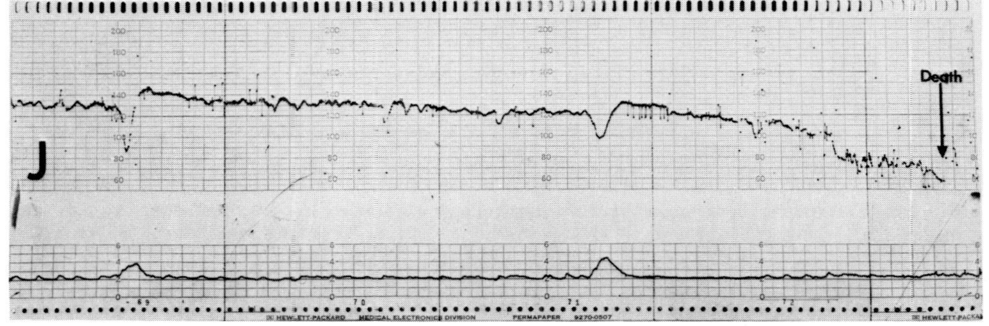

Fig. 1.5   This tracing, from a patient with severe Rhesus isoimmunisation, demonstrates moderate variable decelerations shortly before intrauterine fetal death. The tracing also shows the sinusoidal pattern which is sometimes seen in cases of fetal asphyxia accompanied by hydrops fetalis as in this case.

We also learn from intrapartum monitoring that decelerations complicating severe tachycardia or bradycardia are even more ominous (Beard, 1974). From the preceding discussion we know that the persistently quiescent infant might well be compromised and that the vigorously moving infant has a good prognosis.

As long ago as 1886, Alfred Lewis Galabin, at Guy's Hospital, suggested that a good outcome could be expected if, when the fetus moved, its heart rate increased by 20 beats per minute. This sign has been recently rediscovered and forms the basis of the NST. Acceleration patterns of the FHR in response to fetal movements have been associated with a good fetal outlook, the outcome being generally poorer in those infants not showing this response (Lee et al, 1976; Trierweiler et al, 1976; Flynn & Kelly, 1977).

Thus, it would appear that a healthy infant ought to be characterised by vigorous movement, a normal heart rate with accelerations in response to movements and contractions, whereas a hypoxic fetus should be quiescent, with a very rapid or slow heart rate showing decelerations with contractions. These generalisations seem to be correct, but more detailed interpretation is required in the clinical situation.

Interpretation of antenatal CTGs

Several scoring systems have been described to facilitate the clinical interpretation of records and to allow for better comparison of results. Several such systems have been published by Kubli (1971), Hammacher et al (1974), Fischer et al (1976), Meyer-Menk et al (1976) and Pearson & Weaver (1978). This last evaluation produced data which suggested that there existed a pattern of events which was likely to precede intrauterine fetal death. The healthy fetus was highly reactive with acceleration patterns both with movements and contractions. The earliest evidence of compromise was the presence of deceleration patterns with contractors (see Fig. 1.6).

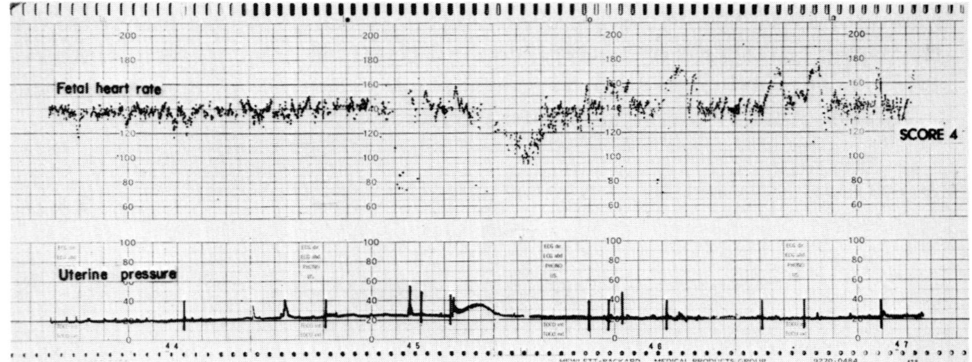

Fig. 1.6   This tracing shows a deceleration pattern following a Braxton-Hicks contraction in the presence of good FHR reactivity to movements. This is probably the earliest CTG sign of intrauterine fetal asphyxia.

Acceleration patterns with fetal movements then disappeared, followed by the cessation of movements, thus indicating that the 'fetal movement alarm signal' of Sadovsky & Yaffe (1973) is when present, really quite a late sign of asphyxia. Eventually, alterations in the baseline FHR were observed, usually in the direction of tachycardia. It was suggested that these acidotic fetuses, who were mostly growth retarded, were probably maintaining cardiac output, and thus their tissue perfusion pressure, by an increase in heart rate. Finally, just before death, severe bradycardia occurred.

Two of these scoring systems will be discussed in some detail, that of Meyer-Menk et al (1976), which is popular on the Continent (Table 1.3), and that of Pearson & Weaver (1978), which is more commonly used in the UK. (Table 1.4.)

The two scoring systems agree in several particulars, the limits for the baseline FHR are identical and in line with tradition. Short-term fluctuation of the FHR is given considerable weight in the Meyer-Menk systems, but is not considered in the Pearson-Weaver score, on the grounds that such an assessment is difficult and does not lend itself easily to numerical definition. Whilst the Meyer-Menk system represents a better quantitative evaluation of the frequency of deceleration patterns, it gives no weight to acceleration patterns with contractions. The latter criticism may be unfair, because such accelerations are probably only manifestations of concurrent fetal activity as explained by Pearson & Weaver (1978). Nevertheless, to be able to differentiate between traces containing more or less than 25 per cent deceleration patterns, as the Meyer-Menk system requires, necessitates a very prolonged period of

Table 1.3 The 10 point scoring system of Meyer-Menk et al (1976)

	0	1	2
BASELINE-LEVEL (bpm)	<100 >180	≥100 <120 >160 ≤180	≥120 ≤160
AMPLITUDE OF FLUCTUATION (Δ bpm)	<5 sinusoidal	>5 <10 (≥25)	>10 <25
FREQUENCY OF FLUCTUATION (cycles/min)	<2 sinusoidal	≥2 ≥4	>4
DECELERATION PATTERN with uterine contractions	late deceleration pattern frequency ≥25% marked variable pattern, severe supine syndrome	late deceleration pattern frequency <25% moderate or mild variable deceleration pattern, early deceleration pattern	lack of deceleration, single mild variable deceleration dip 0
ACCELERATION with arousal test of fetal movements	absolute lack of acceleration (negative response)	atypical shape no spontaneous acceleration	acceleration with fetal movements (positive response)

Table 1.4 The 'six-point' scoring system for antenatal cardiotocographs (Pearson & Weaver, 1978)

	0	1	2
Baseline FHR (beats/minute)	less than 100 or more than 180	100–120 or 160–180	120–160
Movements	none	Present	Present
FHR change	—	No change	Acceleration
Contractions ± FHR change	Deceleration	No change	Acceleration

monitoring in order to obtain sufficient contractions to get a meaningful result. Finally, in the section of the Meyer-Menk score concerned with fetal activity and FHR reactivity, no provision is made for an absence of activity, which frequently has an ominous significance.

The disadvantage of the Pearson & Weaver 'six-point-score' is that the score can be achieved by several combinations of variables. For instance, the score of three is yielded by seven possible combinations. This criticism is even more applicable to the Meyer-Menk score where the maximum score is ten and thus the score of five could be yielded by no less than 51 combinations of variables.

Continued experience of the 'six-point-score' has shown that a good rule is to interpret tracings according to what is known of the order of events preceding death. The measured variables are affected in the following order: (i) FHR response to contractions; (ii) FHR response to movements, and (iii) changes in baseline FHR. Thus, if a fetal tachycardia is the only abnormality observed, then a cause other than asphyxia should be sought for.

Frequency of recording
This generally depends on the indications. These include a low fetal movement count, antenatal bleeding, deterioration of the overall clinical situation and following amniocentesis.

Unfortunately, it is impossible to determine the duration of intrauterine survival of a compromised fetus. The writer has observed two examples where deceleration patterns, a paucity of movements and an unreactive fetus continued for no less than nine and 11 days respectively before death. On the other hand, fetal condition can deteriorate alarmingly rapidly, particularly following antepartum bleeding. Yet it is difficult to make out a case for the frequent routine performance of CTGs, both on logistical and humanitarian grounds. The best compromise seems to be to try to select from the clinic population using clinical and ultrasonic methods, all those women with small poorly grown babies; to use fetal movement charts for the entire antenatal population and to perform adequate CTGs on those other patients with the specific indications outlined in the preceding paragraph.

The technique of recording
The patient lies on a couch with a 15° left lateral tilt to minimise aortocaval compression. The uterine contraction recording head is placed at the point of maximum curvature of the uterine fundus. The FHR recorder is positioned where the fetal heart is best heard with the Pinard's stethoscope. Doppler ultrasound unidirectional transducers give the best results.

A convenient chart speed is 1 cm per minute. The attendant keeps the FHR recorder pointing at the fetal heart, using the oscilloscope display as a guide. Steep, discrete sine waves are ideal. The other hand of the attendant rests lightly on the abdomen as an additional indicator of fetal activity. When fetal movement is felt by the mother she indicates it by pressing an event marker button — frequently there is auditory confirmation of activity and a blip may appear on the uterine pressure tracing. The best and newest monitor available is used for this work and not some veteran machine which has been 'pensioned off' from labour ward duty.

The duration of recording is 30 minutes or until the recognition of at least three adequate Braxton-Hicks contractions.

Management of antepartum asphyxia
Once a diagnosis of antepartum fetal asphyxia has been made the logical treatment is Caesarean section. Whilst preparations are being made for delivery, the administration of pure oxygen by face mask is of benefit as illustrated in Figure 1.7.

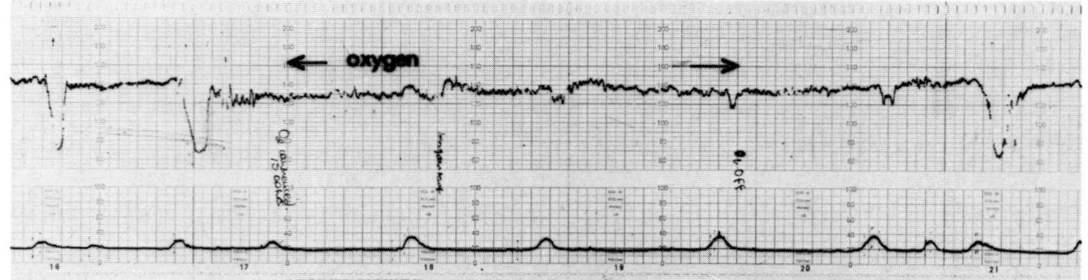

Fig. 1.7 This tracing demonstrates that the administration of oxygen by face-mask may succeed in abolishing deceleration patterns of the FHR. The decelerations reappearing when the oxygen was discontinued.

The use of dextrose infusions in the presence of fetal asphyxia is probably unwise as it may precipitate fetal cerebral oedema and brain necrosis, due to lactate accumulation in the fetal brain (Myers & Yamaguchi, 1977).

ACKNOWLEDGEMENTS

I wish to thank Dr K Boddy, Senior Lecturer, Department of Obstetrics and Gynaecology, Edinburgh University, for permission to reproduce Figure 1.1 and Table 1.1.

REFERENCES

Alberman E 1976 Factors influencing perinatal wastage. In: Beard R W, Nathanielsz P W (eds) Fetal physiology and medicine. Saunders, London, ch 21, pp 415–432

Assali N S, Brinkman E R 1973 The role of circulatory buffers in feral tolerance to stress. American Journal of Obstetrics and Gynecology 117: 643–653

Beard R W 1974 Fetal heart rate patterns and their clinical interpretation. Sonicaid Ltd,

Beazley J M, Underhill R A 1970 Fallacy of the fundal height. British Medical Journal 4: 404–406

Belizan J M, Villar J, Nardin J C, Malamud J, Sainz De Vicuna L 1978 Diagnosis of intrauterine growth retardation by simple clinical method: measurement of uterine height. American Journal of Obstetrics and Gynecology 131: 643–646

Birnholz J C, Stephens J C, Faria M 1978 Fetal movement patterns: a possible means of defining neurologic developmental milestones in utero. American Journal of Roentgenology 130: 537–540

Boddy K, Parboosingh I J T, Shepherd W C 1976 A schematic approach to antenatal care — Published from the Department of Obstetrics and Gynaecology, Edinburgh University

Campbell S 1976 Fetal Growth. In: Beard R W, Nathanielsz P W (eds) Fetal physiology and medicine. Saunders, London, ch 15, pp 271–301

Campbell S, Dewhurst C J 1971 Diagnosis of the small-for-dates fetus by serial ultrasonic cephalometry. Lancet ii: 1002–1006

Fischer W M, Stude I, Brandt H 1976 Ein Vorschlag zur Beurteilung des antepartualen Kardiotokogramms. Zeitschrift Perinatologie 180: 117–123

Flynn A M, Kelly J 1977 Evaluation of fetal wellbeing by antepartum fetal heart monitoring. British Medical Journal 1: 936–939

Galabin A L 1886 A manual of midwifery Churchill, London

Gettinger A, Roberts A B, Campbell S 1978 Comparison between subjective and ultrasound assessments of fetal movement. British Medical Journal 2: 88–90

Goldstein H 1969 High risk predictors at booking and in pregnancy. In: Butler N R, Alberman E D (eds) Perinatal problems. Livingstone, Edinburgh, ch 3, pp 45–46

Gruenwald P 1974 Pathology of the deprived fetus and its supply line. In: Ciba foundation symposium 27: size at birth. Associated Scientific Publishers, Amsterdam, pp 3–19

Hammacher K 1962 New method for the selective registration of the fetal heart beat. Geburtshilfe und Frauenheilkunde 22: 1542–1543

Hammacher K, Brun del Re R, Gaudenz R, de Grandi P, Richter R 1974 Kardiotokographischer Nachweis einer fetalen Gefährdung mit einem CTG-Score. Gynakologische Rundschau 14 Supplement 1: 61–63

Hertogs K, Roberts A B, Cooper D, Griffin D R, Campbell S 1979 Maternal perception of fetal motor activity. British Medical Journal 2: 1183–1185

Hobbins J C, Berkowitz R L, Grannum P A 1978 Diagnosis and antepartum management of intrauterine growth retardation. Journal of Reproductive Medicine 21: 319–325

Holbrooke D, McCurry E, Richards V, Shibata H 1973 Through transmission ultrasonic imaging of intrauterine and fetal structures using acoustical holography. In: Vlieger M de, White D N, McCready V R (eds) Ultrasonics in medicine. Excerpta Medica, Amsterdam, pp 332–344

Hull M G R, Chard T 1976 Hormonal aspects of feto-placental function. In: Beard R W, Nathanielsz P W (eds) Fetal physiology and medicine. Saunders, London, ch 19, pp 371–394

Jarvis G J, MacDonald H N 1979 Fetal movements in small-for-dates babies. British Journal of Obstetrics and Gynaecology 86: 724–727

Keegan K A, Paul R H, Broussard P M, McCart D, Smith M A 1979 Antepartum fetal heart rate testing III the effect of phenobarbital on the nonstress test. American Journal of Obstetrics and Gynecology 133: 579–580

Kubli F 1971 Measurement of placental function. In: Huntingford P J, Beard R W, Hytten R, Scopes J W (eds) Perinatal medicine. Karger, Basel, p 23–42

Kubli F, Boos R, Rüttgers H, Hagens C V, Vanselow H 1977 Antepartum fetal heart rate monitoring. In: Beard R W, Campbell S (eds) The current status of fetal heart rate monitoring and ultrasound in obstetrics. Royal College of Obstetricians and Gynaecologists, London, p 28–47

Lee C Y, Di Loreto P C, Logrand B 1976 Fetal activity acceleration determination for the evaluation of fetal reserve. Obstetrics and Gynecology 48: 19–26

McIlwaine G M, Howat R C L, Dunn F, Macnaughton M C 1979 The Scottish perinatal mortality survey. British Medical Journal ii: 1103–1106

McLean F, Usher R 1970 Measurements of liveborn fetal malnutrition infants compared with similar gestation and with similar birth weight normal controls. Biologia Neonatorum 16: 215–221

Meyer-Menk W, Rüttgers H, Boos R, Würth G, Adis B, Kubli F 1976 A proposal for a new method of CTG evaluation. In: Rooth G, Bratteby L E (eds) Abstracts of the 5th European Congress of perinatal medicine. Almquist and Wicksell Trycheri, Uppsala, p 138

Myers R E, Yamaguchi S 1977 Nervous system effects of cardiac arrest in monkeys. Archives of Neurology 34: 65–74

Neilson J P, Hood V D 1980 Ultrasound in obstetrics and gynaecology. Recent developments. British Medical Bulletin 36: 249–255

Neilson J P, Whitfield C R, Aitchison T C 1980 Screening for the small-for-dates fetus: a two-stage ultrasonic examination schedule. British Medical Journal 280: 1203–1206

Neldam S 1980 Fetal movements as an indicator of fetal wellbeing. Lancet i: 1222–1224

Paul R H, Keegan K A 1979 Nonstress antepartum fetal monitoring. Clinics in Obstetrics and Gynaecology 6: 351–358

Pearson J F 1977 Fetal movements — a new approach to antenatal care. Nursing Mirror 144: 49–51

Pearson J F, Weaver J B 1976 Fetal activity and fetal wellbeing: an evaluation. British Medical Journal 1: 1305–1307

Pearson J F, Weaver J B 1978 A six-point scoring system for antenatal cardiotocographs. British Journal of Obstetrics and Gynaecology 85: 321–327

Quaranta P, Currell R, Redman C W G, Robinson J S 1981 Prediction of small-for-dates infants by measurement of symphyseal-fundal-height. British Journal of Obstetrics and Gynaecology 88: 115–119

Reinold E 1973 Clinical value of fetal spontaneous movements in early pregnancy. Journal of Perinatal Medicine 1: 65

Robinson H P 1973 Sonar measurement of fetal crown-rump length as means of assessing maturity in first trimester of pregnancy. British Medical Journal iv: 28–37

Rosen M G, Hertz R H, Dierker L J, Zador I, Timor-Tritch I E 1979 Monitoring fetal movement. Clinics in Obstetrics and Gynaecology 6: 325–334

Sadovsky E, Yaffe H 1973 Daily fetal movement recording and fetal prognosis. Obstetrics and Gynecology 41: 845–850

Sadovsky E, Polishuk W Z, Mahler Y, Malkin A 1973 Correlation between electromagnetic recording and maternal assessment of fetal movement. Lancet i: 1141–1143

Sadovsky E, Yaffe H, Polishuk W Z 1974 Fetal movements in pregnancy and urinary estriol in prediction of impending fetal death in utero. Israeli Journal of Medical Science 10: 1096–1099

Sadovsky E, Perlman M 1978 Decreased fetal movements and polyhydramnios. Case reports. Acta Obstetricia Gynecologica Scandinavica 57: 177–178

Simmonds S C 1974 Organisation of fetal intensive care. Clinics in Obstetrics and Gynaecology 1: 217–240

Spellacy W N, Cruz A C, Gelman S R, Buhi W C 1977 Fetal movements and placental lactogen levels for fetal-placental evaluation. Obstetrics and Gynecology 49: 113–115

Trierweiler M W, Freeman R K, James J 1976 Baseline fetal heart rate characteristics as an indicator of fetal status during the antepartum period. American Journal of Obstetrics and Gynecology 125: 618–623

Varma T R, Taylor H, Bridges C 1979 Ultrasound assessment of fetal growth. British Journal of Obstetrics and Gynaecology 86: 623–632

Ward H, Rochman H, Varnavides L A, Whyley G A 1973 Hormone and enzyme levels in normal and complicated pregnancy. American Journal of Obstetrics and Gynecology 116: 1105–1113

Westin B 1977 Gravidogram and fetal growth, comparison with biochemical supervision. Acta Obstetricia et Gynecologica Scandinavica 56: 273–282

Winick M 1971 Cellular changes during placental and fetal growth. American Journal of Obstetrics and Gynecology 109: 166–176

Wilds P L 1978 Observations of intrauterine fetal breathing movements — a review. American Journal of Obstetrics and Gynecology 131: 315–338

Wittman B K, Robinson H P, Aitchison T, Fleming J E E 1979 The value of diagnostic ultrasound as a screening test for intrauterine growth retardation: comparison of nine parameters. American Journal of Obstetrics and Gynecology 134: 30–35

2. Fetal monitoring in labour

Anna M. Flynn   John Kelly

Historically, interest in the fetus during labour is a late development. Maubray, in *The Female Physician* published in 1724, shares with us the satisfaction he feels that 'by many happy discoveries and strict enquiries made into the secrets of nature and natural causes, these healing and obstetricious arts are so much improved and advanced that they now seem to have arrived at their very height of perfection'. However, despite the perfection believed to have been obtained, nobody appeared to be particularly interested in the fetus, except so far as its presentation at delivery complicated the mother's prognosis.

Within the next century it became apparent that the duration of labour and the passage of the fetus through the birth canal, represents an acute stress situation for the fetus, carrying a mortality and morbidity unsurpassed over the following four to five decades of life. This realisation spawned the need to monitor the fetus during labour, and the oldest and probably still the most widespread method of monitoring the fetus is periodic auscultation of the fetal heart, either using the Pinard stethoscope or by directly applying the ear to the abdomen.

That this approach has limitations is evident by the occurrence of intrapartum stillbirths in the absence of any early warning signs. Consequently, the past decade has seen the introduction of sophisticated monitoring techniques for a more intensive surveillance of the fetus during labour.

PRESENT-DAY METHODS OF MONITORING

Present-day methods of intrapartum fetal monitoring include:

1. Continuous recording of fetal heart rate by electrocardiography, phonocardiography or ultrasonography.
2. Continuous recording of the stress factor — frequency and strength of the uterine contraction.
3. Fetal blood or tissue sampling for the determination of the acid-base state of the fetus.

Fetal electrocardiography

The first fetal e.c.g. was recorded by Cremer (1906) using external electrodes applied to the abdomen of the pregnant woman. Such a non-invasive technique is ideal but it was not found to be practical as the small amplitude of the fetal complex in comparison to that of the mother, together with the occurrence of extraneous electrical noise, made it impossible to get a sufficiently clear fetal signal to trigger a continuous fetal heart rate recorder. Consequently, external fetal electrocardiography fell into disuse and became superseded by the application of a direct electrode to the fetus. This was found to improve the quality of the fetal e.c.g., making it more reliable and easier to use (Smyth, 1953; Sureau, 1956; Hunter, 1960; Hon, 1963; Hon et al, 1972).

The earliest electrodes had to be held manually on to the fetal head and these were quickly replaced by electrodes which could be clipped on to the fetal scalp through the cervix. A modification of Michel-clips made of silver, silver chloride or stainless steel were used with a second lead in the vagina functioning as a reference electrode. Later a spiral electrode, smaller than the Michel-clip, was introduced (Hon et al, 1972) which had the advantage of being able to pass through a cervix barely dilated. The more recent Copeland electrode which is sufficiently stiff to be applied without any applicator, is both easy and speedy to apply, and can also be used through a very poorly dilated cervix (Showell, 1976; Ghosh & Tipton, 1976; Calvert & Newcombe, 1980).

Using this technique, the fetal heart rate is triggered by the peak of the R wave of the fetal e.c.g. complex. The time interval between each beat is computed into a rate and is then recorded. If no averaging technique is used, this time interval can also be used to give a true beat-to-beat interval variation (BBV) which has been shown to be an important factor in assessing the condition of the fetus, hypoxia and drugs both reducing the BBV.

The chief disadvantages to this method are that the membranes have to be ruptured, the technique is invasive and generally the patient is confined to bed; recent work has shown that for the patient who is ambulant the direct e.c.g. can be recorded using a radio transmitter.

External cardiotocography
The fetal e.c.g. can be recorded from the surface of the maternal abdomen together with the maternal e.c.g. In order to 'clean' the fetal e.c.g. signal sufficiently to enable it to be processed into a continuous heart rate, that of the mother must first be removed. This may be achieved by a 'blanking' technique or a subtraction technique (Wheeler et al, 1978). Nevertheless, despite these techniques the signal-to-noise ratio is small in the fetal e.c.g. and during labour noise is generated from many sources, e.g. fetal e.c.g., maternal electromyogram, as well as mains interference. For practical purposes therefore, external e.c.g. is rarely used during labour because of the poor recording obtained.

Phonocardiography
A phonocardiographic method is based on amplifying with the microphone sounds heard by auscultation and is therefore applied externally to the maternal abdomen. Such a method has to overcome the presence of extraneous noise, which makes it difficult to hear clearly the fetal heart sounds, especially in the obese patient. A further disadvantage and one particularly likely to occur during labour is that the heart signal is very often lost when the fetus or the mother moves, necessitating re-positioning of the microphone head. The method is non-invasive, can be used prior to rupture of the membranes, and has also the great advantage of being completely innocuous to the fetus.

Doppler-ultrasound cardiography
The application of the Doppler shift in association with high frequency sound waves can be used to detect the fetal pulse rate. To achieve this, ultrasound waves are transmitted to the fetus and reflective echoes from the surfaces of the umbilical cord vessels and major fetal vessels are received. The interference due to rhythmic changes of the pulsatile surfaces causes the Doppler shift effect, which can be detected and transformed into a sound wave and by an appropriate machine into a rate. Such a machine may range from a simple one, as the Doptone, to a more sophisticated fetal heart rate monitor, designed for direct e.c.g. recording but possessing also an external ultrasound transducer. This ultrasound transducer may either be a single transmitter/receiver head, or a multiple receiver head. The beam angle is greater with the multiple receiver head transducer, which has the practical advantage in that the fetal pulse can be detected over a wider range, thus accommodating more maternal and fetal movements without signal loss. Ultrasonography can be applied externally without prior membrane rupture, is very simple to apply and can be used successfully by midwives and other para-medical personnel to obtain a continuous record of the fetal heart rate during labour. When the multiple receiver head transducer with the wide beam angle is used, the necessity of having to frequently re-position the transducer head, is greatly reduced. With ultrasonography a true beat-to-beat variation of the fetal heart rate is not possible, and occasionally artifacts may occur, since the ultrasound beam picks up both the fetal and maternal pulses. If a slowing in the fetal heart rate occurs (bradycardia) a check should be made that this is the genuine fetal heart rate and not that of the mother.

The question of the effect of prolonged use of ultrasonic beams on the fetus has never been quite resolved. Experiments with ultrasound seem to suggest some damage (Mackintosh & Davey, 1970). This damage however, has not been substantiated for humans (Abdulla et al, 1971) but again neither has ultrasound been proved innocuous to the fetus. Long-term follow-up studies will be necessary to achieve this.

Tocography
Accurate recordings of uterine activity are now an essential part of fetal monitoring. Each uterine contraction represents a stress for the fetus and in times of stress the fetal heart rate alters. The importance of the relationship between the heart rate patterns and uterine activity is well established (Hon, 1963; Hon, 1968; Caldeyro-Barcia, 1966; Hammacher, 1969; Huntingford & Pendleton, 1969; Wood et al, 1969; Beard et al, 1971a and b).

Measurements of uterine action can be made either by external or internal tocography.

External method of tocography
The uterine contractions can be measured by a displacement transducer, placed on the maternal abdomen close to the fundus. The transducer tip is held against the abdominal wall and as the uterus contracts, the tip moves in proportion to the strength of the contraction. This movement is converted into a measurable electrical signal which indicates the relative intensity of the contraction, i.e. an absolute measurement is not given. Changes in baseline tension also are noted as relative

changes. It is however, an easy to use, non-invasive technique, does not require the membranes to be ruptured and gives a good indication of the duration and frequency of the contractions.

Internal method of tocography

Measurements of amniotic fluid pressure can be obtained by inserting a fluid-filled catheter into the uterus after rupture of the amniotic sac. The amniotic fluid interfaces with the fluid in the catheter and any changes in amniotic fluid pressure are transmitted to the catheter. These changes are detected by an extremely sensitive pressure transducer which converts them into electrical signals. These electrical signals are in turn converted into an exact pressure, expressed in millimetres of mercury. This is a highly efficient method of measuring uterine contractions and there are few problems. Catheter blockage occasionally occurs which can easily be solved by flushing with saline. Uterine perforation and placental separation are potential hazards but are rare and generally associated with the use of introducers to insert the catheter (Trudinger & Pryce-Davis, 1978; Tutera & Newman, 1975). Infection appears to be extremely rare in this country although there are reports from the United States of intrauterine infection associated with an intrauterine pressure catheter (Okada et al, 1977). The problem of infection may be more a reflection of overall infection in the hospital, rather than specifically related to the intrauterine pressure catheters.

INTERPRETATION OF FETAL HEART RATE PATTERNS

Several authors over the past two decades have presented both descriptions and interpretations of fetal heart rate recordings and these classifications are well known (Caldeyro-Barcia, 1966; Hon, 1968; Hammacher, 1969; Huntingford & Pendleton, 1969). There is however, still much subjective interpretation and lack of uniformity on what constitutes a pathological fetal heart rate pattern.

The normal fetal heart rate is characterised by:

1. A rate of 120 to 160 beats/minute
2. No change in the fetal heart rate during uterine contractions
3. A BBV greater than 5 beats/minute.

Abnormalities of the fetal heart rate

Tachycardia

An elevation of baseline fetal heart rate above 160 beats/minute is defined as tachycardia. Tachycardia alone is not indicative of fetal distress, but can reflect several patho-physiological states:

1. *Infection.* Both maternal or fetal infection may result in tachycardia.
2. *Preterm fetus.* The parasympathetic system of the autonomic nervous system is not well developed in the immature central nervous system and the pre-term fetus may manifest a tachycardia. Such a tachycardia may be considered physiological, provided that all ominous potential aetiologies have been ruled out.

3. *Anaemia.* Maternal and fetal anaemias may result in baseline tachycardia. Maternal anaemia of this degree is rare in developed countries. Fetal anaemia can occur in pregnancies complicated by haemolytic disease or fetal bleeding associated with vasa-praevia or amniocentesis.

4. *Acute haemorrhage.* Antepartum maternal bleeding in the latter half of pregnancy can result in fetal tachycardia.

5. *Cardiac failure.* Maternal cardiac failure will produce a fetal baseline tachycardia.

6. *Drug treatment.* Drugs used to arrest premature labour and blocking parasympathetic activity, e.g. β-adrenergic agents, will produce a tachycardia because of unopposed sympathetic activity.

7. *Maternal tachycardia* for whatever reason will result in fetal tachycardia.

8. *Fetal tachycardia* may be just a simple, physiological response of the fetus to exogenous stimulation, whether tactile or auditory.

In general tachycardias can be considered to be a reflection of fetal distress and close observation of the fetal heart rate activity should be maintained. True distressed states will invariably manifest themselves by changes in the BBV and/or the appearance of periodic patterns superimposed on the tachycardia.

Baseline fetal bradycardia
By definition, baseline fetal bradycardia is a heart rate below 120 beats/minute. The baseline bradycardia should be divided into severe, where the rate is less than 100 beats/minute and mild, where the rate is between 100 and 119 beats/minute, since the prognosis for these two gradings is quite different.

A mild bradycardia may occur for which no aetiology is demonstrable and no treatment necessary.

1. Severe bradycardia may be an indication of a conduction defect of the fetal heart with no resulting hypoxia and no operative interference is necessary. The configuration of the fetal e.c.g. helps to substantiate the clinical diagnosis in these cases.

2. All varieties of local anaesthetic drugs (the caine drugs) given to the mother may result in a decrease in the fetal heart rate over a prolonged period. In the case of epidural anaesthesia, the decrease in maternal blood pressure tends to potentiate the bradycardic effect. Preventative treatment by pre-loading the mother's circulation with fluid (Hartman's solution) prior to epidural block has been recommended (Crawford, 1979). When bradycardia occurs, repositioning of the mother, fluid loading and oxygen inhalation should be instigated and are usually sufficient to restore the fetal heart rate to normal.

3. Severe fetal bradycardia is a most ominous sign and indicative of acidosis and/or asphyxia, especially when preceded by a sequence of events which can be correlated with fetal stress and distress. Such a sequence of events might include fetal tachycardia, decreased variability, together with significant decelerative patterns. By the time the bradycardia has occurred, the fetus may be already damaged as the bradycardia reflects incipient fetal death. Therefore, in an optimal situation, therapy or intervention should have been instigated prior to the development of the fetal bradycardia.

Variability of baseline fetal heart rate

The baseline fetal heart rate normally exhibits an oscillating form, reflective of beat-to-beat changes in rate, which produce varying degrees of irregularity and variability in the baseline fetal heart rate. This variability may be further sub-divided into short term and long term variability.

SHORT-TERM VARIABILITY (BBV)

Short-term variability reflects the change in fetal heart rate from one beat to the next. This variability is a measure of the time interval between cardiac systoles, occurring successively and can only be determined by fetal e.c.g. (or fetal phono-cardiographic) techniques. The normal range is between 5 and 15 beats/minute.

LONG-TERM VARIABILITY

This is a term used to describe the oscillatory changes which occur during the course of one minute, and relates to the number of times the long term variability fluctuates during the course of the one minute of observed time. Normally, this is something between two and six shifts in the frequency of oscillatory cycles.

Normal variability both in terms of range and frequency of oscillatory change is associated with good fetal homeostasis and is thought to represent normal autonomic nervous system control of the fetal heart rate as well as an intact circulatory system. Decreases in the baseline fetal heart rate variability (BBV) may be pathologically significant and this is particularly true if the frequency of oscillatory change is also decreased. The most ominous cause of decreased variability is that of fetal hypoxia, distress and potential fetal death. During labour, however, decreased variability is often a reflection of the administration of analgesic, anaesthetic or neurotrophic drugs to the mother, making it sometimes difficult to distinguish these two aetiologies. If decreased variability is not associated with significant decelerative patterns and/or abnormalities in the baseline fetal heart rate, it is probably due to drugs and associated with normal fetal homeostasis.

Fetal heart rate patterns

Fetal heart rate patterns are described as periodic changes in fetal heart rate during uterine contractions, and are of the following types:

EARLY DECELERATIVE PATTERNS (HON) (CALDEYRO-BARCIA — TYPE I DIPS)

This is the fetal heart rate which decelerates early in the contractive phase and returns to baseline at the time the contraction ends. The amplitude of the deceleration is usually moderate (not exceeding 40 beats/minute) and although the patho-physiology of this pattern is not known for certain, it is commonly associated with head compression and is thought to be due to vagal stimulation.

VARIABLE DECELERATIONS (HON) (CALDEYRO-BARCIA — TYPE 0 DIPS)

These are so called because they show variable shapes (U shaped, V shaped) and also a variable temporal relationship to the associated contractions. The variable deceleration is thought to reflect a decreased perfusion of the fetus arising from a disturbance of in-flow anywhere along the course of the umbilical circulation. During the course of normal labour the cord is many times impinged on by fetal extremities or other fetal parts. The transient, fleeting and mild variable decelerations which occur as a result of this fetal movement are generally innocuous. There are, however, moderate and severe decelerations which, if associated with other signs of fetal distress, e.g. reduced BBV and/or tachycardia may be indicative of progressive fetal hypoxia, acidosis and asphyxia. In such severe decelerations, therefore, further investigation to assess the acid base status and/or delivery of the fetus is necessary.

LATE DECELERATIONS (HON) (CALDEYRO-BARCIA — TYPE II DIPS)
A late deceleration is a pattern of uniform shape, being a mirror image of the uterine contraction curve, but in contrast to the early deceleration, is temporarily separated from the contraction. There is a lag time between the onset of the contraction and the onset of the decelerative pattern, and between the return of the contraction to the resting tone and the return of the decelerative pattern to baseline levels. This lag time is usually in excess of 18 seconds (Caldeyro-Barcia, 1968). The mechanism of late decelerations is thought to be utero-placental insufficiency and therefore a late deceleration can never be considered to be normal.

Any entity which interferes with maternal blood supply or placental circulation may result in a late decelerative pattern, e.g.

1. Placental insufficiency in high risk pregnancy states — chronic hypertension, nephrotic syndrome, diabetes, dysmaturity and severe pre-eclampsia.
2. Significant maternal circulatory insufficiency, e.g. hypotension, due to unrecognised caval compression, or to epidural anaesthesia or other maternal pathology, resulting in a decrease in maternal circulating blood.
3. Exaggerated uterine pressures, whether due to hypersystoles (increased frequency of uterine contractions) or baseline hypertonus, or both. Such a tonic uterine state may arise with oxytocin stimulation and cause a late decelerative pattern, or even a prolonged decelerative pattern with resultant bradycardia.

Management. In that uterine contractions are repetitive and represent a recurrent stress to the fetus, late decelerations result in progressive hypoxia and metabolic acidosis in the fetus. The patho-physiology of the late deceleration is impaired placental respiratory function, whether this is caused primarily in the placenta and its vessels, or secondarily by extraneous factors affecting the placental blood flow. Such external factors are generally due to maternal hypotension, secondary to caval compression and/or epidural anaesthesia and hypertonic uterine action. In such cases correction of the external factor responsible, e.g. hypertonus, together with resuscitative measures designed to improve maternal blood pressure and increase the amount of oxygen carried to the fetus, should be instigated without delay. However, an upper optimal maternal PO_2 limit exists beyond which maternal vaso constriction occurs, with no beneficial action on the fetal PO_2. Where there are no responsible external factors or where the above methods are not effective, then delivery should be effected either vaginally or abdominally depending on the condition of the fetus as assessed by the acid base measurement and the clinical stage of the labour.

COMBINED DECELERATION PATTERNS
The classic deceleration patterns just described may occur juxtaposed, imposed or superimposed upon each other. Interpretation of combined patterns is often most

confusing to the examiner. Combinations of all patterns may be seen. Of the various combined patterns, the most frequent and probably the most confusing is the correlation of the variable and late decelerative patterns. Combined patterns should be dissected to ascertain which of the classic patterns is present. Any pattern which does not conform to the above three noted patterns in respect of shape, range and lag time, should be considered as combination patterns. Any combined pattern exhibiting a uniform late deceleration component must be considered to have a hypoxic aetiology and treated identically to that of the late deceleration itself.

PROLONGED DECELERATION PATTERNS

The prolonged deceleration pattern is also known as the unclassified or atypical pattern. The characteristics of the prolonged deceleration are as follows: The pattern is exclusively a deceleration pattern and not associated with acceleration factors. The shape of the pattern may appear to be uniform or non-uniform. During the course of the pattern the wave form may make an attempt to return to baseline or measure a constant depression of rate throughout the pattern.

The onset of the deceleration may occur at any time in relation to the contraction, originating at the onset, the acme, the descending limb of the contraction or independent of the contraction. The pattern may also persist through many uterine contractions. Therefore, lag time criteria cannot be utilised in analysing this pattern.

The range of the pattern is not constant, but for the most part it is of an exaggerated range. The nadir of the pattern is greater than 25 beats from the baseline and in most instances the rate falls well below the 100 beats/minute during the course of the pattern.

The duration of the pattern is dependent upon the aetiologic factor, but by definition it is in excess of two minutes with durations of 8 to 20 minutes being the norm.

The patho-physiology of the prolonged decelerative pattern is usually produced by two mechanisms: (1) the effect of the caine drugs; (2) by hypertonus.

Caine drug effect. Any local anaesthetics (caine drugs) administered to the mother may be absorbed by the maternal circulation and by placental transfer exhibit an effect on the fetus. This was most frequently seen in the utilisation of para-cervical block analgesic techniques. It may occur, however, with the use of caine drugs in epidural and subarachnoid block anaesthetics. The effect of the caine drugs on the fetus appears to be a central effect as opposed to a direct myocardial effect. Because there is no direct myocardial toxicity of the caine drugs on the fetus, there is no morbidity to the fetus during the period of deceleration induced by the caine drug *as long as the fetus remains within the uterus* until the deceleration is resolved; it will be supported by the resuscitative mechanism of the maternal uteroplacental system and fetal homeostasis in regard to an acid balance is sustained. Morbidity will result if the fetus is delivered prior to the time when the caine drug has been metabolised by the fetus (usual eight to 16 minutes). If the fetus is born during the period of deceleration secondary to the caine drug administration, the fetus will be born with a toxic level of drug, with subsequent neonatal effects of cardiovascular collapse and central nervous system overstimulation, as would be seen in an adult receiving toxic levels of caine drug. Once the prolonged deceleration of this nature has been noted it is wise to curtail the further administration of caine drugs to the mother.

Hypertonus. Hypertonus most frequently occurs in situations where drugs are being utilised to stimulate or induce labour. The prolonged deceleration occurring as a result of hypertonus is an ominous, non-assuring pattern and does result in significant biochemical changes after two minutes' duration. The prolonged deceleration of hypertonus, therefore, requires aggressive treatment as opposed to the conservative supportive treatment of the prolonged deceleration secondary to the caine drug effect without hypertonus. The patho-physiology of prolonged deceleration, secondary to hypertonus, is quite similar to that of the late deceleration, in that they both produce hypoxia as a consequence of decreased blood flow to the fetus. The two patterns differ in that the late deceleration reflects an intrinsic defect in utero-placental function in response to normal uterine contractility, whereas the prolonged deceleration arising from excessive contractility is either iatrogenically induced or endogenously produced over-stimulation of uterine activity. If prolonged deceleration is the result of hypertonus, one should immediately initiate procedures such as:

1. immediate curtailment of oxytocic stimulant
2. intravenous fluid loading of the patient
3. oxygen therapy to the mother
4. side positioning of the patient to effect better circulation to the uterus. If the hypertonus does not respond to the above measures, the use of uterine relaxants should be considered though normally they are not necessary.

If these methods are not effective, then delivery should be effected, either abdominally or vaginally, depending on the condition of the fetus and the clinical stage of the labour.

FETAL BLOOD SAMPLING

Continuous cardiotocography is a good indicator of the fetal wellbeing for the 80 per cent of fetuses who go through labour without any problem. The diagnosis of the degree of fetal hypoxia from clinical signs of fetal distress, e.g. pathological fetal heart rate traces and/or the passage of meconium, is as yet not possible in all cases. Yet fetal hypoxia not only results in intrapartum stillbirths, but also contributes substantially to a neonatal morbidity of varying degrees, at its worst resulting in cerebral damage. The diagnosis of fetal hypoxia is, therefore, crucial to monitoring the fetus during labour.

Hypoxia may be acute if caused by partial or complete occlusion of the umbilical cord or by the reduction in uterine blood flow, or it may be chronic if caused by utero-placental insufficiency over a long period. Again, the acute situation may be superimposed on the chronic. In acute hypoxia there is a failure to maintain an adequate passage of oxygen from the mother to the fetus, leading to an accumulation of carbon dioxide, with a respiratory acidosis. Later this leads to an increase in anaerobic glycolysis at the cell level, with an accumulation of lactic acid, superimposing a metabolic acidosis on the respiratory acidosis. The base deficit increases and the pH falls. The PO_2 falls and the PCO_2 rises concurrently, although in the case of chronic placental insufficiency, PO_2 and PCO_2 may not alter significantly. The fall in pH and the increase in base deficit may be the only biochemical changes noted.

Studies showed that for practical purposes, the pH determination is not only the easiest one to measure in the fetus, but also the one with the lowest methodological errors (Kubli, 1967). The fetal blood samples are collected from the fetal scalp capillary blood which has a pH lying midway between that of the umbilical artery and umbilical vein. The original technique described by Saling is still used (Saling, 1964). Normal values have been established for scalp blood pH at 7.33 for the first stage, and 7.29 during the second stage (Paterson et al, 1970; Saling, 1964). Acidosis develops slowly during labour and the present view is that a pH of 7.25 or above is normal, whereas one at 7.20 or below is acidotic. The grey area between 7.20 and 7.25 is inconclusive and can be considered to be in the pre-acidotic range. In such cases repeat pH estimations will be necessary to establish the trend which is emerging — whether an improvement or worsening of the acid base state.

Although fetal blood sampling is widely practised, there are many problems, both with the collection and interpretation of results. It is an invasive technique, necessitating puncture of the fetal scalp each time it is performed, and this has been shown to be not without risk to the fetus, because of haemorrhage and sepsis (Beard et al, 1966; Hull, 1978).

Technical problems in obtaining the samples are encountered when the presenting fetal part is high and there is minimum cervical dilatation. Breech presentations often cause difficulties in sampling, since the breech is not so vascular as the scalp. If the pH of the breech is abnormal it may present difficulty in interpretation, since the blood supply to the head is preferentially oxygenated in comparison with the rest of the body. Consequently, it has been suggested that in the normal breech, fetal blood sampling pH is about 0.05 degrees lower than that of the scalp. Caput formation on the scalp may also produce a lower than normal pH value.

While such technical problems are a decided disadvantage, the major disadvantage with intermittent fetal blood sampling is that the value obtained relates only to the time it has been collected and fetal physiology is in a very dynamic state during labour. Consequently, even when the pH values are collected under optimal conditions, there is a 10 to 15 per cent incidence of false normal values with unexpectedly depressed fetuses at birth, and a 30 to 55 per cent of false abnormal values where apparently operative intervention was not absolutely necessary (Beard et al, 1967). Ideally, therefore, serial samples should be collected, but there is a limit to the number of such samples that can be taken during the course of labour.

Attempts to measure continuous capillary blood pH were a failure because of coagulation problems around the electrode, resulting in significant electrode drift, but research continues to try and develop more reliable methods of detecting acid base changes in the fetus during labour.

RECENT DEVELOPMENTS IN FETAL MONITORING

The most important developments in this field have taken place over the past five years and are:

1. Continuous measurement of fetal tissue pH.
2. Continuous measurement of fetal tissue PO_2 by the transcutaneous route.

3. Intermittent whole blood lactate measurement in the fetus and mother during labour.

Although still in the research stage, these latest monitoring techniques can now be compared with continuous heart rate monitoring and with intermittent acid base studies in the fetus.

Continuous tissue pH

In 1974 Stamm and his co-workers reported for the first time the possibility of continuous tissue pH measurement (tpH) in neonates, using a new micro-electrode where the pH sensitive tip is made of a special Li-Ba-si glass of low electrical

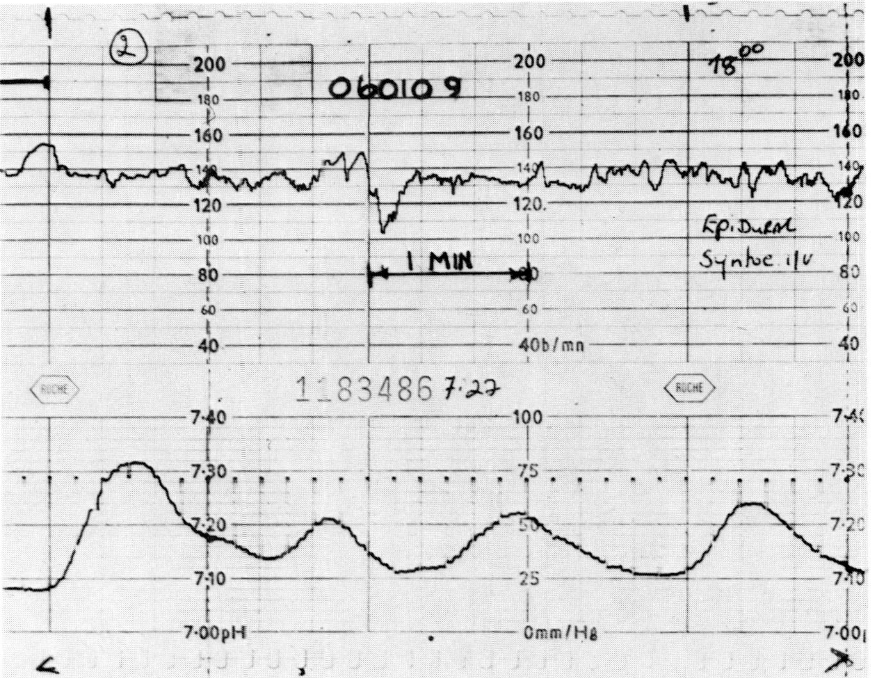

Fig. 2.1   Cardiotocograph record in labour showing: (Top) Fetal Heart Rate and (Bottom) (i) uterine contractions, (ii) continuous tissue pH record each 10 seconds.

resistance and the reference electrode together with the capillary liquid junction is an integral part of the electrode assembly. For use in the fetus during labour, after membrane rupture, the electrode is placed with the sensitive glass tip penetrating for a minimum of 3 mm into the fetal scalp and is attached with the spiral screw electrode, which also serves to record continuously the fetal e.c.g. The tpH values are indicated as vertical bars every 10 seconds on the labour trace, the scale going from 7.00 to 7.40 (Fig. 2.1).

There are two problems associated with the use of continuous tissue pH, which has delayed its introduction as a routine method of fetal monitoring during labour:

Fixation of the electrode to the scalp. In the earlier studies problems were encountered by breakage of the fragile glass electrode at the time of insertion or by the high percentage of electrodes which became dislodged during labour. Further development in the method of fixation have improved the number of successful recordings (Henner et al, 1978; Flynn & Kelly, 1980). (Figs. 2.2 and 2.3.)

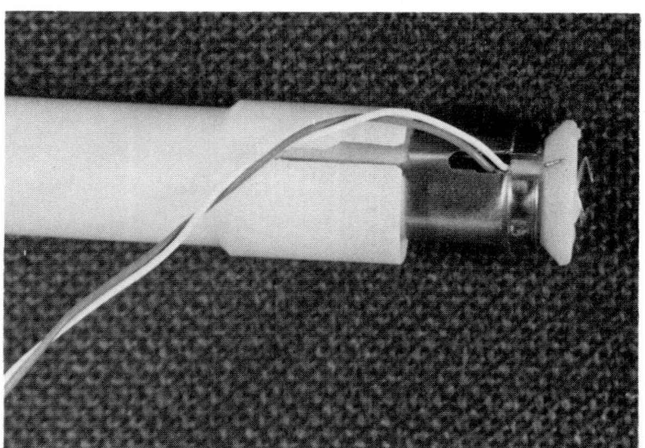

Fig. 2.2   Henner tube for application of e.c.g. double spiral and tpH electrodes.

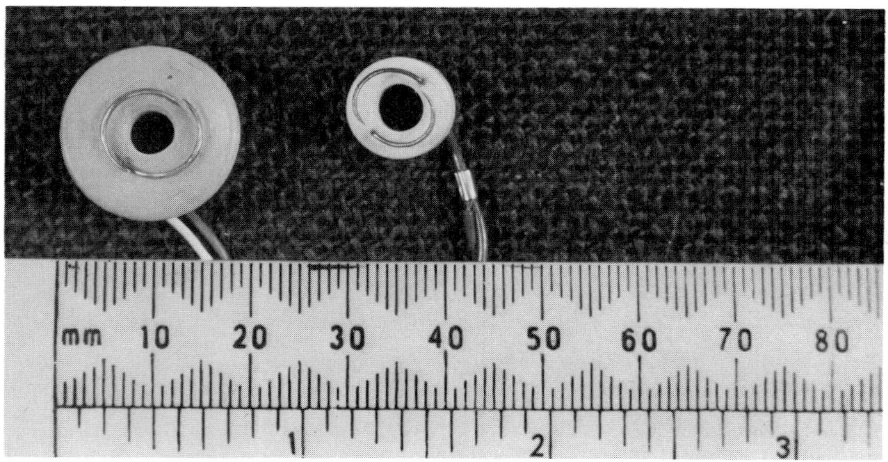

Fig. 2.3   New button double spiral electrode (left) and original one (right).

Despite recent technical improvements in the application ensemble (Henner, 1978) difficulty with fixation of the electrode to the fetal scalp is still its major disadvantage. This, of necessity, limits its use in clinical obstetrics at the present time.

Tissue pH measurement. Workers in the field of tissue pH agree that although it is possible to measure tpH in a given local area with acceptable reliability and reproductibility, our lack of knowledge of tissue pH measurement makes it difficult to know what any particular measurement represents. In the normal situation there is generally a reasonable correlation between scalp capillary blood pH value and that of the tpH reading at that time (R = 0.7) and an excellent correlation between the last tissue pH at the time of delivery in the human fetus and cord arterial blood pH (R = 0.9) with the tpH usually 0.04 pH units lower than that in blood (Sturbois et al, 1978; Hochberg, 1978; Flynn & Kelly, 1978). Studies comparing the tpH changes with different heart rate patterns showed that tpH changes correlated with fetal heart rate patterns in a manner consistent with current concepts of fetal stress and distress, i.e. 93 per cent of late decelerative patterns and 60 per cent of complicated tachycardia showed a fall in tpH, whereas there was no fall in those fetuses with physiological fetal heart rate patterns (Young et al, 1979).

Studies in fetal lambs subjected to measured induced hypoxia by intermittent cord or maternal aortic clamping showed that under conditions of induced hypoxia the

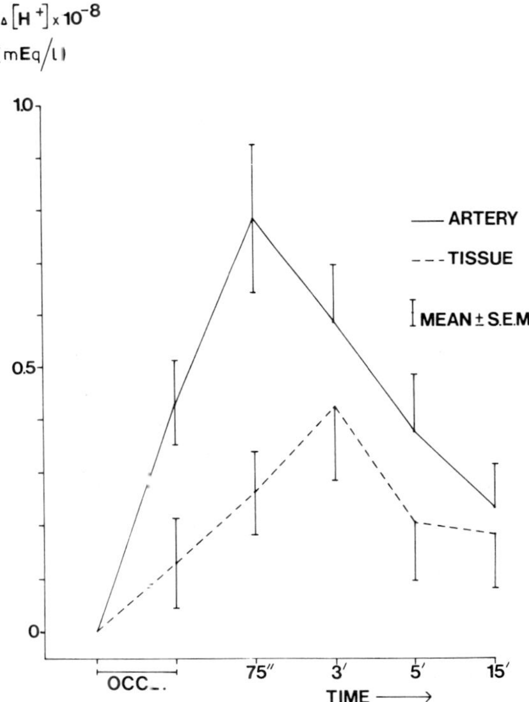

Fig. 2.4 Time relationship between hydrogen-ion concentration in tissue fluid and central arterial blood in fetal lambs during consecutive intermittent maternal aortic occlusions.

tissue pH decreases more slowly than central artery pH and never falls to levels reached by arterial pH. However, both apH and tpH values approximate after 15 minutes recovery from the insult (Fig. 2.4). There is an excellent correlation coefficient (R = 0.91) for tissue pH and arterial artery pH in the steady states (Fig. 2.5) (Flynn et al, 1980).

Continuous tissue PO$_2$ (TCPO$_2$) by the transcutaneous route

Huch (1973) described a Clark-type oxygen electrode (heated to 45°C. in order to produce adequate vaso-dilatation of the skin) which could measure continuously transcutaneous oxygen levels (TCPO$_2$). Further studies showed that in women during labour TCPO$_2$ measured in this way, correlated very closely with arterial oxygen

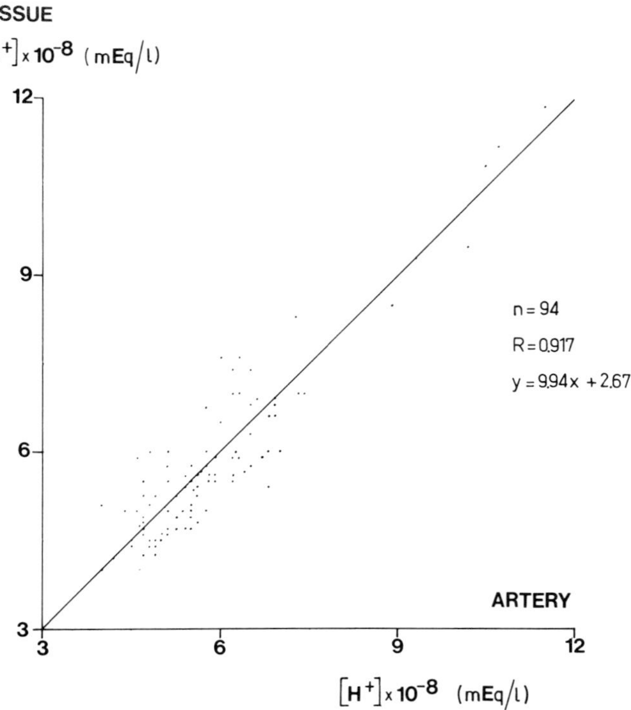

Fig. 2.5 Correlation between hydrogen-ion concentration in tissue fluid and central arterial blood in the steady state in fetal lambs subjected to intermittent cord occlusions.

tensions (PAO_2). Under conditions of hypoxia the $TCPO_2$ lagged behind the intravascular arterial O_2 values by about 30 seconds (Huchs et al, 1974).

In 1977 the same workers described the use of the oxygen electrode for the measurement of transcutaneous PO_2 in the fetus during labour. As with the continuous tpH electrode, fixation to the scalp is critical to good recording. In the case of O_2 electrode, after calibration the fetal scalp must first be shaved to facilitate fixation of the electrode, which is achieved by using a glue paste. One, therefore, requires a minimum cervical dilatation of 3 to 4 cm as well as ruptured membranes. This method of fixation was not found to be wholly satisfactory and modification using a suction technique appeared to give more reliable fixation (Weber & Secher, 1979).

Results show that decreasing levels of $TCPO_2$ have been found to correlate with late decelerative patterns (Huchs et al, 1977; Weber & Secher, 1980). Our knowledge of $TCPO_2$ values in the fetus during labour is imprecise and interpretation of results therefore are difficult. For example, it has been shown that the $TCPO_2$ was zero for periods of 20 minutes several hours before fetal death in utero, and for at least 50 minutes before the fetal heart stopped (Weber & Secher, 1979). More recently, studies have shown that pH and lactate are the only useful biochemical predictors of fetal asphyxia, since all the other biochemical parameters (PCO_2, PO_2 and base excess) show a substantial over-lap between normal and depressed fetuses, with a poor predictive value (Smith & Soutter, 1980). Whether $TCPO_2$ will ever become a clinical tool for routine investigation of fetal asphyxia in the delivery suite, remains for the present, speculative; it has proved, however, to be of value in elucidating the effects on fetal PO_2 of uterine contractions, the administration of anaesthetics and sedative drugs, and oxygen to the mother during labour, thus helping to increase our knowledge of fetal physiology during labour.

Blood lactate levels during labour and delivery

Lactic acid resulting from increased anaerobic glycolysis has been recognised for many years as the most accurate indicator of oxygen deficiency at the tissue or cell level. In adults suffering from shock, studies have shown the superiority of lactic acid measurements over other acid base parameters in predicting the outcome (Peretz et al, 1965; Weil, 1970). The difficulty in measuring lactic acid in the fetus during labour lay in the fact that these conventional methods of assaying lactic acid required at least one ml of blood and a lengthy procedure to make the evaluation. Such factors precluded its systematic use in the fetus during delivery. However, the development in 1975 of a lactate analyser capable of a rapid lactate determination using an electro-chemical enzymatic sensor on a blood sample of 150 μl, allowed the use of this technique to detect changes in lactic acid during labour, both in the normal and depressed fetuses (Soutter et al, 1978).

The results of preliminary studies showed that fetal lactic acid measurement during labour may prove to be useful in the practical clinical management of fetal distress (Smith et al, 1979). A subsequent study has shown that fetal scalp blood lactate measurement is as good an indication of fetal hypoxia as is the pH and both of these measurements are superior in predicting fetal outcome than the other blood acid base parameters (Smith & Soutter, 1980). The advantage of tissue pH is that it is simple to do, being a one stage procedure and giving continuous measurement. The lactate analyser, on the other hand, appears to be more robust, giving less problems with mechanical failures than the electrode. Which of these will develop into a routine clinical tool for the assessment of fetal asphyxia within the next few years depends in great part upon the speed of technological developments.

WHO SHOULD BE MONITORED?

Ideally, all patients should be monitored continuously during labour, yet not all labours require the same intensive care. Recent advances in antepartum monitoring enable the obstetrician to identify a group of 'high risk' patients who will require intensive monitoring during labour, as outlined in the preceding pages. Such a group will include small for dates fetuses, chronic cardiac and renal disease, severe pre-eclampsia, antepartum haemorrhage, rhesus disease and those women who have had a previous Caesarean section or a previous bad obstetric history.

However, consumer groups and sections of the mass media have recently conducted a strong campaign questioning 'intervention' in obstetrics (British Medical Journal Editorial, 5th January, 1980). These trends as well as the economic cost of monitoring patients have obliged obstetricians to re-evaluate the effects of technical obstetrics on the psychological and emotional needs of the mother and the baby.

Between 1975 and 1979 several studies, both retrospective and prospective, were conducted to assess the value of fetal heart rate/pH monitoring, both to the mother and the baby. Four retrospective studies (Tutera & Newman, 1975; Edington et al,

1975; Lee & Baggish, 1976; Hughey et al, 1977) were reviewed by Beard in 1977, who concluded that continuous fetal heart rate monitoring appeared to have a favourable effect on perinatal outcome, although he advocated caution in arriving at this conclusion, because of the lack of standardised management for all patients, and the fact that over the years, improved medical and social services would per se tend to improve perinatal outcome. He considered human error in the interpretation of the fetal heart rate trace to be one of the major problems in fetal monitoring.

In 1978, four prospective randomised controlled trials (Havercamp et al, 1976; Renou et al, 1976; Kelso et al, 1978 and Havercamp et al, 1979) were reviewed by Chalmers (1978). He found that intensive fetal heart rate monitoring alone resulted in an increase in Caesarean sections. When the continuous fetal heart rate monitoring was supplemented with adequate facilities for assessing the fetal acid base status and these techniques were applied to the high risk pregnancy group, they appeared to be associated with a decrease in Caesarean section, when compared with continuous fetal heart rate monitoring alone. There was also a reduced risk of neonatal convulsions and cerebral irritability in this high risk group. From the studies, however, no support was forthcoming to suggest that intermittent auscultation should be replaced by continuous electronic monitoring in a low risk group. Nevertheless, the tendency in some obstetric units towards a liberal policy of induction and acceleration of labour, together with epidural anaesthesia in low risk patients, transfers such patients into the high risk group, and increases the percentage of labour requiring continuous fetal heart rate monitoring. The general conclusion appears to be from these surveys that continuous fetal heart rate supplemented with acid base studies will reliably detect fetal asphyxia. The price to be paid for this is an invasive technique in which patients are confined to bed in the labour ward; risks of maternal infection are increased, and often unnecessary operative intervention and trauma to the mother's psychae and emotions. These disadvantages led to a search for an alternative method to allow 'normal' patients to be as 'normal' as possible in labour, mainly by allowing them to walk around, should they so wish.

Ambulation in labour
Ambulation per se is not an advance, but more a retreat. The most common position throughout the centuries has been some form of upright position, sitting, squatting, standing and kneeling. Birth positions more convenient to the accoucher, came to be preferred during the early part of the 20th century when births became more common in hospitals. Today, labour and childbirth with the woman in the recumbent or semi-recumbent position continues to be employed almost universally, even in developing countries. With the advent of improved fetal monitoring techniques many workers have shown that the supine position, especially in labour, is associated with maternal cardiovascular changes that actively interfere with uterine blood flow. This syndrome — the caval occlusion syndrome — is aggravated by the use of epidural analgesia for pain relief during labour. Although many obstetricians have observed the benefits of ambulation during labour (Krapohl et al, 1970; Mitre, 1974; Mendez-Bauer et al, 1975; Diaz et al, 1978; Flynn et al, 1978) most are reluctant to lose the benefits of direct continuous monitoring with the danger of missing early fetal distress if continuous monitoring is not available. In addition, the architectural layout of the modern delivery suite has little provision for the ambulant patient in labour,

making it difficult for the midwifery staff to find the patient in some part of the hospital every 10 to 15 minutes in order to auscultate the fetal heart. This is inconvenient both for the patient and for the midwife.

Monitoring by radiotelemetry

By means of radiotelemetry the fetal heart rate and intrauterine contractions can be continuously recorded in ambulant patients who are several hundred metres from the labour room (Flynn & Kelly, 1976; Flynn et al, 1978). Further development (Kelly et al, 1980) has allowed continuous monitoring of fetal heart rate and uterine contractions by external techniques to be transmitted by radiotelemetry over a wide radius. This non-invasive continuous fetal heart monitoring can be performed by midwives and allows the patient as much freedom as possible while retaining the benefits of continuous fetal heart rate/uterine contraction monitoring. Since membranes do not have to be ruptured this method is highly acceptable to the patient. Intact membranes until late in labour may have additional physiological benefits as suggested by Dunn (1978). The bag of forewaters is a physiological cervical dilator; the presence of amniotic fluid ensures isometric uterine contractions throughout the first stage of labour, preventing impairment of utero-placental circulation due to retraction of the placental site; the distribution of an even hydrostatic pressure over the whole fetal surface, protects the infant and cord from pressure. In a controlled trial, Caldeyro-Barcia et al (1974) reported an increase in intensity of uterine contractions, in fetal head moulding, in Type I dips and a fall in umbilical artery pH values among infants born to women whose membranes had been ruptured early as opposed to later in labour. Further, the mother and fetus are exposed to the risks of amnionitis and intra-uterine infection when the membranes are ruptured early. It is true that amniotomy has the advantage of revealing unexpected meconium staining of the amniotic fluid, and therefore, possibly a clinical indication of fetal distress. The single non-invasive continuous monitoring of the fetal heart by external methods however, more than balances this last advantage.

We believe in full ambulation for the patient during the early stages of labour. During the later phases or whenever the patient feels more comfortable in bed, she should be placed in a sitting position or the left lateral recumbent position. Studies have shown that ambulation in normal patients is associated with enhanced labour, shorter labour time and healthier babies at birth (Flynn et al, 1978). In addition, fewer analgesic drugs are requested, maternal satisfaction is greater and maternal-infant bonding is enhanced (Broadhurst et al, 1977).

MATERNAL POSITION AT DELIVERY

Recent literature on maternal positioning during the second stage for vaginal delivery shows a tendency to get away from the dorsal position or the Simm's left lateral position. In 1979 Caldeyro-Barcia designed a birthing chair. Other centres, realising the advantages of squatting or sitting during delivery, are experimenting with alternatives to the dorsal recumbent position, by using special beds, chairs and tables. These changes are not easily accomplished and at present are only occasionally used.

The use of computers in intrapartum fetal monitoring

Some modern cardiotocograph machines have incorporated microprocessors capable of recording fetal heart rate variability as an index over periods of two minutes and displaying cumulative uterine action over cycles of 10 to 15 minutes. These microprocessors are also used in some machines to give a clearer and smoother fetal heart trace by an averaging technique. Such averaging techniques, however, may be a disadvantage in that they mask the true beat-to-beat variability of the heart rate which can be an important signal of fetal hypoxia and incipient asphyxia. Apart from such microprocessors the management of fetal heart rate monitoring in labour by computer techniques is rare. Much work however, is being done as an off-line procedure in developing methods of assessing baseline fetal heart rate variability and the classification of the patterns of deceleration. The use of computerised fetal monitoring during labour has, to date, not achieved the rapid development anticipated.

CONCLUSION

The biological data so far available is in favour of fetal heart rate monitoring, although there are disadvantages associated with the procedure. Over the past decade the continuous fetal heart rate has been found to be a good screening system showing when problems are likely to arise in the fetus during labour. Furthermore, improvements in antenatal techniques should allow us to select out the 10 to 20 per cent of high risk pregnancies that require intensive fetal monitoring during labour. In these high risk pregnancies, continuous fetal heart rate patterns require further elucidation by acid base studies — pH being the most reliable and easiest to obtain. At present pH must still be assessed by intermittent capillary sampling, however, continuous tissue pH may become available for such high risk patients within the next few years.

For the normal patient, developments in radiotelemetry using external methods combine the advantages of continuous fetal heart rate screening, with the physiological and emotional advantages to the patient of conditions during labour as near normal as possible. No fetal monitor can substitute for the personal attention and psychological support of the midwife, but the added information from continuous recording of the fetal heart rate and uterine action allows any deviation from the normal to be detected at an early stage. The current situation in many hospitals indicates the need for more intensive training courses in the interpretation of fetal heart rate records for both obstetricians and midwives. This would probably reduce the number of unnecessary operative interventions and lessen both the physical and emotional stress for the mother and baby.

REFERENCES

Abdulla U, Campbell S, Dewhurst C J, Talbert D, Lucas M, Mullarky M 1971 Effect of diagnostic ultrasound on maternal and fetal chromosomes. Lancet ii: p 829

Beard R W 1977 Is intrapartum monitoring worthwhile?. In: Beard R, Campbell S (eds) The current status of fetal heart rate monitoring and ultrasound in obstetrics. Proceedings of the Scientific Meeting of the Royal College of Obstetricians & Gynaecologists, 2nd December, 1977, 2–9, Broadhurst, No 2

Beard R W, Morris E D 1969 Fetal distress — some biochemical considerations. In: Keller R J Modern trends in obstetrics, 4th edn. Butterworths, London, p 273

Beard R W, Morris E D, Clayton S G (1966) Haemorrhage following fetal blood sampling: Journal of Obstetrics and Gynaecology of the British Commonweath 73: 860

Beard R W, Filshie G M, Knight C A, Roberts G M 1971a The significance of the changes in the continuous fetal heart rate in the first stage of labour: Journal of Obstetrics and Gynaecology of the British Commonwealth 78: 865

Beard R W, Brudenell J M, Feroze R M, Clayton S G 1971b Intensive care of the high risk fetus in labour. Journal of Obstetrics and Gynaecology of the British Commonwealth 78: 882

Broadhurst A, Flynn A M, Kelly J, Lynch P F 1977 The effects of ambulation in labour on material satisfaction, analgesia and lactation. Proceedings of International Congress on Psychosomatic Obstetrics and Gynaecology, Rome 1977. 943

Caldeyro-Barcia R 1979 A new birthing chair: International Congress Series No. 572. Gynecology and Obstetrics. Proceedings of the IX World Congress of Gynecology and Obstetrics, Tokyo, 1979. Ed. Shoichi Sakamoto, Shimpei, Tokyo and Tersuya Makayama. Excerpta Medica, Elsevier, North-Holland

Caldeyro-Barcia R, Schwarz R, Belizan J M, Martell M, Nieto F, Sabatino H, Tenzer S M 1974 Adverse perinatal effect of early amniotomy during labour. In: Gluck L (ed) Modern perinatal medicine. Chicago, p 431

Caldeyro-Barcia R, Mendez-Bauer C, Poseiro J J et al 1966 Control of human FHR during labour. In: Cassels D E (ed) The heart and circulation of the newborn and infant. Grune and Stratton, New York City p 7–36

Caldeyro-Barcia R, Casacuberta C, Bustos R, Ginussi, Gulin L, Escerena L, Mendez-Bauer C 1968 Correlation of intrapartum changes in fetal heart rate with fetal blood oxygen. In: Adamson K (ed) Diagnosis and treatment of fetal disorders. Springer Verlag, New York, p 205

Calvert J P, Newcombe R G (1980) Which fetal scalp electrode? Lancet i: 371

Chalmers I 1978 Randomised controlled trials of intrapartum fetal monitoring. In: Thalhammer O, Baumgarten K, Pollack A (eds) Perinatal medicine, 6th European Congress, Vienna, p 260–265

Crawford J S 1979 Continuous lumbar epidural analgesia for labour and delivery. British Medical Journal January 1979

Cremer M 1906 Munchener Medizinische Wochenschrift 53: 811

Diaz A G, Schwarcz R, Fescina R, Caldeyro-Barcia R 1978 Posision materna y trabajo de parto: Separata de la Revista Clinica e Investigacao en Ginecologia y Obstetricia 5(3): 101

Dunn P M 1978 Problems associated with fetal monitoring during labour. In: Thalhammer O, Baumgarten K, Pollack A (eds) Perinatal Medicine, 6th European Congress, Vienna, 1978.

Edington P T, Sibanda J, Beard R W 1975 Influence on clinical practice of routine intrapartum fetal monitoring. British Medical Journal 3: 341

Editorial. British Medical Journal, 5th January 1980

Flynn A M, Kelly J (1978) An evaluation of the continuous tissue pH electrode (tpH) during labour in the human fetus. Archives of Gynecology 22: 105–113

Flynn A M, Kelly J (1976) Continuous fetal monitoring in the ambulant patient in labour. British Medical Journal 2: 842–843

Flynn A M, Kelly J, Hollins G, Lynch P F 1978 Ambulation in labour. British Medical Journal 2: 591

Flynn A M, Martin C B, Van de Wildt B, Jongsma H W 1981 The relationship between arterial and interstitial (subcutaneous tissue) pH in the fetal lamb under conditions of acute hypoxia: Proceedings of the 6th Workshop on Fetal Breathing, University of Oxford, June 1980

Flynn A M, Kelly J 1980 The continuous measurement of tissue pH in the human fetus during labour using a new application technique. British Journal of Obstetrics and Gynaecology 87: 666

Ghosh A K, Tipton R H 1976 Fetal scalp electrodes. Lancet i: 1048

Hammacher K 1969 The clinical significance of cardiotocography. In: Huntingford P J, Huter K A, Saling E (ed) Perinatal medicine, 1st European Congress, Berlin, 1968. Thieme Verlag, Stuttgart

Haverchamp A D, Thompson H E, McFee J G, Murphy J A 1979 A controlled trial of differential effects of intrapartum fetal monitoring. American Journal of Obstetrics and Gynecology 134: 399

Henner H, Ruttgers H, Muliwan D, Haller U, Kubli F 1978 A new application tool for the Roche pH electrode. Archives of Gynecology 226: 75–77

Hochberg H M 1978 Multicentre clinical trials of fetal pH monitoring in the USA. Archives of Gynecology 226: 93–98

Hon E H 1963 The classification of fetal heart rate. No 1. A Working Classification: Obstetrics and Gynecology 22: 137

Hon H E 1968 In: Atlas of Fetal Heart Rate Patterns. Party Press, New Haven, USA

Hon H E, Paul R H, Hon R W 1972 Electronic evaluation of fetal heart rate. XI. Description of a spiral electrode. Obstetrics and Gynecology 40: 362

Huch R 1973 Trancutaneous measurement of blood pcO_2 ($tcPO_2$) — Method and application in perinatal medicine. Journal of Perinatal Medicine 1: 183

Huch A, Huch R, Lindmark G, Rooth G 1974 Maternal hypoxaemia after Pethidine. Journal of Obstetrics and Gynaecology of the British Commonwealth 81: 608

Huch R, Seler D, Salster H, Weinzer K, Lubbers D W 1977 Transcutaneous pcO_2 measurement with a miniturised electrode. Lancet, May 7th, 1977, 982

Hull M G R 1972a Perinatal coagulopathies complicating fetal blood sampling. British Medical Journal 4: 319

Hull M G R 1972b Massive scalp haemorrhage after fetal blood sampling. British Medical Journal 4: 321

Huntingford P J, Pendleton H J 1969 The clinical application of cardiotocography. Journal of Obstetrics and Gynaecology of the British Commonwealth 76: 586

Hunter C A, Lansford K G, Knoebel S B, Braunlin R J 1960 A technique for recording fetal ECG during labour and delivery. Obstetrics and Gynecology 16: 567

Hughey M J, La Pata R E, McElin T W, Lussky R 1977 The effect of fetal monitoring on the incidence of Caesarean section. Obstetrics and Gynecology 49: 513

Kelly J, Flynn A M, Hollins G 1980 Ambulant fetal monitoring. British Journal of Hospital Medicine 24: 449

Kelso I M, Parsons R J, Lawrence G F, Arora S S, Edmonds D K, Cooke I D 1978 An assessment of continuous fetal heart rate monitoring in labour. A randomised trial. American Journal of Obstetrics and Gynecology 131: 526

Krapohl A J, Myers, Grant G, Caldeyro-Barcia R 1970 Uterine contractions in spontaneous labour. American Journal of Obstetrics and Gynecology 106: 378

Kubli F W 1968 Influence of labour on fetal and acid-base balance. Clinical Obstetrics and Gynaecology 11: 168–191

Lee W K, Baggish M S 1976 The effect of unselected intrapartum fetal monitoring. Obstetrics and Gynecology 47: 516

Mackintosh I J C, Davey D A 1970 Chromosome aberrations induced by an ultrasonic fetal pulse detector. British Medical Journal 4: 92

Maubray J 1724 The female physician. Quoted in: Curtis A H (ed) 1973 Obstetrics and gynecology, vol 1, p 11. Saunders, Philadelphia

Mendez-Bauer C, Arroyo C Y, Carcia Ramos A, Mendenay A, Lavilla M, Izquierdo F, Villa Elizaga I, Zammarriogo 1975 Effects of standing position on spontaneous uterine contractions and other aspects of labour. Journal of Perinatal Medicine 3: 89

Mitre I N 1974 The influence of maternal position on duration of the active phase of labour. International Journal of Gynecology and Obstetrics 12: 181

Okado D M, Chow A W, Bruce V T 1977 Neonatal scalp abscess and fetal monitoring: factors associated with infection. American Journal of Obstetrics and Gynecology 129: 185–189

Paterson P, Dunstan M, Trickey N R A, Beard R W 1970 A biochemical comparison of the mature and postmature fetus and newborn infant. Journal of Obstetrics and Gynaecology of the British Commonwealth 77: 390

Peretz D I, Scott H M, Duff J, Dossetor J B, MacLean L D, McGregor M 1965 The significance of lacticacidaemia in the shock syndrome. Annals of the NY Academy of Science 119: 1133

Renou P, Chang A, Anderson I, Wood C 1976 Controlled trial of fetal intensive care. American Journal of Obstetrics and Gynecology 126: 470

Saling E 1964 Technik der endoskopischen Mikrobluhentnahme am Fetus. Geburtshilfe und Frauenheilkunde 24: 464

Showell A W 1976 Surgicraft Copeland Electrode. Lancet p 1075

Smith N C, Quinn M C, Soutter W P, Sharp F 1979 Rapid wholeblood lactate measurements in the fetus and mother during labour. In: Early human development, 3/1, 89–95. Elsevier North-Holland, Biomedical Press

Smith N C, Soutter W P 1980 Intrapartum fetal scalp lactate measurement as an indicator of fetal hypoxia. Abstract. Scientific Programme of the British Congress of Obstetrics and Gynaecology, Edinburgh 1980

Smyth C N 1953 Experimental electrocardiotocography of the fetus. Lancet I: 1124

Soutter W P, Sharp F, Clark D M 1978 Bedside estimation of whole blood lactate. British Journal of Anaesthesia 50: 445

Stamm O 1975 Kontinuierliche subkutane pH-Messung am kindlichen Kopf intra- und postpartum. In: Dudenhausen J W, Saling E, Schmidt E (eds) Perinatale Medizin Vol VI. 7. Thieme, Stuttgart

Sturbois G, Uzan S, Breart S, Rotten D, Salat-Baroux J, Sureau C 1978 Improvements in the results with the continuous tpH electrode due to technical progress. A comparison between two series of cases. Archives of Gynecology 226: 87

Sureau C 1956 Fetal cardiotocogram during gestation and childbirth. Gynecology and Obstetrics (Paris) 551: 21

Trudinger B J, Pryse-Davies J 1978 Fetal hazards of the intrauterine pressure catheter: five case reports. British Journal of Obstetrics and Gynaecology 85: 567

Tutera G, Newman R L 1975 Fetal monitoring: its effects on perinatal mortality and Caesarean section rates and its complications. American Journal of Obstetrics and Gynecology 122: 750

Weber T 1980 Transcutaneous fetal oxygen tension and fetal heart rate patterns preceding fetal death. British Journal of Obstetrics and Gynaecology 87: 165–168

Weber T, Secher N J 1979 Continuous measurement of transcutaneous fetal oxygen tension during labour. British Journal of Obstetrics and Gynaecology 86: 954

Weil M H, Afifi A A 1970 Experimental and clinical studies on lactate and pyruvate as indicators of the severity of acute circulatory failure (shock). Circulation 41: 989
Wheeler T, Murrills A J and Shelly T 1978 Measurement of the fetal heart rate during pregnancy by a new electrocardiographic technique. British Journal of Obstetrics and Gynaecology 85: 12
Wood C, Newman W, Lumley J, Hammond J 1969 Classification of fetal heart rate in relation to fetal scalp blood measurement and Apgar score. American Journal of Obstetrics and Gynecology 105: 942
Young B K, Katz M and Klein S A 1979 The relationship of heart rate patterns and tissue pH in the human fetus. American Journal of Obstetrics and Gynecology, 15th July: 685

3. A critical review of amniocentesis in clinical practice

J. W. K. Ritchie   W. Thompson

INTRODUCTION

Interest in amniotic fluid though sporadic until comparatively recent times is evident throughout medical history. Increasing awareness of the contribution to amniotic fluid made by the fetus and of their unique and intimate relationship has prompted a growing interest in its acquisition and analysis. Advances in the management of complicated antenatal situations have put paid to the obstetrical ethic of non-intervention and stimulated the quest for information to aid intrauterine diagnosis.

Amniocentesis or tapping the amniotic sac transabdominally with a needle for diagnostic or therapeutic purposes was used originally to outline the fetus and placenta radiologically by means of an amniogram (Menees et al, 1930) and later to induce abortion by injection of hypertonic glucose or saline. It was the application of the technique to the field of Rhesus isoimmunisation management by Bevis (1953) and Liley (1961) which ensured that amniocentesis became a commonplace and relatively safe clinical procedure. Further advances in the past decade have led to its widespread use in the assessment of maturity of fetal organs and in the diagnosis of congenital abnormalities and genetic disorders.

The main uses of amniocentesis in modern clinical practice will be considered in this review, namely antenatal genetic diagnosis, Rhesus isoimmunisation management, fetal organ maturity and finally its occasional use for therapeutic purposes. Other related procedures such as fetoscopy and intrauterine fetal transfusion are not included and have been well reviewed elsewhere (Benzie, 1980; Whitfield, 1980).

CLINICAL PHYSIOLOGY OF AMNIOTIC FLUID

Prior to the keratinisation of fetal skin at approximately 20 weeks' gestation the amniotic fluid is isotonic with a composition resembling fetal extracellular fluid (Lind, 1978), and derived chiefly from the fetus, cord and placenta. Secretion by the cells of the amnion is likely to be important only during the embryonic stage of development. In the second half of pregnancy, hypotonic fetal urine is produced at a rate of more than 500 ml/day (Campbell et al, 1973) and becomes an important source of amniotic fluid causing a dilution of its original isotonic state.

Lung fluid probably also contributes to the amniotic fluid volume as the respiratory tract matures and a net outflow of lung fluid of approximately 100 ml/kg/day has been demonstrated in the fetal sheep in the late gestation (Dawes, 1973). Direct evidence for this in humans has not been obtained but surface active phospholipids specific to the lung increase gradually in the amniotic fluid with advancing gestation (Gluck et al, 1971). This suggests that lung fluid from the lower respiratory tract and particularly the alveoli contributes to liquor volume in human pregnancy and is probably dependent upon the presence of fetal chest wall movements. Amniotic fluid is removed by fetal swallowing and the production of amniotic fluid is balanced by its reabsorption through the fetal gastro-intestinal tract; in late pregnancy the human fetus has been shown to swallow on average 475 ml per day (Pritchard, 1966). Fetal abnormalities of the kidney, lung or gastrointestinal tract can disrupt the mechanism of this circulation resulting in a pathological increase in amniotic fluid volume.

In normal pregnancy the volume of amniotic fluid at varying gestations is important to the clinician undertaking amniocentesis. The average volume present at each gestation has been calculated by Abramovich (1970) as shown in Table 3.1 and it

Table 3.1 Average liquor volume at each week in early and mid-pregnancy with the daily and weekly increase in volume (Abramovich D R 1970; reproduced with the permission of the Editor of the British Journal of Obstetrics and Gynaecology).

Menstrual age (weeks)	Average liquor volume (ml)	Average daily increase (ml)
10	34	—
11	44	1.4
12	58	2
13	76	2.6
14	100	3.4
15	130	4.3
16	171	5.9
17	223	7.4
18	292	9.9
19	383	13
20	501	16.9

should be noted that liquor volume virtually doubles between 14 and 16 weeks gestation. At term the average volume falls to around 800 ml having been at a peak of approximately 1000 ml at 34 weeks gestation. After 42 weeks gestation the average volume falls below 500 ml and continues to decrease with prolonged gestation (Queenan et al, 1972).

Amniotic fluid begins to contain cells in significant numbers between 12 and 14 weeks (Wachtel et al, 1969) and the total number of cells rises steadily towards term as shown in Figure 3.1. The number of viable cells rises slowly from 12 weeks to near a maximum at 22 weeks. In clinical practice the timing of amniocentesis for genetic purposes particularly for chromosomal analysis is influenced by amniotic fluid volume and the percentage of viable cells present. As a consequence it is unwise to attempt this procedure before 16 weeks because of the increased risk of failure to obtain fluid and to grow cells from it.

The cells found in amniotic fluid in early gestation are derived mainly from fetal skin and amnion and are of two main types: large polygonal cells and small round cells which predominate. In culture the large polygonal cells disappear and small cells resembling fibroblasts grow progressively. As pregnancy advances epithelial cells of squamous type derived from the fetal skin are increasingly found as well as those from the amnion and other fetal epithelial surfaces such as the buccal mucous membrane, vagina, urinary tract and cord (Wachtel et al, 1969).

Near term the increasing number of cells staining orange with Nile Blue Sulphate has been used to diagnose fetal maturity (Brosens & Gordon, 1966). These cells were

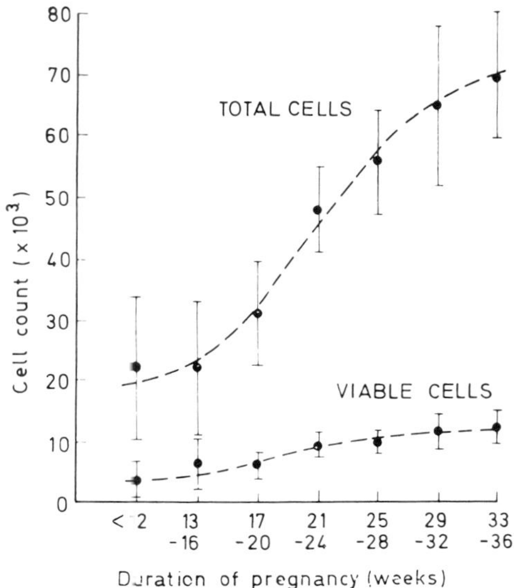

Fig. 3.1   The change in the total number of cells and number of viable cells in amniotic fluid as gestation advances. Emery A E H 1970 Reproduced by courtesy of Butterworths, London, from Emery A E H (1970) Modern Trends in Human Genetics, 1: 257.

thought to contain fat as a feature of maturity but it is considered more likely that the orange stain is taken up due to a covering of vernix (Huisjes, 1978).

TECHNIQUE OF AMNIOCENTESIS

There are minor differences between the technique of amniocentesis performed in early and in late gestation.

Early pregnancy
Initial assessment with ultrasound to demonstrate the number of fetuses, viability, gestational age and the position and depth of the placenta is an essential prerequisite and may be facilitated by the patient having a full bladder. Using real-time ultrasound a full bladder is not always essential and occasionally can make the amniocentesis more difficult by changing the angle of the uterus to the abdominal wall. The operator localises the pool of liquor of maximum depth; the transducer head placed first in the horizontal and then vertical position and gently rocked to give the angle of approach and depth of entry. The latter technique is not possible using a static compound B-scan machine. Most real-time scanners incorporate centimetre markers on the screen which aid depth localisation. The site should be fixed either visually in relation to other abdominal landmarks or with an indelible marker and amniocentesis performed without moving the patient using a 20 gauge spinal needle with a stilette, the latter preventing contamination of the fluid with maternal cells. A formal sterile technique involving drapes and gown has been described (Mellows, 1980) but is not necessary. For several years we have used a 'no touch technique' without local anaesthetic and have found it entirely satisfactory. The quantity of amniotic fluid removed is usually between 10 and 20 ml as this is sufficient to complete full

investigations. If there is doubt about the origin of the fluid, urine may be excluded simply by testing immediately for the presence of protein using a dip-stick. If heavily blood-stained fluid is obtained, it may not be suitable for genetic analysis; a further attempt at amniocentesis should be avoided for at least two weeks.

If a patient with an indication for genetic amniocentesis is found to have a multiple pregnancy some advocate that an attempt should be made to obtain fluid from each sac since the overall risk of abnormality is double that in singletons (Hunter & Cox, 1979). This is not only technically more difficult but probably increases the risk of abortion and may present a difficult ethical decision should abnormality be diagnosed in only one fetus. It is perhaps wiser not to undertake genetic amniocentesis in multiple pregnancy and the patient counselled accordingly.

Late pregnancy
The technique of localising the liquor pool with ultrasound is similar but where the pool is small or the placenta thick and anterior, the indication must be reviewed and

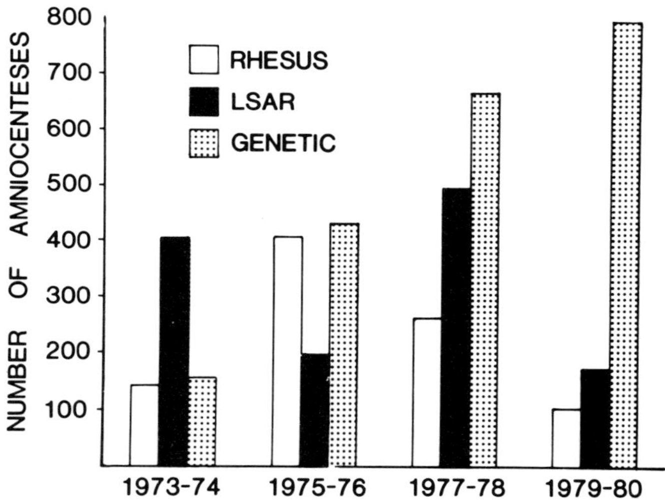

Fig. 3.2   A comparison of the number of amniocenteses for various indications, Royal Maternity Hospital, Belfast 1973–80.

the risk weighed before proceeding. There are fewer indications for amniocentesis in late pregnancy because of rapid simple pregnancy dating using ultrasound and better perinatal care. This is reflected in the change in our own clinical practice where it can be seen from Figure 3.2 that amniocentesis for Rhesus isoimmunisation and fetal lung maturity have decreased while genetic amniocenteses have increased substantially.

When amniocentesis cannot be performed with the help of ultrasonic localisation of the placenta and the liquor pool, then the technique of displacing the presenting part out of the pelvis has been employed with relative success (Gordon & Deukmedjian, 1975). An occasional complication is the subsequent leak of liquor from the puncture created in membranes so near to the cervix (Gunston & Davey, 1978).

COMPLICATIONS OF AMNIOCENTESIS

Complications following amniocentesis are similar whether the procedure is performed in early or in late gestation and they have been reviewed by Fairweather (1978). Serious complications were reported more frequently in the early days of amniocentesis but the availability of ultrasound together with better technique seems to have reduced these problems since the procedure is now in widespread use in clinical practice.

Maternal complications

Infection

Infection is an obvious but, fortunately, rare complication which on occasions in the past has led to maternal death (Fairweather, 1978) although this has not been reported in recent literature. In our own experience only one case of serious maternal infection has occurred after genetic amniocentesis in the past ten years; a normal fetus was lost and the mother survived after intensive antibiotic therapy.

Haemorrhage

Serious maternal bleeding from uterine or abdominal wall is rare and maternal death as a result is extremely unlikely.

Isoimmunisation

Amniocentesis may cause or increase isoimmunisation, the most serious of which is Rhesus. Sensitisation is more likely to occur when the placenta is anterior or when blood or blood stained fluid is obtained since both these complications are associated with a high incidence of feto-maternal transfusion (Curtis et al, 1972; Wang et al, 1967). The risk can be reduced by accurate localisation of the placenta at amniocentesis and considering carefully the value of amniocentesis in each case. It is now advocated that Rhesus Anti-D immuno-globulin should be given to all non-sensitised Rhesus negative women undergoing amniocentesis increasing the dose if feto-maternal transfusion is proven (Benzie, 1980). The Department of Health and Social Services in the United Kingdom has recommended using $50\,\mu$g of Rhesus Anti-D immuno-globulin before 20 weeks' gestation and $100\,\mu$g thereafter, in the absence of antibodies (DHSS, 1976).

Leakage of liquor and preterm labour

This may occur occasionally but is rarely serious and is usually transient, the risk being greater after suprapubic amniocentesis (Gordon & Deukmedjian, 1975). Preterm labour has been reported after amniocentesis but the risk is minimal and in reviewing the literature Fairweather (1978) considered it a more theoretical than practical complication.

Fetal complications

Haemorrhage

This complication may have serious consequences and has been reported in most large series of amniocentesis. More disturbing is that it continues to occur despite improvements in ultrasound equipment and in technique. It is more likely after amniocentesis in late pregnancy and has occurred in our own hospital practice three times in the past ten years leading to fetal exsanguination and death on two occasions. The most recent instance occurred when amniocentesis was being performed in the usual manner in late pregnancy where the amount of liquor was reduced. A bloody tap was followed some eight hours later by emergency delivery for fetal bradycardia. At Caesarean section the liquor was heavily blood stained and the infant died soon after birth due to exsanguination. Where a clinical reduction in liquor volume is suspected and ultrasound is not available, it is probably unwise to attempt amniocentesis.

Direct injury

Injury to the fetus is not common after amniocentesis in the third trimester and although puncture of the eye, lung, heart and spleen have been reported (Fairweather, 1978) these complications seem less likely today. In early pregnancy amniocentesis may occasionally cause linear skin lacerations or dimple-like scars and their incidence appears to be directly related to the number of attempts at amniocentesis and the experience of the operator (Epley et al, 1979).

Abortion and premature labour

Spontaneous abortion is a definite but small risk after mid-trimester amniocentesis occurring in 3.5 per cent of cases in the collaborative study of the National Institute of Child Health and Human Development (1976) while in controls the rate was 3.2 per cent. However, the incidence of abortion is known to be greater in women at risk of having a fetus with a neural tube defect (Nevin & Johnston, 1980a) and in those aged 35 years and over.

The risk of abortion due to amniocentesis is important in genetic counselling and has been calculated for our own population as follows. In a series of 1290 consecutive mid-trimester amniocenteses performed during 1970–1978 at the Royal Maternity Hospital, Belfast, abortion occurred on 27 occasions, a rate of 2.2 per cent (Ritchie et al, 1980). The timing of the abortions in relation to amniocentesis is shown in Table 3.2 and it is likely that at least some were unrelated to the procedure. If it is assumed

Table 3.2 Distribution of interval between spontaneous abortion and genetic amniocentesis in 1290 patients, Royal Maternity Hospital, Belfast 1970–78.

	Number	Percentage of total
Less than 48 hours	1 ⎫	
Between 2 and 6 days	4 ⎬	0.7
Between 1 and 2 weeks	4 ⎭	
Between 2 and 4 weeks	5 ⎫	1.5
More than 4 weeks	13 ⎭	
	27	2.2

that the test is unlikely to cause a spontaneous abortion after an interval or more than two weeks then the 'excess' risk involved in mid-trimester amniocentesis in our hands is in the region of 0.7 per cent. A somewhat higher figure (1.0 to 1.5 per cent excess risk) was quoted by the Working Party on Genetic Amniocentesis of the Medical

Research Council (1978) as a result of a multicentre study in nine centres in the United Kingdom. It should be noted that this multicentre study was carried out at a time when ultrasonic localisation of the placenta and liquor pool was not performed routinely.

Neonatal morbidity

The Medical Research Council's collaborative study in the United Kingdom (1978) suggests that there may be a risk of idiopathic respiratory distress, talipes and congenital dislocation of the hip after mid-trimester amniocentesis all of which are theoretically possible results of a reduction in liquor volume. The evidence is statistically significant and is sufficient to stimulate careful paediatric assessment at birth of all such infants with a view to the diagnosis of these specific complications.

INDICATIONS FOR AMNIOCENTESIS

Genetic disease and congenital abnormalities

Fuchs & Riis (1956) were first to use amniotic fluid examination in the prevention of hereditary disease by determining fetal sex from the chromatin in the nuclei of the cells in the fluid. In this way, although they were unable to diagnose the disease itself, they were able to identify fetuses at risk and to terminate such pregnancies selectively. During the past decade mid-trimester amniocentesis for the diagnosis of a variety of genetic disorders has become well established in many centres (Nadler & Gerbie, 1970), its use increasing as more and more conditions can be specifically diagnosed in utero.

Skilled genetic counselling is essential before embarking on an amniocentesis for the diagnosis of a genetic disorder since the patient must understand the full implications of the investigations. Expectations regarding the test should not be unrealistic and patients should be fully informed of the risks of amniocentesis and the procedure involved for the termination of pregnancy if the latter should be indicated.

The objects of antenatal diagnosis are either:

1. To exclude an abnormal fetus in a high-risk situation. The diagnostic accuracy of amniocentesis for genetic disease is extremely good (at least 99.4 per cent, Table

Table 3.3   Results of genetic amniocentesis.

	U.S. Study[1] 1971–3	British[2] Study 1973–6	Toronto[3] Study 1971–9	Belfast Study 1970–9
No. of amniocenteses	1041	2428	3323	1290
Abnormal fetuses detected	3.3%	4.6%	3.2%	3.9%
Errors	0.6%	0.6%	0.2%	0%
Accuracy rates	99.4%	99.4%	99.8%	100%

(1) NICHD Amniocentesis Registry
(2) The assessment of the hazards of amniocentesis (1978)
(3) Benzie R J (1980)

3.3) and the vast majority of patients can be reassured and relieved of the anxiety of bearing an abnormal child.
2. To identify an abnormal fetus and proceed to termination of the pregnancy. It

must be appreciated that some women will wish to have an amniocentesis but will not be prepared to have termination even in the presence of an abnormal baby. Some couples wish simply to be prepared in the event of an abnormal fetus being diagnosed.

The decision to embark on a further pregnancy or to continue a pregnancy when a fetal abnormality has been diagnosed or to have a therapeutic abortion rests with the parents alone and it is important that there should be no medical pressure on them to act in a certain way. The general practitioner or obstetrician providing antenatal care should be aware that failure to initiate genetic counselling may be construed as negligence and if necessary the patient should be referred to the appropriate centre for further assessment. On the other hand termination of pregnancy may not be acceptable to some couples or may be illegal and antenatal screening tests should not be carried out without informed consent.

The genetic-obstetric clinic
Ideally the expertise required in genetic counselling, ultrasound, obstetrics, cytogenetics and biochemistry should be concentrated in a few major centres where the genetic-obstetric clinic can provide a balanced and comprehensive evaluation for couples who have been referred with a potential problem. Patients may be referred to the clinic by obstetricians, general practitioners or the geneticist who has interviewed the patient following the birth of an abnormal baby and requested attendance in a subsequent pregnancy. Patients are best seen jointly by a medical geneticist and an obstetrician when the extent and limitations of genetic diagnosis can be explained to the couple. A particularly anxious couple who do not have an increased risk of a congenital abnormality may request amniocentesis. Each case must be dealt with individually on its own merits and not dismissed without careful consideration; the risks of the procedure should be understood by the parents before a decision is made. Careful counselling will dissuade the majority of such parents particularly after real-time ultrasonic examination has revealed to them the moving fetus in utero and its outline. If genetic amniocentesis is undertaken then tests to detect a neural tube defect together with chromosomal analysis should be performed though this is an expense beyond some laboratories.

A genetic-obstetric clinic was established in the Royal Maternity Hospital, Belfast in 1970 and now provides a service for Northern Ireland, a Province with a population of 1.5 million (total births approximately 30 000 per annum). Approximately 15 couples per week are interviewed and around 400 amniocenteses performed per year. Experience at this clinic highlights the advantages of the team approach providing optimum communication between the obstetrician, geneticist and laboratory. The same clinicians can give important psychological support for those patients who require termination of pregnancy by providing this service and subsequent detailed examination of the fetus. The importance of this approach cannot be over-emphasised in the light of recent reports concerning mothers' attitudes to termination in these circumstances (Donnai et al, 1981).

In the course of screening for trisomy, the fetus may be shown to have an XXY chromosome constitution. In these circumstances should the obstetrician tell the patient or recommend termination? The answer is probably no to both these questions. The condition is compatible with normal life and although the techniques for termination of pregnancy in the mid-trimester have improved since the introduction of prostaglandins it is not without hazard to the mother (Ritchie & Traub, 1979).

After chromosomal analysis the obstetrician will know the sex of the fetus and the question arises whether or not the mother should be informed. It has been suggested that she should not be told as occasionally an error may be made when a normal female is reported but followed by the birth of a normal male; this can occur because of contamination of the amniotic sample with maternal cells. Rarely a male chromosome constitution is found but is complicated by androgen insensitivity (testicular feminising syndrome); in this situation the fetus will appear female at birth. In Benzie's view (1980) these events are so unlikely that they should not alter a general policy of giving patients all the information obtained from testing.

Neural tube defects
Neural tube defects which include anencephaly and spina bifida with or without hydrocephalus are the most common serious congenital abnormalities in the United Kingdom. The incidence of these disorders has a marked geographical variation ranging from 3.5 per 1000 in the South of England to 7.7 in parts of Wales and 8.7 in Northern Ireland (Elwood & Elwood, 1980). In 1972, Brock & Sutcliffe demonstrated that amniotic fluid contains excessive amounts of alpha-fetoprotein (AFP) in the presence of a neural tube defect. Amniocentesis during the mid-trimester leading to detection of raised AFP levels provides an effective means of detecting neural tube defects; the advantage of this biochemical test being that the result is rapidly available. Normally small but increasing amounts of AFP are present in amniotic fluid during the first trimester of pregnancy; the level falls during the second trimester to undetectable amounts mirroring the fetal serum concentration and reflecting production by the fetal liver. At 16 weeks' gestation when amniocentesis is usually performed the normal mean level of AFP in amniotic fluid is approximately $17 \mu g/ml$ (Nevin et al, 1974). Anencephalic fetuses and those with 'open' neural tube defects which account for 95 per cent of all cases have consistently raised amniotic fluid levels (Fig. 3.3).

The remaining 5 per cent of neural tube defects which have closed lesions may not have a raised amniotic AFP level and thus cannot be detected by biochemical analysis of amniotic fluid. More recently additional tests on amniotic fluid have been described; qualitative electrophoresis of acetylcholinesterase (Smith et al, 1979; Buamah et al, 1980) has proved a most valuable adjunct to AFP and a combination of both tests yields more information than either test alone. Diagnosis is assisted further by the examination of the fluid for rapidly adhering cells (Brock & Gosden, 1977). These recently described additional tests on the fluid improve the accuracy of the diagnosis since several other pathological conditions have been reported with raised amniotic fluid levels. These conditions include missed abortion (Milunsky et al, 1974), Turner's syndrome (Seller et al, 1974), Sacrococcygeal teratoma (Schmid & Muhlethaler, 1975), Exomphalos (Nevin & Armstrong, 1975), Meckel's syndrome (Nevin et al, 1979), congenital nephrosis (Kjessler et al, 1975), severe Rhesus isoimmunisation (Seppala & Ruoslahti, 1973), tetralogy of Fallot (Seppala, 1975) and absence of the fetal urethra (Nevin et al, 1978).

Parents who have had a child with a neural tube defect have a recurrence rate of

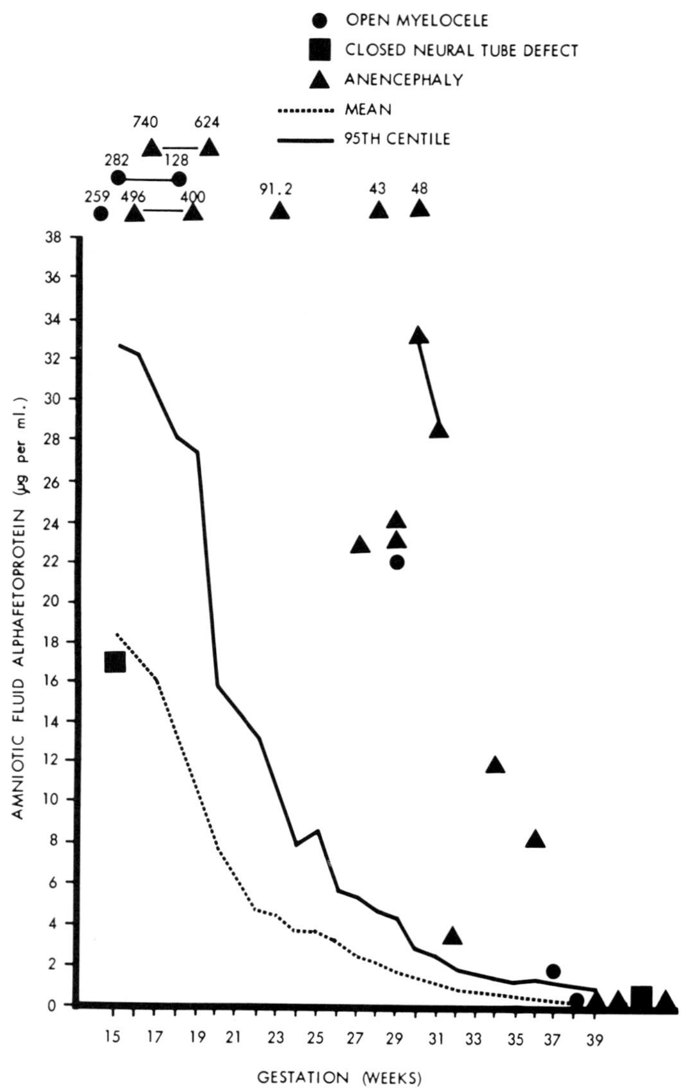

Fig. 3.3 Amniotic fluid AFP concentration at different gestational ages. Fetuses with anencephaly or an open neural tube defect have consistently raised levels. (Nevin N C et al, 1974; Reproduced by permission of the Editor of the British Journal of Obstetrics and Gynaecology).

about 1 in 20 in any further pregnancy; a couple who have two children with neural tube defects have a recurrence rate of 1 in 10 rising to 1 in 5 in an area of high incidence (Nevin & Johnston, 1980b); with three children this rises to more than 1 in 4. An affected adult with a neural tube defect has a recurrence rate of 1 in 20 in his or her children and a family history of neural tube defects gives a 1 in 60 risk.

Unfortunately about 90 per cent of neural tube defects occur in mothers who are not known to be at risk. Low but measurable AFP concentrations occur in maternal serum during the second trimester in normal pregnancy while in the presence of an open neural tube defect it is markedly elevated and increasingly so after the 13th week of gestation. This has provided a useful method of screening all pregnancies to pick up an 'at risk' group of women who can then be offered amniocentesis (Brock, 1976). The optimum time for maternal screening is 16 to 18 weeks gestation when those patients with a serum AFP concentration of 2.5 times the normal median are considered for further investigation. If the concentration is high a repeat serum test with an ultrasonic scan may be performed and if the level is still raised the patient offered detailed assessment with a view to amniocentesis. Where skilled interpretation of an ultrasonic scan is available this procedure may suffice after a single raised serum AFP.

The proportion of women referred for amniocentesis by these criteria is about 2 to 3 per cent, and of these, about 1 in 10 will be found to have a neural tube defect. The number of unnecessary amniocenteses varies with the local incidence of neural tube defects and is decreased in areas with a higher incidence (MRC Working Party, 1978). Although pilot studies have shown that screening is capable of identifying about 90 per cent of neural tube defects, a widespread programme is likely to identify only 75 per cent. The duration of pregnancy if wrongly estimated can lead to error in the interpretation of the serum AFP results, which also can be high in multiple pregnancy (Wald et al, 1975), and in missed or threatened abortion (Garoff & Seppala, 1975). Furthermore, about 20 per cent of women present after 20 weeks' gestation, by which time it is too late to initiate a screening programme due to decreased specificity of the test and unacceptability of termination of pregnancy after 20 weeks.

Since the introduction of maternal serum AFP there has been a strong lobby for antenatal population screening and its implementation in some areas of the UK has been associated with a dramatic fall in the birth of infants with neural tube defects; for example, in the West of Scotland the incidence has fallen from 3.7 per 1000 to 0.8 per 1000 births (Ferguson-Smith, 1981). Studies showing that screening is cost-effective support this approach, the annual cost being similar to that of hospitalisation and treatment of surviving infants with spina bifida during the first year of life (Glass & Cove, 1978).

The cost effectiveness of population screening is dependent upon a high natural incidence of neural tube defects and also a high patient acceptance of pregnancy termination. Recent evidence suggests that the natural incidence may be falling (Bradshaw et al, 1980; Scott et al, 1981). The financial implications, organisation difficulties and maternal psychological stress (Stirrat et al, 1979) involved in a screening programme have led many to question its value (Harris et al, 1980; Farrant, 1980). Ultrasonic screening in early pregnancy using much improved high resolution equipment has provided an increasingly important alternative to screening by maternal AFP (Christie et al, 1980) but the expertise required may be beyond all but a few centres. This method is reported to diagnose more than 90 per cent of neural tube defects with a false negative rate of less than 20 per cent which compares favourably with maternal serum AFP. The additional information obtained about the pregnancy and the considerable reduction in the number of unnecessary amniocenteses are major advantages of this approach.

Chromosomal abnormalities
The indications for amniocentesis to diagnose fetal chromosomal abnormalities are listed in Table 3.4. With advancing maternal age there is an increased risk of

Table 3.4   Indications for genetic amniocentesis

Chromosomal
    Parent with balanced translocation
    Advanced maternal age
    Previous infant with chromosomal defect
    Parental mosaicism

X-Linked Condition
    Duchenne muscular dystrophy
    X-Linked mental retardation
    Mucopolysaccardosis

Inborn Error of Metabolism
    Galactosaemia
    Congenital adrenal hyperplasia
    Homocystinuria

Neural Tube Defect
    Previous delivery of one or more infants with neural tube defects
    Parental neural tube defect
    A family history of neural tube defect
    A raised maternal serum alpha fetoprotein not due to multiple pregnancy

non-disjunction leading to a trisomic fetus, the most common being trisomy 21 which causes Down's syndrome (mongolism). Other rarer conditions are trisomy 18 (Edward's syndrome) and trisomy 13 (Patau's syndrome). The incidence of Down's syndrome in the general population in the UK is about 1 to 2 per 1000 live births but the risk increases with maternal age (Fig. 3.4). Under the age of 20 the risk is 1 in

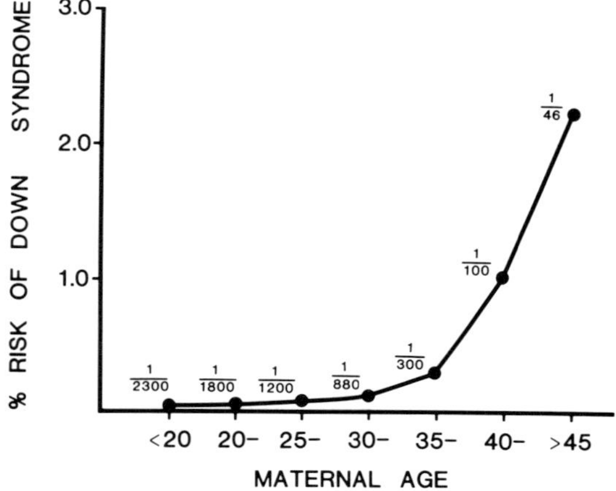

Fig. 3.4   The risks of Down Syndrome according to give year periods of maternal age (After Nevin, 1981).

2300 rising to 1 in 46 over the age of 45; half the children with trisomy 21 are born to mothers over the age of 35. The incidence of Down's syndrome and other chromosomal abnormalities is usually recorded at birth but since the introduction of amniocentesis and antenatal diagnosis these disorders have been found to occur more frequently at 15 to 16 weeks gestation than in the newborn (Ferguson-Smith 1976). Down's syndrome appears to have twice the incidence at 15 to 16 weeks' gestation than that reported at birth and this large discrepancy, though difficult to explain, may be due partially to the demise of trisomic fetuses between 16 weeks and term and to underestimates of Down's syndrome at birth. These facts indicate that it is wiser to use the somewhat higher estimates of risk when genetic counselling is undertaken.

Increased maternal age is also associated with a higher incidence of the other autosomal trisomies. The incidence of all chromosomal abnormalities at birth for women of 40 to 45 is about one in 45; recent figures derived from amniocentesis have again shown a higher incidence at 15 to 16 weeks, the total risk at this maternal age perhaps being as high as one in 25. Most agree that genetic amniocentesis should be performed in all women who are 40 years or over. Hagard & Carter (1976) using a cost benefit analysis have shown that antenatal diagnosis for women over the age of 35 would be economical but under that age would not. If the risk of abortion due to amniocentesis is taken as less than 1 per cent (Ritchie et al, 1980) then it can be argued that the incidence of the condition must exceed this before amniocentesis is justified and on this basis most centres now recommend the procedure for women of 38 years and over. In younger patients who request amniocentesis after full discussion an ultrasonic scan should be performed and the technical difficulties of amniocentesis assessed. Most patients would accept advice against amniocentesis where occasionally the risk of the procedure may outweigh the low detection rate.

Regardless of age, a history of having had a child with Down's syndrome indicates the requirement for genetic assessment prior to embarking on a further pregnancy. A small proportion (probably less than 5 per cent) of Down's syndrome have a different aetiological mechanism. Here one or another parent is a carrier of a balanced translocation and there is a considerable risk of recurrence in future children born to the couple. The risk in a mother with a 14/21 translocation is approximately 1 in 10 while if the father is the carrier of the translocation the risk is less: probably about 1 in 30. The reason for this difference is unknown.

Apart from familial Down's syndrome due to translocation there is also a small but significant familial incidence of the ordinary trisomy 21 variety thought to be due to mosaicism in one or other parent. The risk of a recurrence of the defect in a subsequent pregnancy is relatively high in all types of familial Down's syndrome and amniocentesis should be advised.

A patient who has a history of habitual abortion should be investigated for a chromosomal defect before embarking on a further pregnancy. Provided the parental chromosomes are normal, it is probably not justifiable to perform an amniocentesis except in the older patient because of the increased risk of abortion.

Amniocentesis in pregnant women over 38 and in those with familial chromosomal disorders will detect only about 30 per cent of chromosomally abnormal fetuses but it is hoped that better methods of screening the general population might become available. For example, ultrasonic measurement of the cephalic index (ratio of occipito-frontal to biparietal diameter) at 16 to 20 weeks may help to identify fetuses with Down's syndrome (Buttery, 1979) and the presence of a 'double bubble' is suggestive of duodenal atresia also associated with the condition. If chromosomal analysis was performed consistently on the products of conception of every woman who had more than one spontaneous abortion, it would be possible to detect a high risk group (MacHenry et al, 1979) and there is also a good case for chromosomal analysis of every unexplained perinatal death.

Inborn errors of metabolism

Jeffcoate and his colleagues (1965) were the first to report the value of amniocentesis for the antenatal diagnosis of metabolic diseases when a greatly increased concentration of steroids was demonstrated in the amniotic fluid surrounding a fetus who was found at birth to be suffering from the adrenogenital syndrome. Today an ever increasing list of inborn metabolic errors can be diagnosed antenatally (Burton & Nadler, 1980; Siggers, 1978) encompassing the majority of the inborn errors of carbohydrate, lipid and protein metabolism; these are generally autosomal or occasionally X-linked recessive disorders and result in varying degrees of mental and physical handicap. Severe disability often leads to death in early childhood. Unfortunately, two of the commonest disorders, cystic fibrosis and phenylketonuria are not included although the detection of methylumbelliferyl-guanidinobenzoate (MUGB) reactive proteases in amniotic fluid in the former condition may prove helpful (Nadler & Walsh, 1980).

Parents of an affected child have a one in four risk that a subsequent infant will have the disease. Where no treatment is available, and this is the position in the majority of cases, antenatal diagnosis offers the parents an opportunity to have a normal unaffected infant by allowing them the option of termination when an affected infant has been identified. In a minority of cases such as galactosaemia, congenital adrenal hyperplasia and vitamin B12 responsive methylmelonic acidaemia antenatal diagnosis may offer the advantage of early antenatal or immediate postnatal treatment of the disorder. Early treatment of the salt-losing variety of the adrenogenital syndrome can be life-saving.

The majority of inborn errors of metabolism are extremely rare though certain disorders are found to occur with greater frequency in selected populations. The gene of Tay-Sachs disease is carried by almost one in 27 individuals in the Ashkenazi Jewish population. Carriers can be accurately identified by assay of the serum hexosaminidase-A activity and offered an option of antenatal diagnosis (Kaback, 1977). With more refined biochemical methods it may be possible to develop this principle and apply it to other metabolic disorders.

The underlying defect in the majority of metabolic disorders is a deficiency of activity of a specific enzyme that mediates a normal metabolic process. Provided the enzymatic deficiency is demonstrated in cultivated skin fibroblasts it can be detected from an analysis of the amniotic fluid or the cellular contents. The disorders associated with a tissue-specific enzyme deficiency not demonstrated in fibroblasts cannot be diagnosed antenatally by this method; examples are phenylketonuria and glycogen storage disease. Cultivated amniotic fluid cells provide the most reliable method for antenatal diagnosis of inherited metabolic disorders though cell free amniotic fluid and cultivated amniotic fluid cells can be used.

Amniotic fluid samples are best obtained at 16 weeks' gestation when optimum cellular growth can be expected; the reliability of diagnosis is good but is dependent on the expertise of the individual laboratory. Disorders which are biochemically different often present similar clinical findings and it is essential to make the correct biochemical diagnosis: otherwise antenatal diagnosis is impossible. Biochemical tests should be completed as quickly as possible because of the extreme patient anxiety encountered during the waiting period. Until recently the biochemical analysis of cultured cells took four to six weeks because large numbers of cells had to be harvested but microchemical analysis has made it possible within three weeks of amniocentesis (Niermeijer et al, 1975).

In recent years there has been a rapid development of gene mapping. If the locus for a particular gene is known to be closely linked to that for a genetic marker such as blood group or HLA is may be possible to determine from the presence of the marker whether the fetus has inherited the gene for the disease. Myotonic dystrophy and congenital adrenal hyperplasia have been predicted antenatally through linkage of the gene with secretor status and HLA locus respectively. A further exciting development has been the use of DNA polymorphisms to predict genetic disorders in the fetus. This has actually been achieved for sickle cell disease. Clearly this approach will be applicable to other genetic disorders.

X-linked recessive disorders

Antenatal determination of sex from amniotic fluid can be used for the diagnosis of certain X-linked disorders such as Duchenne muscular dystrophy and mucopolysaccaridosis Type II. In some situations such as Duchenne muscular dystrophy the method does not permit a direct diagnosis but a selective therapeutic abortion of male fetuses can be undertaken since only the male fetus suffers from the disease. In some situations such as haemophilia and mucopolysaccharidosis Type II it is possible to determine if the male fetus is affected. It must also be appreciated by the mother that 50 per cent of her female children will carry the disease into the next generation.

A method of antenatal determination of sex, based upon the presence or absence of sex chromatin in the nuclei of amniotic fluid cells, was developed following its discovery by Barr & Bertram (1949) but Nadler & Gerbie (1971) reported that suitable preparations for such analyses could only be obtained from 73 per cent of patients. Better accuracy can be achieved by the identification of the Y-chromatin with fluorescence microscopy after staining with quinacrine dihydrochloride. Detection of both X and Y chromatin is more reliable than either alone (Ju et al, 1976) but most laboratories consider these methods not sufficiently accurate and advise a full chromosome analysis.

Rhesus incompatability

In 1953 Bevis reported that the severity of haemolytic disease in the newborn correlated with the amount of bilirubin-like pigments in the amniotic fluid and since then management of the condition has been based on quantifying bilirubin in liquor samples obtained at amniocentesis rather than on the more unreliable method of maternal serum antibody titres used previously. Biochemical methods of estimating bilirubin have been used but are unsatisfactory because its concentration in amniotic fluid is very low. The most successful method described uses spectrophotometry and depends upon the observed and the expected optical density difference (ODD) recorded at 450 nm, a variety of procedures being used to compensate for the presence of blood or meconium. The ratio between bilirubin and protein in amniotic fluid has been the most commonly used alternative method of assessing the severity of the disease (Cherry et al, 1965) but its alleged accuracy has not been reproducible (Walker et al, 1969).

A variety of charts to facilitate prediction of the course of the disease have been suggested but the most common in use is that originally reported by Liley (1961) and later modified (Liley, 1963). A number of zones are used to indicate the likely cord haemoglobin concentration and hence the severity of the disease. The timing of delivery is indicated when the bilirubin ODD at 450 nm is plotted on a semi-logarithmic graph against weeks of gestation. The lines dividing the zones slope downwards with increasing gestation reflecting normal reduction in bilirubin concentrations.

Examination of amniotic fluid has become established as the corner stone of management in Rhesus haemolytic disease and Liley (1961) indicated that such tests

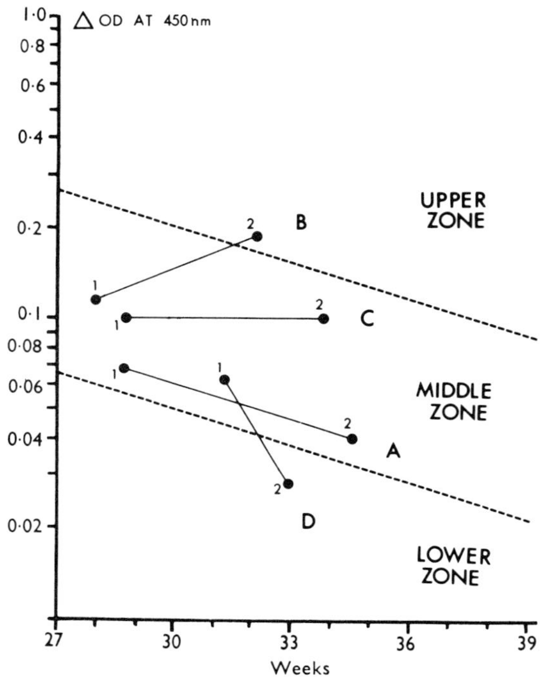

Fig. 3.5   Liley's prediction zones, with the △OD at 450 nm plotted against gestational age. In each of the four examples shown the initial estimation was in the middle zone, giving a prediction of probably mild or moderately severe haemolytic disease. In Case A the usual gradual reduction in amniotic fluid bilirubin occurred, with the △OD at 450 nm remaining low in the middle zone and with an unchanged prediction. The upward trend in Case B resulted in a second estimation being in the upper zone, giving a revised prediction of probably severe haemolytic disease. In Case C the static bilirubin trend approached (and could be extrapolated into) the upper zone, indicating that severe haemolysis would have become likely if the pregnancy had been continued to term. The steeply falling bilirubin trend in Case D reached the lower zone, giving a revised prediction of an unaffected or only very mildly affected baby. (Reproduced by courtesy of W B Saunders Co Ltd, from Whitfield C R (1974), Clinics in Obstetrics and Gynecology, 1: 69).

performed on two or more occasions gave even more useful information. This was confirmed by Whitfield and his colleagues (1968) when they demonstrated that major prediction errors could be minimised using two or more tests to establish a trend of bilirubin concentration in the liquor (Fig. 3.5). The possibility that this trend would not only correlate with the condition of the fetus at a given gestation but by extrapolation might also be used to plan obstetrical management, led Whitefield to develop the concept of the Action Line (Whitfield, 1970) as shown in Figure 3.6. The Action Line, derived from past experience of fetal outcome, starts at 24 weeks and if the extrapolated ODD at 450 nm, estimated on two or more occasions, crosses the Action Line before 31 weeks then intrauterine fetal transfusion is indicated while if the line is crossed at a later date immediate delivery is undertaken if fetal lung maturity is confirmed (Fig. 3.6). Although the fetal condition does not always follow the predicted course the method has been used successfully at the Royal Maternity Hospital, Belfast, for over a decade.

Recently, the need for amniocentesis has diminished (Table 3.2) not least because the number of severely affected cases has been reduced by anti-D immunoglobulin and because of the voluntary curtailment of family size. Also the indications for

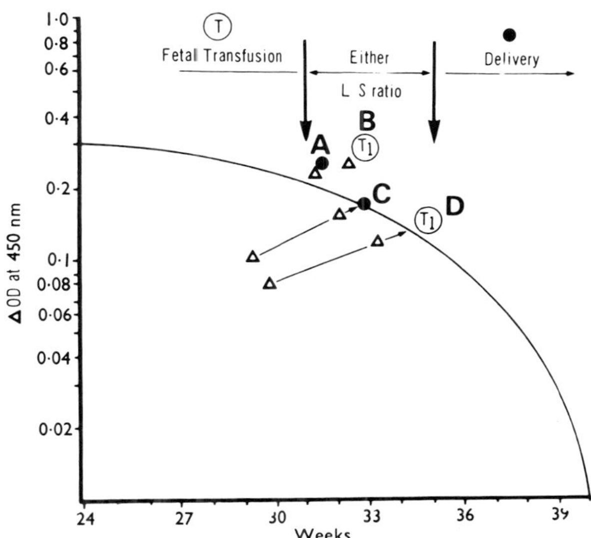

Fig. 3.6   The revised action line (ΔOD at 450 nm values plotted against gestational age) with four illustrative cases showing the use of AF surfactant tests (LSAR) when intervention is indicated between 31 and 35 weeks. Because there was adequate fetal pulmonary surfactant (LSAR > 2.0) immediate delivery was indicated in Case A (during 32nd week) and in Case C (33 weeks). Because there was insufficient surfactant (LSAR < 2.0) intrauterine transfusion was performed to allow postponement of delivery in Case B (32 weeks) and Case D (35th week). (Reproduced by courtesy of Journal of Clinical Pathology, from Whitfield C R 1976, 29, Suppl., 55).

amniocentesis and the number performed in each case have altered in the past five years further reducing the number of amnioceteses performed in this condition. Previously amniocentesis was indicated in all Rhesus negative women with serum antibodies and repeated two or three weeks later to determine a trend. The introduction of an automated method of measuring maternal serum concentration of anti-D antibody protein permits a more selective approach. This test described by Rosenfield et al (1968) has not only altered the requirement for amniocentesis but when sudden increases in antibody protein occur has helped detect a rapid increase in the fetal haemolytic process (Fraser et al, 1972). If the antibody protein remains below 0.3 μg per ml of maternal serum throughout the first affected pregnancy or below 0.5 μg per ml when antibodies have already been detected amniotic fluid analysis is not undertaken (O'Sullivan, 1981). Also amniocentesis is not repeated if the liquor bilirubin ODD is less than 0.035 at the first tap.

It is important to note that the Rhesus antibodies anti-c and anti-E require to be managed in a similar fashion using amniocentesis since they can be associated with severe haemolytic disease, although less frequently. The anti-D antibody protein provides no information in these cases. Other immune antibodies usually carry no significant risk of haemolytic disease apart from anti-Kell, the risk of which can be minimised by delivery at term. Determination of amniotic fluid volume occasionally alters the prediction of the severity of the fetal haemolytic process (Thompson et al, 1971) and, although providing more accurate information, the procedure has been abandoned in routine clinical practice of Rhesus management.

Maturity studies

Estimates of gestational age have been sought by investigating the maturation of various fetal organs such as the skin, kidney and lung; the popularity of such methods grew with the increasing use of amniocentesis but more recently has declined with the advent of simple and readily available real-time ultrasound (Table 3.2).

The assessment of gestation using the cytological appearance of desquamated fetal cells stained with Nile Blue Sulphate (Brosens & Gordon, 1966) was disappointing (Chan et al, 1969) even though other stains such as haematoxylin and eosin or Papanicolaou were shown to be superior (Lind & Billewicz, 1971). The amniotic fluid content of creatinine and urea have been shown to be the best indicators of fetal kidney development and hence gestational age (Lind, 1978) although the 'true' creatinine must be measured by sensitive techniques and the maternal serum concentration should be subtracted from the amniotic fluid concentration to increase the accuracy of both methods. The assessment of gestational age was most accurate when a scoring system was used combining amniotic fluid cytology and creatinine and urea content (Lind & Billewicz, 1971). Although much more promising this combined method required good biochemical laboratory services which limited its use in small hospitals and in developing countries. However, the techniques of estimating lung maturity and the increasing use of fetal measurement using ultrasound has superceded the method.

Gluck and his colleagues (1971) made an important contribution to obstetrical and neonatal management when they showed that the idiopathic respiratory distress syndrome (IRDS) and thus lung maturity could be anticipated by measuring the relative amount of the surface active phospholipid lecithin. The method of comparing this phospholipid, which increases rapidly as gestational age advances, with the more constant levels of another phospholipid sphingomyelin (Gluck & Kulovich, 1973) has stood the test of time although many other methods of quantitatively estimating the presence of surfactant have been reported. The simple practical method of measuring the area ratio of phospholipid spots (LSAR) separated by thin layer chromatography using planimetry (length by width) has been adopted by many centres (Whitfield, 1978) although when the fluid is contaminated by meconium, chlorhexidine antiseptic cream or heavily blood stained the method is unreliable (Whitfield & Sproule, 1974). The LSAR is highly predictive of severe IRDS when less than 1.5 while the disease is most uncommon or very mild when over 2.0; between these values IRDS may occur in up to 20 per cent of cases (Whitfield & Sproule, 1974). More recent information (Kulovich et al, 1979; Whittle et al, 1981) suggests that the presence of phosphatidyl glycerol indicating the formation of mature surface active phospholipid may increase the accuracy of prediction when the LSAR value falls in this range.

If a rapid and simple test is required to predict lung maturity the foam stability (shake or bubble) test devised by Clements et al (1972) has been shown when accurately performed to be nearly as reliable as the LSAR (Keniston et al, 1975). It has the advantage of not requiring sophisticated and expensive biochemical techniques and is therefore useful as a side-room procedure and in developing countries (Sutton, 1977). Amniotic fluid is serially diluted in normal saline into five test tubes and an equal volume of 95 per cent ethanol is added. The tubes are shaken for 15 seconds and allowed to stand for 15 minutes and then examined in a good light against a black background for the presence of a complete ring of bubbles at the level of the miniscus (Clements et al, 1972). If no bubbles are present in any tube, the test is negative, while a positive result can be graded according to the number of tubes in which bubbles persist (Fig. 3.7).

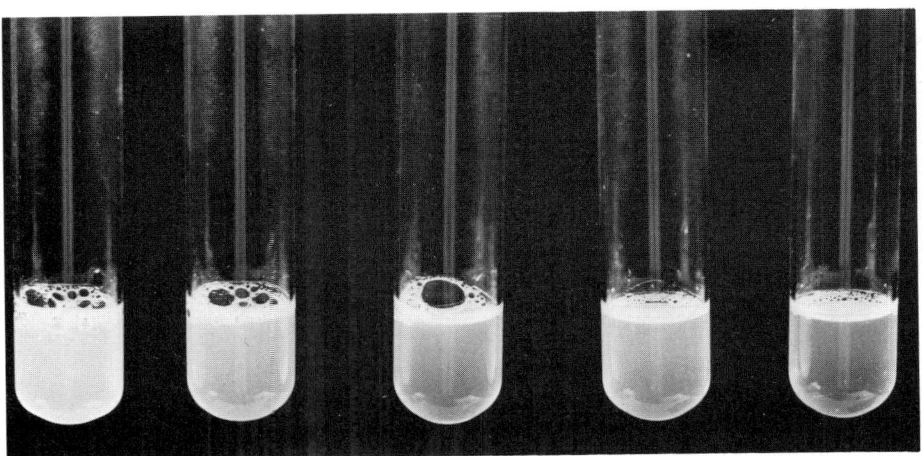

Fig. 3.7   A positive shake test. A complete ring of bubbles is present in all five tubes at 15 minutes (After Clements, 1972).

The prediction of fetal lung maturity has made an important contribution to reducing perinatal mortality and morbidity in clinical practice particularly when elective delivery has to be carried out before term or when menstrual dates are uncertain (Rome et al, 1975). However, information provided by ultrasound measurements in early pregnancy has reduced the need for amniocentesis in these clinical situations. Additional information in late pregnancy such as the presence of predominantly regular fetal breathing movements (Boddy et al, 1980) and the ultrasonic architecture of the placenta indicate the likelihood of a mature LSAR (Grannum et al, 1979) although neither are totally reliable (Patrick, 1981). Also neonatal care is such that it is rare to encounter serious life-threatening respiratory problems in neonates weighing more than 2.5 kg. Estimation of the LSAR is still preferable when information concerning accurate gestational dating is not available and neonatal care is not optimal. It should be remembered that the LSAR is less reliable in the presence of maternal diabetes and severe Rhesus disease (Whitfield & Sproule, 1974).

The LSAR can provide vital information when elective preterm delivery is contemplated except when events occur so rapidly as to make amniocentesis impracticable. This information may not only influence the place and timing of delivery but will help the neonatologist in preparing for the infant and may alter management since early intervention with assisted ventilation is now being used more frequently in the smaller neonate (McClure, 1981). The presence of phosphatidyl glycerol together with an LSAR result of more than 2.0 suggests mature lungs and should reduce the need for maternal steroids and tocolytic drugs. Also when the membranes rupture spontaneously before 34 complete weeks added information can be gained from amniocentesis by carrying out a gram stain of amniotic fluid and culture for aerobic and anaerobic bacteria (Garite et al, 1979). In the absence of antenatal information, the LSAR may be performed on the gastric aspirate of the newborn since it correlates well with that in amniotic fluid (McClure et al, 1976).

Amniocentesis for polyhydramnios

The withdrawal of liquor amnii after penetration of the amniotic sac has been used therapeutically in polyhydramnios for a century or more. In clinical practice today, the majority of cases of severe polyhydramnios can be managed by hospitalisation and bed rest without intervention until labour starts or until the membranes rupture spontaneously. If severe abdominal pain or dyspnoea develops it may be necessary to remove some of the excessive amniotic fluid by amniocentesis, particularly when the fetus is apparently normal but premature and it is advantageous to allow the pregnancy to continue. The very slow release of liquor helps obviate the dangers of premature separation of the placenta which sometimes follows the escape of massive quantities of amniotic fluid (Gough, 1959). Amniocentesis with controlled release of liquor can also be useful prior to artificial rupture of the membranes for induction of labour as it assists in the stabilisation of the fetal lie and decreases the risk of prolapsed cord.

Amniography

Although amniography was originally described over 50 years ago (Menees et al, 1930) as one of the first uses of amniocentesis, the procedure is not widely used today. It consists of the injection into the amniotic cavity of radio-opaque dyes followed by radiological examination of the abdomen two to 12 hours later. Its most important use is to outline the fetal bowel prior to intrauterine fetal transfusion in the management of severe Rhesus isoimmunisation. An aqueous radio-opaque contrast media is injected into the amniotic cavity and the iodinated fluid is swallowed by the fetus; the gastrointestinal tract can be demonstrated using image intensification and a needle can be introduced into the fetal peritoneal cavity. Lack of fetal swallowing indicated by absence of dye in the bowel suggests an obstruction in the upper gastrointestinal tract.

In early pregnancy the rapid injection of a water soluble contrast media followed by an immediate radiograph may assist in the diagnosis of molar pregnancy; the latter condition producing a characteristic honeycomb appearance. This technique has been superceded by ultrasound which has the obvious advantage of being non-invasive.

A variant of amniography, called fetography, utilises an opaque contrast media which has a lipid affinity; this coats the vernix-covered skin of the fetus and can assist in the identification of soft tissue lesions such as an encephalocele. In early pregnancy, when this technique would provide most useful information there is no vernix and the contrast material does not adhere to the skin.

Amiography carries the additional risk of maternal allergy to the iodine containing contact media and increased myometrial irritability leading to abortion or premature labour.

SUMMARY

During the past decade amniocentesis has become a routine procedure and provided much added information about the fetus. There has been a change in the relative indications for the test in clinical practice with greater emphasis on the diagnosis of genetic disease and congenital abnormalities; a trend which is likely to continue. Amniotic fluid analysis remains the mainstay of Rhesus isoimmunisation management but the decreasing number of amniocenteses performed for this reason reflects the declining incidence of the condition. In current practice the estimation of pulmonary maturity from amniotic fluid while useful has less application in late pregnancy because of alternative methods of assessing gestational age. On the other hand refined biochemical analysis of lung phospholipids has increased the usefulness of amniocentesis in problems occuring in preterm pregnancy.

In evaluating the benefits of amniocentesis it should not be forgotten that the indications are relative and the risks not insignificant.

ACKNOWLEDGEMENTS

Our thanks are due to our colleague Professor Norman Nevin for his valuable help and advice in the preparation of the manuscript and to Miss Patricia Thompson for typing it.

REFERENCES

Abramovich D R 1970 Fetal factors influencing the volume and composition of liquor amnii. Journal of Obstetrics and Gynaecology of the British Commonwealth 77: 865–877

Barr M L, Bertram E G 1949 Morphological distinction between behaviour of the nuclear satellite during accelerated nucleoprotein synthesis. Nature 163: 676

Benzie R J 1980 Amniocentesis, amnioscopy and fetoscopy. In: MacGillivray I (ed) Clinics in obstetrics and gynaecology, vol 7, ch 1, p 439

Bevis D C A 1953 The composition of liquor amnii in haemolytic disease of the newborn. Journal of Obstetrics and Gynaecology of the British Empire 60: 244–251

Boddy K, Cole R A, Thomson P G, McDicken W N, Anderson T 1980 Human fetal breathing movements and newborn respiratory distress. Proceedings of the 22nd British Congress of Obstetrics and Gynaecology, Edinburgh, p 118

Bradshaw J, Wesler J, Weatherall J 1980 Congenital malformations of the central nervous system. Population trends 19: 13–18

Brock D J H 1976 Prenatal diagnosis — clinical methods. British Medical Bulletin 32: 16–20

Brock D J H, Gosden C 1977 Early antenatal diagnosis of small open spina bifida lesions. British Medical Journal 2: 934

Brock D J H, Sutcliffe R G 1972 Alpha-fetoprotein in the antenatal diagnosis of anencephaly and spina bifida. Lancet 2: 197–199

Brosens I, Gordon H 1966 The estimation of maturity by cytological examination of the liquor amnii. Journal of Obstetrics and Gynaecology of the British Commonwealth 73: 88–90

Buamah P K, Evans L, Milford Ward A 1980 Amniotic fluid acetylcholinesterase isoenzyme pattern in the diagnosis of neural tube defects. Clinica Chimica Acta 103: 147–151

Burton B K, Nadler H L 1980 Antenatal diagnosis of metabolic disorders. In: Gerbie A B (ed) Clinics in obstetrics and gynaecology, vol 7, ch 3, p 29

Buttery B 1979 Occipitofrontal biparietal diameter ratio: an ultrasonic parameter for the antenatal evaluation of Down's syndrome. Medical Journal of Australia 2: 662–664

Campbell S, Wladimiroff J W, Dewhurst C J 1973 The antenatal measurement of fetal urine production. Journal of Obstetrics and Gynaecology of the British Commonwealth 80: 680–686

Chan W H, Willis J, Wood J 1969 The value of Nile Blue Sulphate stain in the cytology of the liquor amnii. Journal of Obstetrics and Gynaecology of the British Commonwealth 76: 193–195

Cherry S H, Kochwa S, Rosenfield R E 1965 Bilirubin-protein ratio in amniotic fluid as an index of the severity of erythroblastosis fetalis. Obstetrics and Gynecology 26: 826–832

Clements J A, Platzker A C, Tierney D F, Hobel C J, Creasy R K, Margolis A J et al 1972 Assessment of the risk of the respiratory distress syndrome by a rapid test for surfactant in amniotic fluid. New England Journal of Medicine 286: 1077–1081

Christie A D, Millar W G, Donald J D 1980 Ultrasound screening for neural tube defects. Proceedings of the 22nd British Congress of Obstetrics and Gynaecology, Edinburgh, p 82

Curtis J D, Cohen W N, Richerson H B, White C A 1972 The importance of placental localisation preceding amniocentesis. Obstetrics and Gynecology 40: 194–198

Dawes G S 1973 Breathing and rapid eye movement sleep before birth. In: Comline K S, Cross K W, Dawes G S, Nathanielsz P W (eds) Foetal and neonatal physiology Proceedings of Sir Joseph Barcroft Centenary Symposium Cambridge University Press, Cambridge, ch 6, p 49

Department of Health and Social Services, Standing Committee 1976 Haemolytic disease of the newborn. Revised version London DHSS par 4. 7

Donnai P, Charles N, Harris R 1981 Attitudes of patients after 'genetic termination of pregnancy. British Medical Journal 282: 621–626

Elwood J M, Elwood J H 1980 Epidemiology of anencephalus and spina bifida. Oxford University Press, Oxford, ch 10, p 87

Emery A E H 1970 Antenatal diagnosis of genetic disease In: Emery A E H (ed) Modern trends in human genetics I, Butterworths, London, ch 9, p 267

Epley S L, Hanson J W, Cruikshank D P 1979 Fetal injury with mid-trimester diagnostic amniocentesis. Obstetrics and Gynecology 53: 77–80

Fairweather D V I 1978 Techniques and safety of amniocentesis. In: Fairweather D V I, Eskes T K A B (eds) Amniotic fluid — Research and clinical application, 2nd edn. Excerpta Medica, Amsterdam, ch 2, p 19

Farrant W 1980 Stress after amniocentesis for high serum alpha-fetoprotein concentrations. British Medical Journal 281: 452

Ferguson-Smith 1976 Prospective data on risk of Down Syndrome in relation to maternal age. Lancet 2: 252

Ferguson-Smith M A 1981 Personal communication

Fraser I D, Tovey G H, Lockyer W J, Sobey D F 1972 Antibody protein levels in the maternal serum in Rhesus iso-immunization. Journal of Obstetrics and Gynaecology of the British Commonwealth 79: 1074–1079

Fuchs F, Riis P 1956 Antenatal sex determination. Nature 177: 330

Garite T J, Freeman R K, Linzey E M, Braly P 1979 The use of amniocentesis in patients with premature rupture of membranes. Obstetrics and Gynecology 54: 226–230

Garoff L, Seppala M 1975 Prediction of fetal outcome in threatened abortion by serum placental lactogen and alpha fetoprotein. American Journal of Obstetrics and Gynecology 121: 257–261

Glass N J, Cove A R 1978 Cost effectiveness of screening for neural tube defects. In: Scrimgeour J B (ed) Towards the prevention of fetal malformation. Edinburgh University Press, Edinburgh, p 217

Gluck L, Kulovich M V 1973 Lecithin/sphingomyelin ratios in amniotic fluid in normal and abnormal pregnancy. American Journal of Obstetrics and Gynecology 115: 639–546

Gluck L, Kulovich M V, Borer R C, Brenner P H, Anderson G G, Spellacy W N 1971 Diagnosis of respiratory distress syndrome by amniocentesis. American Journal of Obstetrics and Gynecology 109: 440–445

Gordon H R, Deukmedjian A G 1975 Suprapubic vs periumbilical amniocentesis. American Journal of Obstetrics and Gynecology 122: 287–292

Gosden C, Buckton K, Fotheringham Z, Brock D J H 1981 Prenatal fetal karyotyping and maternal serum alpha-fetoprotein screening. British Medical Journal 282: 257–282

Gough H M 1959 Accidental haemorrhage following rupture of the membranes in cases of hydramnios. Journal of Obstetrics and Gynaecology of the British Empire 66: 473–476

Grannum P A T, Berkowitz R L, Hobbins J C 1979 The ultrasonic changes in the maturing placenta and their relation to fetal pulmonic maturity. American Journal of Obstetrics and Gynecology 133: 915–922

Gunston K D, Davey D A 1978 The safety of amniocentesis in relation to site and method. South African Medical Journal 54: 492–493

Hagard S, Carter F A 1976 Preventing the birth of infants with Down's Syndrome: a cost-benefit analysis. British Medical Journal 1: 753–756

Harris S, Read A P, Donnai D, Donnai P 1980 Stress after amniocentesis for high serum alpha-fetoprotein concentrations. British Medical Journal 281: 807

Huisjes H J 1978 Cytology of the amniotic fluid and its clinical applications. In: Fairweather D V I, Eskes T K A B (eds) Amniotic fluid — research and clinical application, 2nd edn. Excerpta Medica, Amsterdam, ch 7, p 93

Hunter A G W, Cox D M 1979 Counselling problems when twins are discovered at genetic amniocentesis. Clinical Genetics 16: 34–42

Jeffcoate T N A, Fliegner J R H, Russel S H, Davis J C, Wade A P 1965 Diagnosis of the adreno genital syndrome before birth. Lancet 2: 553–555

Ju K S, Park I J, Jones H W, Winn K J 1976 Prenatal sex determination by observation of the X-chromatin and the Y-chromatin of exfoliated amniotic fluid cells. Obstetrics and Gynecology 47: 287–290

Kaback M M 1977 Tay-Sachs disease: prenatal diagnosis and heterzygote screening 1969–1976. Pediatric Research 2: 458

Keniston R C, Pernoll M L, Buist N R M, Lyon M, Swanson J R 1975 A prospective evaluation of the L/S ratio and the RST in relation to fetal pulmonary maturity. American Journal of Obstetrics and Gynecology 121: 324–332

Kjessler B, Johansson S G O, Sherman M, Gustavson K-H, Hultquist G 1975 Alpha fetoprotein in antenatal diagnosis of congenital nephrosis. Lancet 1: 432–433

Kulovich M V, Hallman M B, Gluck L 1979 The lung profile I Normal Pregnancy. American Journal of Obstetrics and Gynecology 135: 57–63

Liley A W 1961 Liquor amnii analysis in management of pregnancy complicated by Rhesus sensitization. American Journal of Obstetrics and Gynecology 82: 1359–1370

Liley A W 1963 Intrauterine transfusion of fetus in haemolytic disease. British Medical Journal 2: 1107–1109

Lind T 1978 The biochemistry of amniotic fluid. In: Fairweather D V I, Eskes T K A B (eds) Amniotic fluid — Research and clinical application, 2nd edn. Excerpta Medica, Amsterdam, ch 5, p 59

Lind T, Billewicz W Z 1971 A point scoring system for estimating gestational age from examination of amniotic fluid. British Journal of Hospital Medicine 5: 631–685

Medical Research Council 1978 An assessment of the hazard of amniocentesis. Medical Research Council Working Party. British Journal of Obstetrics and Gynaecology 85: suppl 2, p 37

Mellows H J 1980 How to do an amniocentesis. British Journal of Hospital Medicine 24: 268–271

Menees T O, Millar J D, Holly L E 1930 Amniography. Preliminary Report. American Journal of Roentgenology 24: 353–366

Milunsky A, Alpert E, Charles D 1974 Amniotic fluid alpha-fetoprotein in anencephaly. Obstetrics and Gynecology 43: 592–594

McClure B G 1981 Personal communication

McClure G, Mock G, Hicks E, Reid M, Greene E 1976 Study of neonatal gastric aspirate related to amniotic fluid and to the occurrence of idiopathic respiratory distress syndrome. Journal of Perinatal Medicine 4: 163–167

MacHenry J C R M, Nevin N C, Merrett J D 1979 Comparison of central nervous system malformations in spontaneous abortions in Northern Ireland and South-east England. British Medical Journal 1: 1395–1397

Nadler H L, Gerbie A B 1970 Role of amniocentesis in intrauterine detection of genetic disorders. New England Journal of Medicine 282: 596–599

Nadler H L, Walsh M M J 1980 Intrauterine detection of cystic fibrosis. Pediatrics 66: 690–692

Nevin N C 1981 Personal communication

Nevin N C, Armstrong M J 1975 Raised alpha-fetoprotein in amniotic fluid and maternal serum in a triplet pregnancy in which one fetus had an exomphalocoele. British Journal of Obstetrics and Gynaecology 82: 826–828

Nevin N C, Johnston W P 1980a A family study of spina bifida and anencephalus in Belfast, Northern Ireland 1964–1968. Journal of Medical Genetics 17: 203–211

Nevin N C, Johnston W P 1980b Risk of recurrence after two children with central nervous system malformations in an area of high incidence. Journal of Medical Genetics 17: 87–92

Nevin N C, Thompson W, Nesbitt S 1974 Amniotic fluid alpha-fetoprotein in the antenatal diagnosis of neural tube defects. Journal of Obstetrics and Gynaecology of the British Commonwealth 81: 757–760

Nevin N C, Ritchie A, McKeown F, Roberts G 1978 Raised alpha-fetoprotein levels in amniotic fluid and maternal serum associated with distension of the fetal bladder caused by absence of the urethra. Journal of Medical Genetics 15: 61–63

Nevin N C, Thompson W, Davison G, Horner W T 1979 Prenatal diagnosis of the Meckel's syndrome. Clinical Genetics 15: 1–4

NICHD National Institute for Child Health and Development 1976 National registry for amniocentesis study group mid-trimester amniocentesis for prenatal diagnosis: safety and accuracy. Journal of the American Medical Association 236: 1471–1476

Niermeijer M F, Koster J F, Jahodova M, Fernandes J, Heukels-Dully M J, Glajaard H 1975 Prenatal
    diagnosis of type II glycogenesis (Pompe's disease) using microchemical analysis. Pediatric Research 9:
    498–503
O'Sullivan J F 1981 Personal communication
Patrick J 1981 Personal communication
Pritchard J A 1966 Fetal swallowing and amniotic fluid volume. Obstetrics and Gynecology 28: 606–610
Queenan J T, Thompson W, Whitfield C R, Shah S I 1972 Amniotic fluid volumes in normal pregnancies.
    American Journal of Obstetrics and Gynecology 114: 34–38
Ritchie K, McClure G 1979 Prematurity. Lancet 2: 1227–1229
Ritchie J W K, Traub A I 1979 Rupture of the uterus during prostaglandin-induced abortion. British
    Medical Journal 25: 496
Ritchie J W K, Thompson W, Nevin N C 1980 Pregnancy outcome following genetic amniocentesis.
    Proceedings of the 22nd British Congress of Obstetrics and Gynaecology, Edinburgh p 81
Rome P M, Glover J I, Simmons S C 1975 The benefits and risk of amniocentesis for the assessment of fetal
    lung maturity. British Journal of Obstetrics and Gynaecology 82: 662–668
Rosenfield R E, Cherry S H, Goodman A, Rubinstein P, Haber G V 1968 Assay of prenatal antibodies to
    determine the need for amniotic fluid studies. Bibliotheca Haematologica 29: 968–972
Schmid V, Muhlethaler J P 1975 High amniotic fluid alpha-fetoprotein in a case of fetal sacrococcygeal
    teratoma. Human genetics 26: 353–354
Scott M, Elwood H, Nevin N C, Ritchie J W K 1981 A change in the natural incidence of ancencephaly
    (letter) Lancet, in press
Seller M J, Craesy M R, Alberman E D 1974 Alpha-fetoprotein levels in amniotic fluids from spontaneous
    abortions. British Medical Journal 2: 524–525
Seppala M 1975 Fetal pathophysiology of human alpha-fetoprotein. Annals of the New York Academy of
    Science 259: 59–73
Seppala M, Ruoslahti E 1973 Alpha-fetoprotein in Rh-immunized pregnancies. Obstetrics and Gynecology
    42: 701–706
Siggers D C 1978 Prenatal diagnosis of genetic disease. Blackwell Scientific Publications, Oxford, ch 3, p 20
Smith A D, Wald N J, Cuckle M S, Stirrat G M, Bobrow M, Lagercrantz H 1979 Amniotic fluid
    acetylcholinesterase as a possible diagnostic test for neural tube defects in early pregnancy. Lancet 1:
    686–688
Stirrat G M, Turnbull A C, Bennett M J, Bobrow M, Lindenbaum R H, Wald N J, Cuckle H S 1979
    Clinical dilemmas arising from the antenatal diagnosis of neural tube defects. British Journal of
    Obstetrics and Gynaecology 86: 161–166
Sutton C 1977 Practical approach to problems of the parturient diabetic in developing countries. British
    Medical Journal 2: 1069–1072
Thompson W, Lappin T R G, Elder G E 1971 Liquor volume by direct spectrophotometric determination
    of injected PAH. British Journal of Obstetrics and Gynaecology 78: 341–344
Wachtel E, Gordon H, Olsen E 1969 Cytology of amniotic fluid. Journal of Obstetrics and Gynaecology of
    the British Commonwealth 76: 596–602
Wald N J, Cuckle H S 1980 Alpha-fetoprotein in the antenatal diagnosis of open neural tube defects.
    British Journal of Hospital Medicine 23: 473–489
Wald N, Barker S, Peto R, Brock D J H, Bonnar J 1975 Maternal serum alpha-fetoprotein levels in
    multiple pregnancy. British Medical Journal 1: 651–652
Walker W, Landon M J, Oxley A 1969 Protein content of liquor amnii in prediction of severity of
    haemolytic disease of the newborn. British Medical Journal 1: 605–607
Wang M Y F W, McCutcheon E, Deforges J F 1967 Feto-maternal haemorrhage from diagnostic
    transabdominal amniocentesis. American Journal of Obstetrics and Gynecology 97: 1123–1128
Whitfield C R 1970 A three year assessment of an action line method of timing intervention in Rhesus
    immunization. American Journal of Obstetrics and Gynecology 108: 1239–1244
Whitfield C R 1978 Prediction of fetal pulmonary maturity clinical application. In: Fairweather D V I,
    Eskes T K A B (eds) Amniotic fluid — research and clinical application, 2nd edn. Excerpta Medica,
    Amsterdam. ch 18, p 393
Whitfield C R 1980 Prediction of Rhesus haemolytic disease. In: Barson A J (ed) Laboratory investigation
    of fetal disease. Wright, Bristol, ch 13, p 299
Whitfield C R, Sproule W B 1974 Fetal lung maturation. British Journal of Hospital Medicine 12: 678–690
Whitfield C R, Neely R A, Telford M E 1968 Amniotic fluid analysis in Rhesus isoimmunisation. Journal
    of Obstetrics and Gynaecology of the British Commonwealth 75: 121–127
Whittle M J, Wilson A I, Whitfield C R, Paton R D, Logan R W 1981 Amniotic fluid phospholipid profile
    determination by two-dimensional thin-layer chromotography as an index of fetal lung maturation.
    British Medical Journal 282: 428–430

4. Renal disease in pregnancy

John M. Davison   Adrian Katz   Marshall D. Lindheimer

Clinicians may be consulted on the advisability of conception, or continuing a pregnancy, in women with renal disease and advice is too often based on anecdotal clinical experience. Consequently, many incline towards therapeutic termination of pregnancy regardless of the type and severity of the disease. This is unfortunate, because recent evidence suggests that in most cases in which disease is mild and hypertension absent, pregnancies will end successfully. This chapter focuses on the changes that occur in the urinary tract during normal gestation, the detection and management of renal disease in pregnancy, the effect of pregnancy on the remote prognosis in women with underlying renal disease and acute renal failure in pregnancy. Space limitations preclude any discussion of infectious renal complications which have been detailed elsewhere (Lindheimer & Katz, 1977; Davison & Lindheimer, 1978).

THE KIDNEY IN NORMAL PREGNANCY

Cognisance of the changes which affect the urinary tract during normal gestation is important if the early signs of renal dysfunction are to be detected in pregnant women.

Anatomical changes

Kidney length increases approximately 1 cm during normal pregnancy. More striking, however, are the anatomic changes in the calyces, renal pelvis, and ureter, which dilate markedly, often giving the erroneous impression of obstructive uropathy (Bailey & Rolleston, 1971; Roberts, 1976). These anatomical changes have important clinical implications: urinary stasis within the ureters may contribute to the propensity of gravidas with asymptomatic bacteriuria to develop frank pyelonephritis, and dilatation of the urinary tract may lead to collection errors in tests based on timed urine volume (e.g. 24-hour oestriol, creatinine, or protein excretion). Furthermore, acceptable norms of kidney size should be increased by 1 cm if estimated during pregnancy or immediately after delivery. Since dilatation of the ureters may persist until the 12th to 16th postpartum week, elective radiologic examination of the urinary tract during this period should be deferred.

Functional changes

RENAL HAEMODYNAMICS
Glomerular filtration rate (GFR) and effective renal plasma flow (ERPF) increase to levels about 50 per cent above non-pregnant values. These increases occur shortly

after conception (Davison & Noble, 1981), and all increments are present in the second trimester (Davison & Hytten, 1974; Dunlop, 1981). There is a reduction in GFR of some 15 per cent during the third trimester (measured as 24-hour creatinine clearance) and this is of more than academic interest especially when assessing the course of pregnancy in a woman with known renal disease (Davison et al, 1980).

Since GFR increases without substantial alterations in the production of creatinine and urea, plasma levels of these solutes decrease. Creatinine levels fall from a non-pregnant level of 73 μmol/l to 65 μmol/l in the first trimester, to 51 μmol/l in the second trimester and to 47 μmol/l in the third trimester (Kuhlback & Widholm, 1966). Some of the fall in plasma urea may be due to reduced protein degradation as well as increased clearance of this solute. Average plasma urea levels of 3.5, 3.3 and 3.1 mmol/l in successive trimesters, rising to 4.3 mmol/l six weeks postpartum, have been described (Robertson & Cheyne, 1972). It should be remembered that urea levels can be reported in a number of different ways. Results may be given as either plasma (or serum) or whole blood levels, the latter being 10 per cent below plasma levels.

Awareness of these physiological changes is important since values considered normal in non-pregnant women may reflect decreased renal function during pregnancy. Plasma levels of creatinine and urea exceeding 75 μmol/l and 4.5 mmol/l respectively, should alert the clinician to investigate renal function further.

A number of other changes in normal pregnancy may be due to altered renal haemodynamics, including excretion of nutrients and protein. With regard to nutrient excretion, particularly glucose, there is evidence that tubular reabsorption is in fact, less efficient (Davison & Dunlop, 1980). The increase in urinary protein excretion might be due to increased glomerular plasma flow. However, proteinuria is not to be considered abnormal until it exceeds 500 mg in 24 hours and increasing proteinuria in women with known chronic renal disease does not necessarily signify deterioration.

VOLUME HOMEOSTASIS

Most healthy women gain approximately 12.5 kg during the first pregnancy and 1 kg less during subsequent pregnancies. This increment in weight consists largely of fluid, as total body water increases six to eight litres, four to six of which are extracellular. There are also increases in plasma volume (which is greatest during the second trimester when increments approach 50 per cent) and in fluid within fetal and maternal interstitial spaces, which are greatest in late pregnancy. During most normal pregnancies there is also a gradual cumulative retention of about 900 mmol of sodium, distributed between the products of conception and the maternal extracellular space. The alterations in maternal intravascular and interstitial spaces produce a 'physiological' hypervolaemia. Nevertheless, the mother's volume receptors sense these changes as normal, and when salt restriction or diuretic therapy limits this physiological expansion, the maternal response resembles that of salt-depleted non-pregnant subjects. The meaning or importance of these changes is unknown, but Gibson (1973) reported that multigravidas considered 'poor reproducers' have smaller increments in both plasma volume and GFR when compared to multigravidas who have delivered normal sized babies. In this respect, we too have noted a failure of GFR to increase early in the pregnancies of women who subsequently aborted (Davison & Noble, 1981), as shown in Figure 4.1.

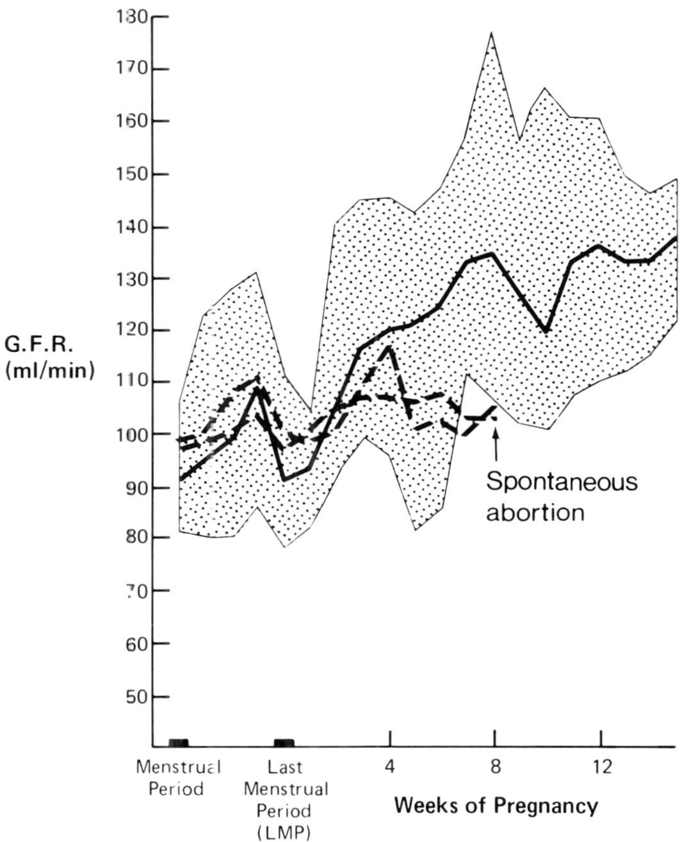

Fig. 4.1   Weekly 24-hour creatinine clearances (GFR) over conception and in early pregnancy in two women who had spontaneous uncomplicated abortions. Solid line represents the mean and stippled area the range for eight healthy women over same period of time.

The influence of humoral changes during normal pregnancy on renal sodium handling and volume regulation is also incompletely understood. Aldosterone secretion and excretion and levels of plasma desoxycorticosterone, cortisol, estrogen, and prolactin all increase during normal gestation. These and other factors which may influence renal sodium handling during gestation have been discussed in detail elsewhere (Lindheimer et al, 1978; Nolten & Ehrlich, 1980; Lindheimer & Katz, 1981).

Blood pressure regulation

Mean blood pressure decreases early in pregnancy and, by the second trimester, diastolic levels are 10 to 15 mmHg lower than before the patient became pregnant. Blood pressure then increases slowly, approaching pre-pregnancy values shortly before delivery. Since cardiac output rises quickly in the first trimester (reaching values that are 40 per cent greater than those before pregnancy) and remains relatively constant thereafter, the decline in blood pressure must be due to a marked decrease in peripheral vascular resistance. This is greatest in the uterine vasculature, which eventually develops into a large, low resistance shunt. However, other organ systems, especially the kidneys and skin, participate in the generalised vasodilatation which is characteristic of normal pregnancy. The rise of blood pressure toward non-pregnant levels after the second trimester suggests that increasing vasoconstrictor tone is a feature of late normal pregnancy, and if the clinician is not aware of this pattern of change diagnostic errors may ensue. For instance, most women with mild essential hypertension show a fall in blood pressure early in pregnancy and display normal levels at that time. When frankly elevated pressures are then noted in late pregnancy they may be erroneously labelled as pre-eclamptic.

RENAL DISEASE AND PREGNANCY

Pathophysiology of renal dysfunction
In order to assess pregnancy and its altered homeostasis in the context of coexisting renal disease it is important to mention some of the events that occur when nephron

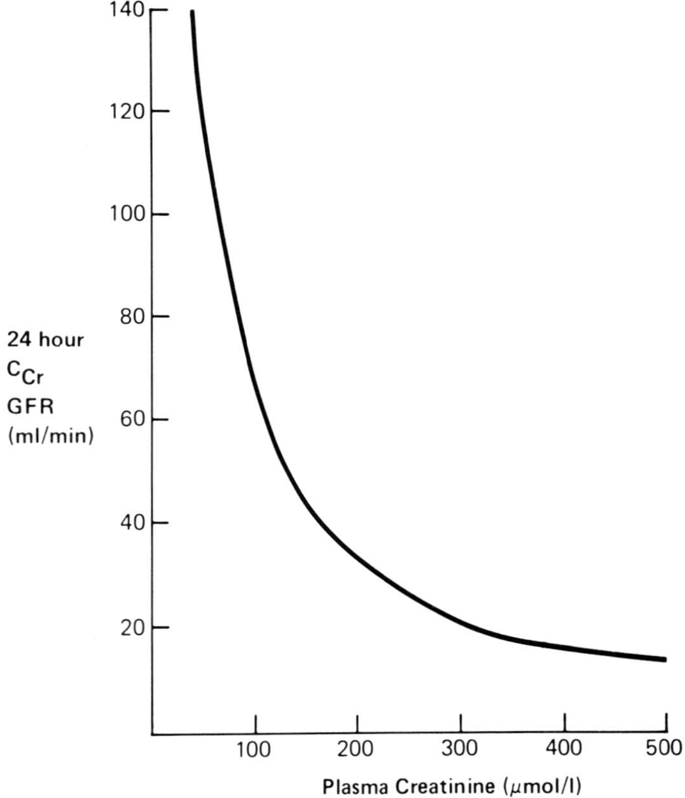

Fig. 4.2   Relationship of clearance of creatinine (ml/min) to plasma creatinine concentration (µmol/l) assuming a constant creatinine excretion of about 11.5 mmols per 24 hours

mass has been lost. Figure 4.2 demonstrates the relation between plasma creatinine and renal clearance of creatinine. It can be seen that an individual may lose approximately 50 per cent of function and yet maintain a plasma creatinine level of less than 130 μmol/l. But if renal function is more severely compromised then small decreases in GFR cause plasma creatinine to increase markedly. Furthermore, loss of renal mass evokes a compensatory increase in the function of the remaining nephrons. For instance, removal of one kidney in a healthy individual immediately halves the total number of nephrons, but within one to two weeks the GFR in the remaining kidney attains a level only slightly below the pre-operative value for both kidneys. This compensatory increase in function also occurs in certain renal diseases so that GFR itself may not decrease until a substantial part of the renal mass has been destroyed. Thus a patient who has lost 75 per cent of her nephrons may have lost only 50 per cent of function and may have a deceptively normal plasma creatinine. This emphasises that evaluation of renal function should be based on the clearance of creatinine rather than on its plasma concentration.

In patients with renal disease, pathology may be both chemically and clinically silent: most individuals remain symptom free until their GFR falls to one third of its original level and many plasma constituents are frequently normal until a late stage of the disease. However, it is now apparent that many biochemical events (which are not commonly tested in clinical laboratories) become abnormal early in the course of renal disease, even when GFR has decreased only slightly. In the long term some of these changes are detrimental to the individual. Bricker et al (1976) have dubbed these mechanisms 'trade-offs'; their effects on the outcome of pregnancy are unknown, but there is no doubt that women with even mild renal insufficiency may enter pregnancy with an internal milieu that is already vastly different from that of a woman with normal kidneys.

Renal function during pregnancy
As renal disease progresses and function declines, the ability to conceive and to sustain a viable pregnancy decreases. Normal pregnancy is rare when renal function decreases to a degree that non-pregnant plasma creatinine and urea levels exceed 275 μmol/l and 10 mmol/l, respectively. One author (Bear, 1976) advises that pregnancy should not be undertaken when non-pregnant plasma creatinine exceeds 150 μmol/l. These increments above normal non-pregnant levels appear trivial, but they represent decrements of greater than 50 per cent in function. Moreover, degrees of functional impairment that do not cause symptoms or appear to disrupt homeostasis in non-pregnant individuals, do jeopardise pregnancy. The importance of the remarkable increment in GFR that occurs during normal pregnancy is unclear. It is of interest that women with poor reproductive histories (including small-for-dates pregnancies) who are otherwise healthy, manifest smaller increments in GFR than control women who have normal pregnancies (Gibson, 1973). The question therefore arises as to what happens to renal haemodynamics in women with underlying renal disease especially if their non-pregnant values suggest a decrease in functioning mass. Sporadic observations suggest that such patients experience variable but definite increments in GFR during pregnancy.

The course of pregnancy
There are conflicting views concerning the course of pregnancy in women with renal disorders. The cause of these divergent views is uncertain, but may reflect the variability of the populations studied and the lack of large prospective series in which

diagnosis was established by biopsy and the pathology correlated with observations of fetal outcome.

Most investigators believe that, with the exception of an increased frequency of exacerbation of pyelonephritis, pregnancy has no adverse effect on the natural history of established renal parenchymal disease with the proviso that renal function is preserved or only moderately compromised and hypertension is absent (Werko & Bucht, 1956; Kaplan et al, 1962; Felding, 1969; Strauch & Hayslett, 1974; Bear, 1976; Klockars et al, 1980; Katz et al, 1980 and 1981). Others maintain that pregnancy frequently results in progression of the renal lesions and further deterioration of renal function (Tenney & Dandrow, 1961; Kincaid-Smith et al, 1967; Fairley et al, 1973). These latter authors also believe that fetal outlook is poor primarily because many of these pregnancies are complicated by the early appearance of pre-eclampsia. It appears, however, that in certain instances the decline in renal function in women with pre-existing renal disease may have resulted from dehydration and reduced renal perfusion secondary to stringent sodium restriction and/or inadvertent diuretic therapy.

IMPORTANT PROBLEMS IN PREGNANT WOMEN WITH RENAL DISEASE

Our own experience agrees with the majority view, and stems from a collaborative study between three medical centres which comprised 121 pregnancies in 89 women with a variety of renal disorders which had been diagnosed by renal biopsy (Katz et al, 1980 and 1981). From our study the answers to a number of important questions have emerged.

The effect of pregnancy on blood pressure
Hypertension, usually of a mild degree, was noted in 23 per cent of all pregnancies, but in half of them blood pressure had been elevated prior to conception. Hypertension was both more common and more severe in women with diffuse glomerulonephritis, but there was also a substantial incidence in women with focal glomerulonephritis and, not surprisingly, arteriolar nephrosclerosis.

The effect of pregnancy on renal function
Increased proteinuria was the most common renal effect of pregnancy, reflecting in part the tendency to increased protein excretion seen in normal pregnancy as well. Severe or substantially increased proteinuria was evident in almost 50 per cent of pregnancies, and occurred in nearly all types of renal disease, although it was uncommon in women with chronic interstitial nephritis (predominantly of infective origin). Protein excretion was massive, exceeding 3 g per 24 hours in 30 per cent of pregnancies, and led frequently to nephrotic oedema.

Serial measurements of 24-hour creatinine clearance over conception and in each trimester of 33 pregnancies indicated that although GFR in women with renal disease was approximately one standard deviation below that of normal pregnant women, the increment produced by pregnancy was essentially identical in the two groups (Fig. 4.3). The substantial increment in GFR during pregnancy compared with measurements postpartum was confirmed with inulin clearances, and a similar rise in effective

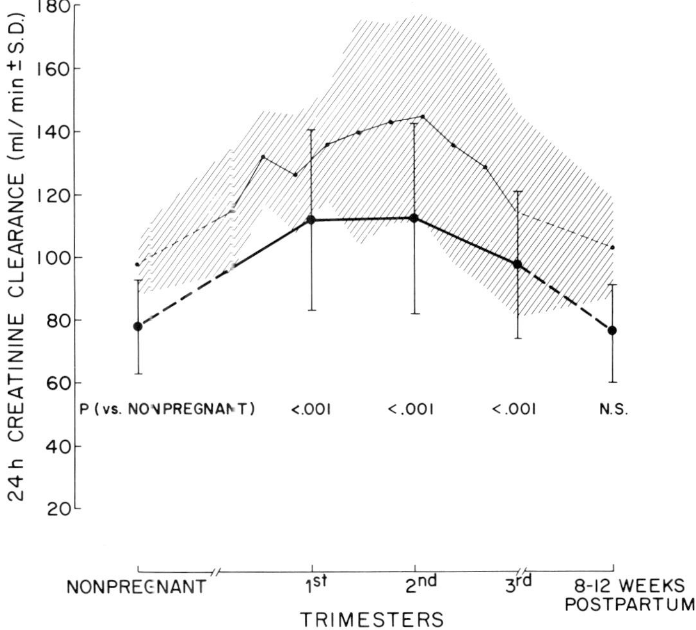

Fig. 4.3 Serial 24-hour creatinine clearances (mean ± 1SD) during 33 pregnancies of 26 women with renal disease studied before conception, in each trimester and 8–12 weeks postpartum (solid line). Measurements from 10 healthy women (mean ± 1SD) are shown in hatched area. (From Katz et al, 1980)

renal plasma flow (C_{PAH}) was noted in a smaller number of pregnant women (Table 4.1).

Table 4.1 Renal haemodynamics in patients with renal disease during pregnancy and postpartum

	During pregnancy		>6 weeks postpartum (ml/min ± SE)		P
GFR (C_{inulin})	124.5 ± 5.9	(26)	76.5 ± 3.6	(26)	<0.001
ERPF (C_{PAH})	612.8 ± 75.5	(7)	379.3 ± 42.3	(7)	<0.02

(Number of patients in parentheses)

Renal function decreased in 16 per cent of all pregnancies, most often in women with diffuse glomerulonephritis. The decrement was usually mild to moderate, and reversed after delivery. In two women deterioration of renal function was due to acute tubular necrosis during pregnancy. In one woman with sickle-cell nephropathy GFR decreased markedly postpartum due to renal vein thrombosis, which was treated successfully with anticoagulants. About 20 per cent of the women with chronic pyelonephritis had one or more episodes of acute urinary tract infection during pregnancy.

The incidence of pre-eclampsia
There is controversy about the incidence of pre-eclampsia in women with pre-existing renal disease. Our observations may help explain this situation: 'Superimposed pre-eclampsia' was diagnosed on clinical grounds in 13 women and eclampsia in one, although only 4 of these women were normotensive and were without proteinuria

before conception. Thirteen of the women had renal biopsy performed postpartum and the characteristic glomerular changes of pre-eclampsia were evident in only seven, including the one with eclampsia. These results emphasise that the diagnosis of pre-eclampsia cannot be made with certainty on clinical grounds alone and this is particularly true in women with coexistent renal disorders, in whom hypertension and proteinuria may be manifestatious of the underlying disease.

The effect on obstetric outcome

Despite the fact that the group had potentially serious disease, there were 116 live births from a total of 123 offspring. Perinatal mortality and the incidence of preterm deliveries and small-for-dates infants were, however, moderately higher than in healthy pregnancies (Table 4.2). As the data span a period of 20 years it is possible that the perinatal morbidity might have been reduced if current standards of fetal surveillance and perinatal care had been available. More encouraging, and contrary to a widely held view, is that a large majority (75 per cent) of the newborns' weights were adequate for gestational age (Fig. 4.4).

It must be emphasised that none of the women in our survey had overt renal insufficiency before pregnancy and therefore the favourable prognosis described above obviously applies only to women with preserved renal function at conception and may not be valid for women who have greater impairment of function. Occasionally women with moderately severe renal disease have borne viable infants and there are also reports in the literature of live births in a few pregnant women who were on maintenance haemodialysis or who experienced sudden deterioration in renal function and were managed with haemodialysis (Goldsmith et al, 1971; Marwood et al, 1977; Registration Committee of the European Dialysis and Transplant Association, 1980).

The effect of pregnancy on long-term renal prognosis

Follow-up data ranging from three months to 23 years postpartum were available in 80 of those women. The prevalance of hypertension or renal function abnormalities, as well as their severity, were considerably less than during pregnancy and the postpartum period (Fig. 4.5). Only five women had progressed to endstage renal disease, the onset of which bore no consistent temporal relationship to the pregnancy. These patients had renal disorders that carried a poor prognosis and there was no evidence that the intervening pregnancy had accelerated the progression of their diseases. Only one woman had severe hypertension and seven had mild hypertension, four having been hypertensive prior to the index pregnancy. Decrements in renal function were also mild, the highest creatinine level being 150 μmol/l. Abnormal proteinuria was present in 33 women, but in contrast to the situation in pregnancy the amount excreted was small in most instances, exceeding 3 g per 24 hours in only five women.

Summary

Our study has shown that in the absence of overt renal insufficiency or significant hypertension prior to conception, women with renal disease should not be discouraged from becoming pregnant and in such patients there is no evidence that pregnancy accelerates the progress of their disease.

Table 4.2 Classification of renal disease and outcome of pregnancy[a]

Diagnosis	Gravidas	Pregnancies	Fetal deaths[a]	Neonatal deaths	Preterm deliv's	Small-for-gestational-age infants	Birthweight live infants[b]			
							1500g	1500–2000g	2000–2500g	>2500g
Diffuse glomerulonephritis	26	33	3	3	13	9	6	3	6	13
Focal glomerulonephritis	12	26	2	2	1	6	0	1	7	18
Membranoproliferative glomerulonephritis	4	4	0	0	0	1	0	0	1	3
Membranous nephropathy	7	10	0	0	1	1	0	0	2	5
Lipoid nephrosis	3	6	0	0	1	4	0	0	4	2
Focal glomerulosclerosis	1	1	0	0	0	0	0	0	0	1
Interstitial nephritis	21	26	1	1	4	2	0	1	4	20
Arteriolar nephrosclerosis	8	8	0	0	3	3	2	2	0	4
Others[d]	7	7	1	0	1	1	1	0	1	4
Totals	89	121[c]	7	6	24	27	9	7	25	70
Per cent			5.7%	4.9%	20.0%	24.3%	8.1%	6.3%	22.5%	63.1%

[a] Stillbirths and 2nd trimester spontaneous abortions
[b] Birthweight available for only 111 of the 116 live infants
[c] Two sets of twins
[d] Includes sickle cell nephropathy, two patients; one each of polycystic kidney disease, IgA nephropathy, diabetic glomerulosclerosis, renal amyloidosis, and bilateral renal artery stenosis

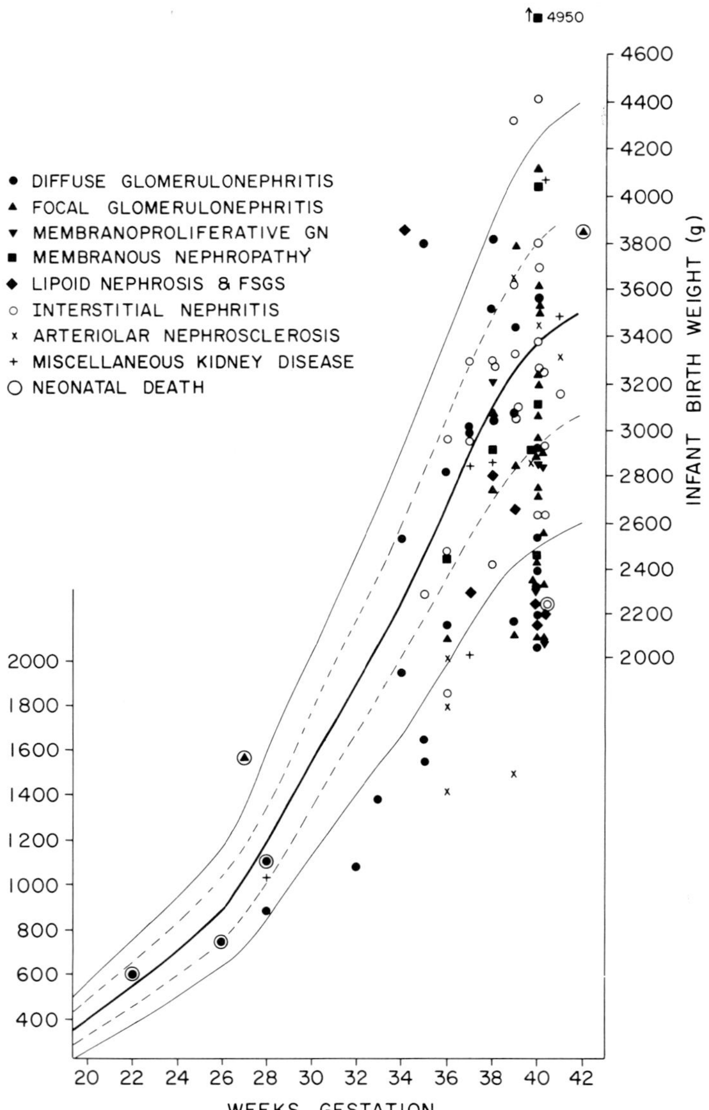

Fig. 4.4   Birthweight in relation to gestational age for 111 live births. Lines represent mean weight ± 1 and 2 SD of 25 608 live births at University Hospital of Cleveland, Ohio, USA compiled by Dr C. H. Hendricks between 1958 and 1968. (From Katz et al, 1980)

SPECIFIC RENAL DISEASES AND PREGNANCY

Table 4.3 summarises the course of pregnancy in a number of specific diseases. From the literature and our own studies a number of generalisations can be made regarding these conditions.

Acute and chronic glomerulonephritis

Acute post-streptococcal glomerulonephritis complicating pregnancy is very rare, but

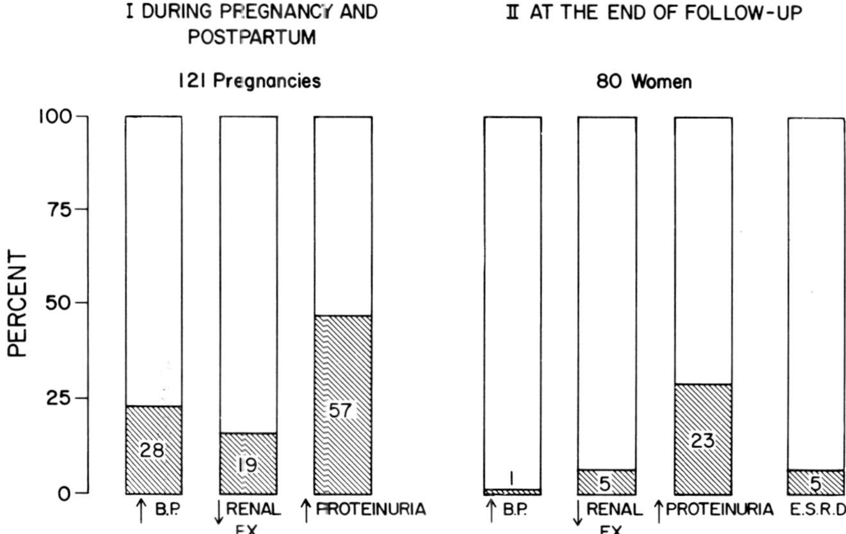

Fig. 4.5   Course of renal disease in 89 women during gestation and the puerperium (3 bars on the left) and in 80 women followed-up after pregnancy (4 bars on the right). Numbers within bars are individual pregnancies (on the left) and individual women (on the right). ESRD = end-stage renal disease. Fx = function.

Table 4.3   Summary of effects of pregnancy on pre-existing renal disease

Chronic glomerulonephritis, non-infectious tubulointerstitial disease (e.g. polycystic kidneys)	Usually no adverse effect in the absence of hypertension. Urinary tract infections may occur more frequently. Some believe that glomerulonephritis is adversely affected by coagulation changes in pregnancy.
Lupus nephropathy	Controversial; prognosis most favourable if disease in remission >6 months prior to conception. Steroid dosage should be increased in the puerperium.
Diabetic nephropathy	Probably no adverse effect on the renal lesion, although frequency of leg oedema, pre-eclampsia and infection higher.
Nephrotic syndrome	Tolerated well, infants may have low birth weight. Diuretics should not be used.
Chronic pyelonephritis	Bacteriuria during pregnancy leads to more frequent exacerbation.
Urolithiasis	Infections may be more frequent otherwise ureteral dilatation and stasis do not seem to affect the natural history.
After nephrectomy; solitary and pelvic kidneys	Pregnancy usually well tolerated. Dystocia has been attributed to pelvic kidneys.
Transplanted kidneys	Most pregnancies succeed, but hypertensive and infectious problems are more frequent than in normal pregnancy. Immuno-suppressive therapy may cause fetal adrenal failure, congenital anomalies and intrauterine growth retardation.

(Adapted from Lindheimer and Katz, 1977)

does occur, and has been mistaken for pre-eclampsia. In the earlier literature, cases occurring during pregnancy were marked by irreversible declines in maternal renal function and poor fetal outcome. These reports, however, probably describe exacerbations of a chronic process or another disease, for in the several instances where documentation of the diagnosis was appropriate, recovery of maternal function was complete and the pregnancy usually had a successful outcome. The prognosis of chronic glomerulonephritis during pregnancy is hard to evaluate primarily because most authors have documented poorly the cases they reported, often failing to list the degree of functional impairment and the blood pressure prior to conception. In addition, the histology of the 'glomerulonephritis' was rarely detailed. Ferris (1975) reviewed eight series published between 1956 and 1969 that comprised 365 women presumed to have chronic glomerulonephritis. The incidence of 'toxemia' was slightly increased but there were no maternal deaths during 424 pregnancies and fetal survival was 93 per cent in 196 normotensive patients. In contrast, 45 per cent of the fetuses of the women who had both renal disease and hypertension died. The Melbourne group (Kincaid-Smith et al, 1967 and 1980; Fairley et al, 1973) have stated that pregnancy tends to aggravate most glomerular diseases due to the hypercoagulable state that accompanies pregnancy, claiming that crescentic glomerular lesions occur more readily. They also indicate that such patients are more prone to superimposed pre-eclampsia or hypertensive crises early in pregnancy. In our own series, renal function decreased most often in patients with diffuse glomerulonephritis (11 out of 19) in whom hypertension was both more common and severe; nonetheless, most of the pregnancies were successful (27 out of 33) (see Table 4.2).

Hereditary nephritis is an uncommon disorder which may first manifest or exacerbate during pregnancy (Gill & Hayslett, 1969; Grunfeld et al, 1973). A variant of hereditary nephritis in which the patients have disordered platelet morphology and function can occur. Pregnancy in these women has been successful from a renal viewpoint but can be complicated by bleeding problems.

Collagen diseases

There are differing opinions regarding the effects of pregnancy on lupus nephropathy and transient improvement, no change and a tendency to relapse have all been reported. Of importance though is that some of these patients have a tendency towards relapse (occasionally severe) in the puerperium and therefore it may be prudent to prescribe or increase the use of steroids during this period. Lupus nephropathy may sometimes become manifest during pregnancy and when accompanied by hypertension and renal dysfunction in late pregnancy may be mistaken for pre-eclampsia. Placental transmission of lupus serum factors also occurs, which may relate to the high frequency of spontaneous abortions in these women (Bresnihan et al, 1977). Placental arteritis (Abramowsky et al, 1980) and an increased incidence of congenital cardiac anomalies (Chameides et al, 1977; Berute et al, 1978) have been described in the infants of women with systemic lupus even though the maternal disease appeared quiescent.

Patients with lupus nephropathy were not included in our previously described survey (Katz et al, 1980) as the case histories of 9 of our patients were incorporated into another multicentre study involving 65 pregnancies in 47 patients (Hayslett & Lynn, 1980). The majority of these gestations succeeded, especially if the maternal disease was in remission for at least 6 months prior to conception, even if the patient had severe histopathologic changes in her renal biopsy and heavy proteinuria in the early stages of her disease. However, continued signs of disease activity or increasing renal dysfunction reduced the likelihood of an uncomplicated pregnancy. Similar findings in women with longstanding lupus nephropathy have recently been published (Houser et al, 1980).

In contrast to lupus nephropathy, the outcome of pregnancy in women with renal involvement due to periarteritis nodosa and scleroderma is very poor, largely because of the associated hypertension which is frequently of a malignant nature. Not only is fetal prognosis dismal, but many of the cases reported ended with maternal deaths.

Diabetes mellitus

Since many diabetic pregnant women are juvenile diabetics, they probably harbour early microscopic changes in their kidneys. During pregnancy diabetic women have an increased prevalence of bacteriuria and may be more susceptible to symptomatic urinary tract infection. They also have an increased frequency of leg oedema and pre-eclampsia. Some authorities believe that diabetic nephropathy worsens during pregnancy, presumably based on observations in women with considerable functional impairment prior to conception. Some of these reports, however, are from centres where antenatal care included vigorous salt restriction, an approach which decreases renal haemodynamics in patients with renal parenchymal disease. In contrast, most of a group of women with diabetic nephropathy studied serially during pregnancy demonstrated the normal increments in renal function (Sims, 1961). A recent study has revealed that pregnancy does not accelerate deterioration of diabetic nephropathy (Kitzmiller et al, 1981). Fetal outcome in diabetics is discussed elsewhere in this book.

Tubulointerstitial diseases

The prognosis of pregnancy in women with 'chronic pyelonephritis' seems similar to that of patients with glomerular disease, in that its outcome is most favourable in normotensive patients with adequate renal function. Women whose disease is of infectious nature have a propensity to exacerbate during pregnancy, which may be minimised if the patient is well hydrated and rests frequently positioned in lateral recumbency (ureteral obstruction by the enlarged uterus does not occur in this position). Some have suggested that these patients are more prone to hypertensive complications during gestation but in our study (Katz et al, 1980) gravidas with interstitial nephritis had a more benign prenatal course than women with glomerular disease.

Polycystic kidney disease

This entity may remain undetected during pregnancy, but careful questioning of gravidas for a history of familial problems and the use of ultrasonography may lead to earlier detection. These patients do well when functional impairment is minimal and hypertension absent, which is often the case during childbearing years.

Urolithiasis

Urolithiasis during pregnancy has a prevalence of between 0.03 to 0.35 per cent and most of the stones contain calcium. The older literature tended to stress the dramatic complications which occur when calculi cause obstructive uropathy and infection supervenes. However, a study of nonselected stone formers indicated that the course of the disease is unaffected by pregnancy, although urinary tract infections were more common in such patients (Coe et al, 1978). Similar findings have been noted in recent retrospective investigations (Cumming & Taylor, 1979; Lattanzy et al, 1980). If nephrectomy has been performed because of nephrolithiasis the remaining kidney may be infected and such patients should be carefully scrutinised by means of frequent urine cultures throughout pregnancy.

Lastly, renal calculi are one of the most common causes of non-uterine-related abdominal pain severe enough to require hospitalisation of pregnant patients (Folger, 1955). When complications suggest the need for surgical intervention, then pregnancy should not be a deterrent to intravenous urography.

Miscellaneous renal disease

Renal tuberculosis does not seem to be affected by pregnancy. Women with solitary but normally situated kidneys seem to tolerate pregnancy well (Davison, 1978). Pelvic kidneys are associated with decreased fetal salvage because of an association with other malformations of the urogenital tract.

NEPHROTIC SYNDROME AND PREGNANCY

The most common cause of nephrotic syndrome in late pregnancy is pre-eclampsia (Fisher et al, 1977; First et al, 1978). This form has a poorer fetal prognosis than pregnancy-induced hypertension with less heavy proteinuria, but maternal prognosis is similar (Studd, 1973).

Other causes of nephrotic syndrome in pregnancy include membranous nephropathy, proliferative or membranoproliferative glomerulonephritis, lipoid nephrosis, lupus nephropathy, hereditary nephritis, diabetic nephropathy, renal vein thrombosis, amyloidosis and secondary syphilis. Some of these conditions do not respond to, and may even be aggravated by, corticosteroids, which underscores the importance of establishing a tissue diagnosis before initiating therapy.

If renal function is adequate and hypertension is absent, there should be few complications during pregnancy; however, several of the 'physiological changes' occurring during gestation may simulate aggravation or exacerbation of the disease. For example, increments in renal haemodynamics as well as increases in renal vein pressure may enhance protein excretion. Levels of serum albumin usually decrease by 5 to 10 g/l in normal pregnancy, and the further decreases that can occur in the nephrotic syndrome may enhance the tendency toward fluid retention. Therefore a high protein diet (3 g/kg day) is important in these patients. Despite oedema, diuretics are to be avoided as these patients have a decreased intravascular volume and saliuretic therapy could further compromise uteroplacental perfusion or aggravate the increased tendency to thrombotic episodes.

While the majority of these pregnancies succeed and are maintained to term, there is evidence that the hypoalbuminaemia and the associated decreased intravascular volume may cause small-for-dates infants. Furthermore, there is a report that infants of normotensive mothers who had heavy proteinuria during pregnancy manifested impaired neurologic and mental development (Rosenbaum et al, 1969) and this requires further study.

Table 4.4 outlines the problems in pregnant women with heavy proteinuria (literature summarised by Lindheimer & Katz, 1977 and 1981).

MANAGEMENT OF PREGNANT WOMEN WITH RENAL DISEASE

Several points regarding management in specific cases have already been made. The following comments apply to management in general.

Maternal surveillance

RENAL FUNCTION
Serial data on renal function are needed to supplement routine antenatal observations.

Table 4.4 Manifestations and management of nephrotic syndrome in pregnancy

Manifestation	Effect of Pregnancy	Management
1. Proteinuria	Increments in renal haemodynamics as well as increases in renal vein pressure may enhance protein excretion and simulate aggravation of disease. Protein loss may also lead to intrauterine fetal growth retardation.	Prescribe high protein diet (3 g/kg body weight). The infusion of salt-poor albumin is recommended for patients wth decreasing renal function secondary to marked oligaemia, and for those with postural hypotension.
2. Hypoalbuminaemia	Levels of serum albumin usually decrease 5–10 gm/l in normal pregnancy. The further decrease in nephrotic patients may enhance the tendency towards fluid retention.	
3. Oedema	Usually increases during pregnancy.	Avoid diuretics, which may increase the intravascular oligaemia and compromise uteroplacental perfusion.
4. Infectious complications	There may be a high incidence of infectious complications in nephrotic pregnant women.	Screen frequently for asymptomatic bacteriuria.
5. Thrombotic episodes	Pregnancy in a hypercoagulable state and some have claimed that there are more frequent episodes of thrombotic episodes in pregnant patients with nephrosis.	Not anticoagulated prophylactically, but if anticoagulation is required, heparin, which does not cross the placenta, is the preferred mode of therapy.
6. Hyperlipidaemia	Cholesterol and free fatty acids normally increase during pregnancy.	Treatment rarely required in pregnancy and most lipid lowering agents have not been tested in this situation.

(Adapted from Lindheimer and Katz, 1977).

Specialised tests involving infusion procedures are usually not available and their use is primarily for clinical research. Tests that are available for use in routine clinical practice include the estimation of plasma urea and electrolytes, creatinine and urea clearance determination, concentration and dilution procedures and urinary pH testing after acid loading. It should always be remembered that the functions assessed by clinical tests are usually influenced by multiple mechanisms. For example, urea and creatinine clearances do not measure absolute GFR: urea is reabsorbed and creatinine secreted by the renal tubules, so that the clearance of either gives only an approximation of the GFR. Nevertheless, these tests have generated a great deal of empirical information and provide adequate, if not precise, assessments of renal function in numerous clinical situations.

In the last analysis the management of pregnant women with renal disease requires serial surveillance of creatinine clearance. If renal function deteriorates during any stage of pregnancy, reversible causes such as urinary tract infection or obstruction, subtle dehydration or electrolyte imbalance (perhaps secondary to inadvertent diuretic therapy) should be sought. Near term, a 15 per cent decrement in function (which affects plasma creatinine minimally) is permissible (Davison et al, 1980). If hypertension accompanies any observed decrease in renal function the outlook is usually more serious: immediate decisions and action may be required and the patient should be hospitalised. Failure to detect a reversible cause of the decrease in renal function is grounds for recommending termination of pregnancy.

THE ROLE OF RENAL BIOPSY IN OBSTETRIC PRACTICE

There is no doubt that the introduction of percutaneous renal biopsy in the 1950s has revolutionised our understanding of kidney pathology. Experience with renal biopsy in pregnancy is sparse, mainly because clinical circumstances rarely justify the minimal risks of biopsy at this time and the procedure is usually deferred to the postpartum period. Another reason for this dearth of information is that reports of excessive bleeding and other complications of gravidas have led some to consider pregnancy a relative contra-indication to renal biopsy (Schewitz et al, 1965), although other clinicians have not observed an increased morbidity of this procedure in gravidas (Lindheimer et al, 1975). In general, if the biopsy is performed in the immediate puerperium in subjects with well-controlled blood pressure and normal coagulation indices, the morbidity is similar to that reported in non-pregnant patients.

Indications for antepartum biopsy are few, one example being the nephrotic syndrome of unknown aetiology occurring late in the second or early in the third trimester. Diagnosis of pre-eclampsia may influence decisions concerning termination of pregnancy, while demonstration of other pathology by biopsy is helpful in selecting therapy. Renal biopsies should not be performed after 34 weeks' gestation since by this time the fetus will probably be delivered regardless of biopsy results.

Fetal surveillance

Determinations of fetal status are important because renal disease is associated with intrauterine growth retardation. Also, when complications do arise the judicious moment for intervention may be influenced by fetal status. Use of modern techniques for fetal surveillance minimises death in utero, preventable neonatal morbidity and mortality, and the hazards of prematurity.

The usefulness of 24-hour total urinary estriol excretion in patients with renal disease is controversial, primarily because the main urinary estriol metabolite oestriol-16-glucosiduronate is removed by glomerular filtration and tubular excretion (Marwood et al, 1977). A more useful parameter is measurement of free or unconjugated oestriol.

The remainder of the current antenatal armamentarium, i.e. ultrasound, antepartum electronic monitoring and amniotic fluid assessment of gestational age should be utilised in these pregnancies. There is presently little information regarding the correlation of lecithin-sphingomyelin ratios with clinical outcome in renal disease, but our personal experience indicates that false-positive results are uncommon.

PREGNANCY IN RENAL TRANSPLANT RECIPIENTS

Reproductive function is abnormal in haemodialysed women who manifest a variety of menstrual irregularities, often fail to ovulate and have difficulty conceiving (Emmanouel et al, 1981). Recent studies suggest that the abnormality may be due to impairment of positive oestradiol feedback on the hypothalamus which is responsible for the normally occurring cyclic release of LH at mid-cycle in healthy premenopausal women (Lim et al, 1980). Hyperprolactinaemia occurs and this may also account for the poor fertility in these women. Renal transplantation usually reverses these problems, the resumption of regular menstruation and ovulation correlating closely with the level of function achieved by the graft (Merkatz et al, 1971). As the number of transplanted women of childbearing age continues to increase clinicians are more likely to be faced with the task of counselling such patients as to whether or not they should conceive as well as managing the pregnancies of those already pregnant. Indeed, it has been estimated that one of every fifty women of childbearing age having a functional renal transplant becomes pregnant (British Medical Journal, 1976). We have reviewed this topic combining our own experiences with the many reports in the literature (Davison and Lindheimer, 1981), bringing together the experience of 697 such pregnancies. Inevitably it is difficult to assess the exact incidence of the various problems because some of the data in the literature are incomplete and many more pregnancies than those reported have occurred. Excluding the large Denver series (Penn et al, 1980), where 75 per cent of patients had received kidneys from living related donors, only 20 per cent of births occurred in recipients of living donor grafts. Despite publication of numerous case reports, several series and registry data from North America and Europe, little has been done to establish guidelines on standards of care for the transplant recipient who conceives. In some instances pregnancy was not diagnosed until the second or even the third trimester and many patients were under the impression that they could not conceive. Medical concern seems to have been limited to the advisability of allowing pregnancy to continue rather than the advisability of the initial conception, and only recently have appeals for closer cooperation between nephrologists and obstetricians been made.

Pregnancy management

Patients must be monitored as high-risk cases. Management requires attention to blood pressure control, renal function, anaemia, urinary tract infection and bone disease. Meticulous assessment of fetal growth is needed and this is best performed by serial ultrasound assessment. Measurement of maternal urinary oestriol excretion is of no value because the administration of steroids suppresses the synthesis of fetal adrenal steroid precursors and the transplanted kidney may not excrete oestriol normally. Where there is evidence of intrauterine growth retardation the possibility of congenital cytomegalo virus infection should be considered (Evans et al, 1975).

Maternal complications include serious infection, septicaemia, steroid-induced hyperglycaemia and uterine rupture.

Allograft function during pregnancy
Even though a transplanted kidney is ectopic, denervated, potentially damaged by previous ischaemia and immunologically different from both recipient and her fetus the augmentation of GFR characteristic of early pregnancy in healthy women is invariably evident (Davison, 1978) (see Fig. 4.6). The better the renal function before

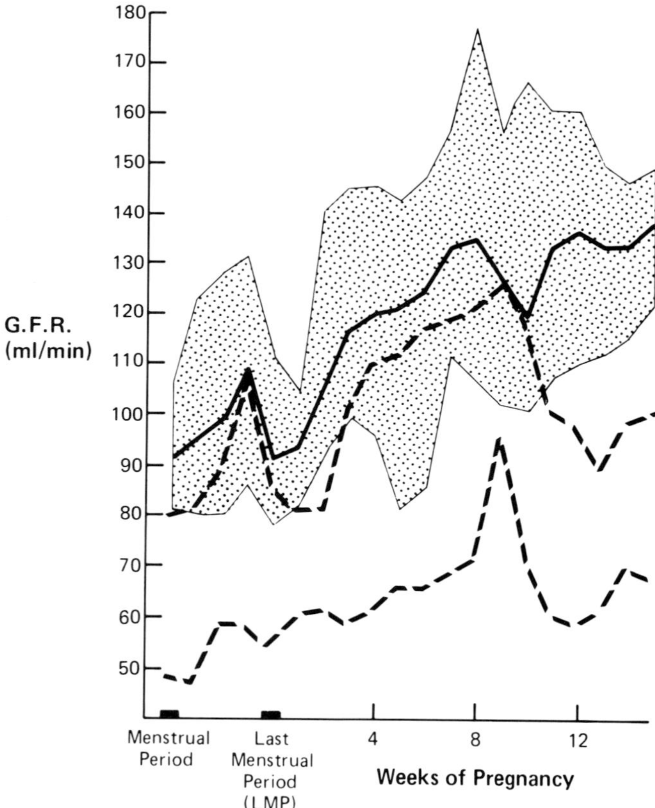

Fig. 4.6 Weekly 24-hour creatinine clearance (GFR) over conception and in early pregnancy in two renal transplant patients. Solid line represents the mean and stippled area the range for eight healthy women at same period of time.

pregnancy the more satisfactory the obstetrical outcome. Permanent impairment of renal function is occasionally seen especially where renal function is already compromised prior to conception. In patients with satisfactory renal function before pregnancy, there may be some deterioration during the third trimester, with or without proteinuria, but this is usually transient with normal function returning in the postpartum period. Renal transplant patients have a 30 per cent chance of developing pre-eclampsia. Occasionally plasma urate levels and 24-hour urinary protein excretion are well above the physiological norm for pregnancy, and yet do not herald the onset of pre-eclampsia.

Allograft rejection during pregnancy
It has been reported that serious rejection episodes occur in 9 per cent of women with pregnancies lasting into the third trimester (Rudolph et al, 1979). While this incidence is no greater than that expected for non-pregnant transplant patients it must be considered unusual because it has always been assumed that the privileged immunological state of pregnancy would benefit the transplant. Furthermore, there are reports (Kaufman et al, 1967; Rifle & Traeger, 1975) of reduction or cessation of immunosuppressive therapy during pregnancy without rejection. Rejection occasionally occurs in the puerperium due, perhaps, to a return to a normal immune state (despite immunosuppression) or possibly a rebound effect from the altered immunoresponsiveness associated with pregnancy. When patients who show functional declines are analysed no relationship to prior rejection episodes, transplant to pregnancy time interval, problems in previous pregnancies or HLA types is apparent.

Rejection in the non-pregnant patient is often a difficult diagnostic problem and in the absence of a renal biopsy cannot be distinguished from acute pyelonephritis and recurrent glomerulopathy. Its clinical hallmarks are fever, decreasing urinary output and deteriorating renal function often associated with renal enlargement and tenderness. In pregnancy the differential diagnosis will also include severe pre-eclampsia.

Management of delivery
The transplanted kidney is not lodged in the true pelvis and usually does not produce any mechanical dystocia during labour. During vaginal delivery there is no apparent mechanical injury to the transplanted kidney. Caesarean section is usually necessary only for purely obstetrical reasons. Augmentation of steroids is necessary to cover the stress of delivery.

Neonatal problems
There are substantial hazards to the neonate. Pre-term delivery occurs in 50 per cent and intrauterine growth retardation in 15 per cent. One or more complications occur in about 35 per cent, including respiratory distress syndrome, leucopenia, thrombocytopenia, adrenocortical insufficiency and infection. There are no predominant or frequent developmental abnormalities. It is imperative that any child exposed to immunosuppressive therapy have a careful evaluation of the immune system and long-term follow-up.

Pregnancy counselling
Couples who want a child should discuss all the implications of pregnancy and long-term prospects. We assess our patients on the basis of the following general guidelines:

1. Good general health for two years after transplantation.
2. Stature compatible with good obstetric outcome.

3. No proteinuria.
4. No significant hypertension.
5. No evidence of graft rejection.
6. No evidence of pelvicalyceal distension on a recent excretory urogram.
7. Plasma creatinine of 180 μmol/l or less.
8. Drug therapy: prednisone, 15 mg/day or less and azathioprine, 2 mg/kg/day or less.

After full pre-pregnancy assessment has been undertaken advice can then be given (Davison et al, 1976). It can only be advice, since patients must ultimately decide for themselves what degree of risk is acceptable. If the situation is tackled prospectively the final decision is in the nature of an agreement rather than a judgement. Major concern is that the mother may not survive or remain well enough to raise the child she bears. Average survival figures of large numbers of patients from all over the world (Advisory Committee to Renal Transplant Registry, 1977; UK Transplant, 1980) indicate that between 60 to 80 per cent of recipients of kidneys from related living donors are alive five years after transplantation and with cadaver kidneys the figure is 40 to 50 per cent. Functional survival of the allograft at five years is 45 to 65 per cent in recipients of living donor kidneys and 30 to 35 per cent in recipients of cadaver organs. Despite these statistics many patients will choose parenthood in an effort to renew a normal life and possibly in defiance of their anxious families and the sometimes negative attitudes of the medical establishment.

ACUTE RENAL FAILURE IN PREGNANCY

Acute renal failure occurs once in 10 000 pregnancies (Lindheimer et al, 1982); its frequency of distribution is bimodal, with one peak in early pregnancy (12 to 18 weeks) and the second during the 35th to 40th gestational week. Cases occurring in early pregnancy are primarily due to septic abortion, while those in late gestation are associated with pre-eclampsia and with hemorrhagic complications, particularly abruptio placentae (Smith et al, 1965; Emmanouel & Katz, 1973; Chugh et al, 1976).

By far the majority of patients with acute renal failure have acute tubular necrosis, and on rare occasion, glomerular or obstructive nephropathy occurs. However, in contradistinction to the aetiologic breakdown in non-pregnant populations, a substantial number of cases are due to acute cortical necrosis. Such cases are apt to occur late in pregnancy and seem to be frequently associated with pre-eclampsia and abruptio placentae. The reasons pregnant women are so susceptable to acute cortical necrosis, its relationship to coagulopathy, and the management of acute renal failure are detailed elsewhere (Lindheimer and Katz, 1977 and 1981).

While necrosis may involve the entire renal cortex causing irreversible anuria, it is usually the 'patchy' variety that occurs more often in pregnancy. The latter is characterised by an initial episode of severe oliguria followed by a variable return of function and a stable period of moderate renal insufficiency (Grünfeld et al, 1980). Years later, for reasons still obscure renal function decreases again often approaching terminal renal failure (Kleinknecht et al, 1973).

There are two rare forms of acute renal failure peculiar to pregnancy (Sun et al,

1975; Lindheimer and Katz, 1977; Williams, 1977). One, acute fatty liver of pregnancy (also called obstetric pseudo-acute yellow atrophy) is characterised by jaundice and severe hepatic dysfunction in late pregnancy or the early postpartum period. The renal failure appears to be due to hemodynamic factors, as in the 'hepatorenal syndrome', but some cases have been associated with intravascular coagulation. Recently reversible urea cycle enzyme abnormalities resembling those seen in Reye's syndrome have been described (Weber et al, 1979). The mortality rate in obstetric pseudo acute yellow atrophy is high with death resulting primarily from hepatic rather than renal failure.

The second form of renal failure peculiar to pregnancy goes by a variety of names including idiopathic postpartum renal failure or haemolytic uraemic syndrome. The patient usually has an uncomplicated pregnancy and delivery but three to six weeks into the puerperium develops severe hypertension and uraemia, often accompanied by microangiopathic haemolytic anaemia (Segonds et al, 1979). The pathophysiology and recent theories of management of the syndrome are discussed elsewhere (Lindheimer & Katz, 1977; Remuzzi et al, 1979; Webster et al, 1980). Unfortunately, to date, most women have died and those who have survived had severely reduced renal function.

CONCLUSIONS

Coexistence of pregnancy and renal disease worries clinicians who in the past have been quick to terminate such pregnancies regardless of the type and severity of the patient's disease. We have reviewed this topic and have concluded that most women with mild and moderate renal disease tolerate pregnancy well. The key to success is close scrutiny of the antenatal course with cooperation between obstetrician, nephrologist, and eventually paediatrician. Finally, the ability to detect and understand renal disease during pregnancy requires an understanding of the striking alterations occurring in the urinary tract during normal pregnancy.

REFERENCES

Abromowsky C R, Vegas M E, Swinehart G, Guyves M T 1980 Decidual pathology of the placenta in lupus erythematosus. New England Journal of Medicine 303: 668–672
Advisory Committee to the Renal Transplant Registry 1977 The 13th report of the human renal transplant registry. Transplant Proceedings 9: 9–26
Bailey R R, Rolleston G L 1971 Kidney length and ureteric dilatation in the puerperium. Journal of Obstetrics and Gynaecology of the British Commonwealth 78: 55–61
Berube S, Lister G, Toews W H, Creasy R K, Heymann M A 1978 Congenital heart block and maternal systemic lupus erythematosus. American Journal of Obstetrics and Gynecology 130: 595–596
British Medical Journal Editorial 1976 Pregnancy after renal transplantation 1: 733–734
Bear R A 1976 Pregnancy in patients with renal disease: A study of 44 cases. Obstetrics and Gynecology 48: 13–18
Bresnihan B, Grigor R R, Oliver M, Lewkonia R M, Hughes G R V, Lovins R E, Faulk W P 1977 Immunological mechanism for spontaneous abortion in systemic lupus erythematosus. Lancet 2: 1205–1207
Bricker N S, Bourgoignie J J, Weber H 1976 The renal response to progressive nephron loss. In: Brenner B M, Rector F C, Jr (eds) The kidney. Philadelphia. vol 1
Chameides L, Truex R C, Vetter V, Rashkind W J, Galioto F M, Jr, Noonan J A 1977 Association of maternal systemic lupus erythematosus with congenital complete heart block. New England Journal of Medicine 297: 1204–1207
Chugh K S, Singhal P C, Sharma B K, Pal Y, Mathew M T, Dhall K, Datta B N 1976 Acute renal failure of obstetrics origin. Obstetrics and Gynecology 48: 642

Coe F C, Parks J H, Lindheimer M D 1978 Nephrolithiasis during pregnancy. New England Journal of Medicine 298: 324–326

Cumming D C, Taylor P J 1979 Urologic and obstetric significance of urinary calculi in pregnancy. Obstetrics and Gynecology 53: 505–509

Davison J M, Hytten F E 1974 Glomerular filtration during and after pregnancy. Journal of Obstetrics and Gynaecology of the British Commonwealth 81: 588–595

Davison J M, Lind T, Uldall P R 1976 Planned pregnancy in a renal transplant recipient. British Journal of Obstetrics and Gynaecology 83: 518–527

Davison J M 1978 Changes in renal function in early pregnancy in women with one kidney. Yale Journal of Biological Medicine 51: 347–349

Davison J M, Lindheimer M D 1978 Renal Disease in Pregnant Women. Clinical Obstetrics and Gynecology 21: 411–427

Davison J M, Dunlop W 1980 Renal hemodynamics and tubular function in normal human pregnancy. Kidney International 18: 152–161

Davison J M, Dunlop W, Ezimokhai M 1980 Twenty-four hour creatinine clearance during the third trimester of normal pregnancy. British Journal of Obstetrics and Gynaecology 87: 106–109

Davison J M, Lindheimer M D Gynaecological and Obstetrical Problems after Renal Transplantation. Nieren und Hochdruckkrankheiten. In press

Davison J M, Noble M C B 1981 Serial changes in 24-hour creatinine clearance during normal menstrual cycles and the first trimester of pregnancy. British Journal of Obstetrics and Gynaecology 88: 10–17

Emmanouel D S, Katz A I 1973 Acute renal failure in obstetric septic shock: Current views on pathogenesis and management. American Journal of Obstetrics and Gynecology 117: 144–159

Emmanouel D S, Lindheimer M D, Katz A I Endocrine abnormalities in chronic renal failure. Seminars in Nephrology. In press

Evans T J, McCollum J P K, Valdimasson H 1975 Congenital cytomegalovirus infection after maternal renal transplantation. Lancet 1: 1359–1360

Fairley K F, Whitworth J A, Kincaid-Smith P 1973 Glomerulonephritis and pregnancy. In: Kincaid-Smith P, Mathew T H, Becker E L, (eds) Glomerulonephritis, Part II, p 997–1011

Felding C F 1969 Obstetric aspects in women with histories of renal disease. Acta Obstetrica et Gynecologica Scandinavica 48: Suppl 2–43

Ferris T F 1975 Renal Disease. In: Burrow G N, Ferris T F (eds) Medical Complications during Pregnancy, W B Saunders, Philadelphia, p 1–52

First M R, Ooi B S, Wellington J, Pollak V E 1978 Pre-eclampsia with the nephrotic syndrome. Kidney International 13: 166–177

Fisher K A, Ahuja S, Luger A, Spargo B H, Lindheimer M D 1977 Nephrotic proteinuria with pre-eclampsia. American Journal of Obstetrics and Gynecology 129: 643–646

Folger G K 1955 Pain and pregnancy: treatment of painful states complicating pregnancy, with particular emphasis on urinary calculi. Obstetrics and Gynecology 5: 513–515

Gibson H M 1973 Plasma volume and glomerular filtration rate in pregnancy and their relationship to fetal growth. Journal of Obstetrics and Gynaecology of the British Commonwealth 80: 1067–74

Gill G N, Hayslett J P 1969 Hereditary nephritis and pregnancy. American Journal of Obstetrics and Gynecology 104: 19–24

Goldsmith H J, Menzies D N, De Boer C H, Caplan W 1971 Delivery of healthy infants after five weeks' dialysis treatment for fulminating toxaemia of pregnancy. Lancet ii: 738–740

Grünfeld J P, Boise E P, Hinglais N 1973 Progressive and non-progressive hereditary chronic nephritis. Kidney International 4: 216–220

Grünfeld J P, Ganeval D, Bournerias F 1980 Acute renal failure in pregnancy. Kidney International 18: 179–191

Houser M T, Fish A J, Tegatz G E, Williams P P, Michael A F 1980 Pregnancy and systemic lupus erythematosus. American Journal of Obstetrics and Gynecology 138: 409–413

Hayslett J P, Lynn R I 1980 Effect of pregnancy in patients with lupus nephropathy. Kidney International 18: 207–220

Kaplan A L, Smith J P, Tillman A J B 1962 Healed acute and chronic nephritis in pregnancy. American Journal of Obstetrics and Gynecology 83: 1519–1525

Katz A I, Davison J M, Hayslett J P, Singson E, Lindheimer M D 1980 Pregnancy in women with kidney disease. Kidney International 18: 192–206

Katz A I, Davison J M, Hayslett J P, Lindheimer M D 1981 Effect of Pregnancy on the Natural History of Kidney Disease. Contributions to Nephrology 1981, 25: 53–60

Kaufmann J J, Dignam W, Goodwin W E, Martin D C, Goldman R, Maxwell M H 1967 Successful normal childbirth after kidney homotransplantation. Journal of the American Medical Association 200: 162–165, 167

Kincaid-Smith P, Fairley K F, Byllen M 1967 Kidney disease and pregnancy. Medical Journal of Australia 2: 1155–1159

Kincaid-Smith P, Whitworth J A, Fairley K F 1980 Mesandial IgA nephropathy in pregnancy. Clinical and Experimental Hypertension 2 821–838

Kitzmiller J L, Brown E R, Philipe M, Stark M R, Acker D, Kaldany A, Hare J W 1981 Diabetic nephropathy and perinatal outcome. American Journal of Obstetrics and Gynecology. In press

Kleinknecht D, Gainfeld J P, Gomez P C, Moreau J F, Garcia-Torres R 1973 Diagnostic procedures and long-term prognosis in bilateral renal cortical necrosis. Kidney International 4: 390–400

Klockars M, Saarikoski S, Ikonen E, Kuhlback B 1980 Pregnancy in patients with renal disease. Acta Medicine Scandinavica 207: 207–214

Kuhlback B, Widholm O 1966 Plasma creatinine in normal pregnancy. Scandinavian Journal of Clinical and Laboratory Investigation 18: 654–658

Lattanzy D R, Cook W A 1980 Urinary calculi in pregnancy. Obstetrics and Gynecology 56: 462–470

Lim V S, Henriquez C, Sievertsen G, Frohman L A 1980 Ovarian function in chronic renal failure: Evidence suggesting hypothalaemic anovulation. Annals of internal medicine 57: 7–12

Lindheimer M D, Spargo B H, Katz A I 1975 Renal biopsy in pregnancy-induced hypertension. Journal of Reproductive Medicine 15: 189–194

Lindheimer M D, Katz A I 1977 Kidney function and disease in pregnancy. Lea and Febiger, Philadelphia

Lindheimer M D, Katz A I, Nolten W, Oparil S, Ehrlich E N 1978 Sodium and minerocorticoids in normal and abnormal pregnancy. In: Hamburger J, Crosnier J, Mazwell M H (eds) Advances in nephrology 7: 33–59

Lindheimer M D, Katz A I 1981 The renal response to pregnancy. In: Brenner B M, Rector F C, Jr (eds) The kidney, 2nd edn. W B Saunders, Philadelphia, p 1762–1815.

Lindheimer M D, Katz A I, Gareval D, Grünfeld J P 1982 Renal failure in pregnancy. In: Brenner B M, Lazarus J H, Mayers B D (eds) Acute renal failure W B Saunders, Philadelphia. In press.

Marwood R P, Ogg C S, Coltart T M, Klopper A I 1977 Plasma oestrogens in a pregnancy associated with chronic hemodialysis. British Journal of Obstetrics and Gynaecology 84: 613

Merkatz I R, Schwartz G H, David D S, Stenzel K H, Riggio R R Whitsell J C 1971 Resumption of female reproductive function following renal transplantation. Journal of the American Medical Association 216: 1749–1757

Nolten W E, Ehrlich E N 1980 Sodium and mineralocorticoids in normal pregnancy. Kidney International 18: 162–172

Penn I, Makowski E L, Harris R 1980 Parenthood following renal transplantation. Kidney International 18: 221–233

Registration Committee of the European Dialysis and Transplant Association 1980 Successful pregnancies in women treated by dialysis and kidney transplantation. British Journal of Obstetrics and Gynaecology 87: 839–845

Remuzzi G, Misiani R, Marchesi D, Livio M, Mecca G, de Gaetano G, Donati M B 1979 Treatment of hemolytic uremic syndrome with plasma. Clinical Nephrology 12: 279–284

Rifle G, Traeger J 1975 Pregnancy after renal transplantation: an international review. Transplantation Proceedings, Suppl 1, 7: 723–728

Roberts J 1976 Hydronephrosis of pregnancy. Urology 8: 1–5

Robertson E G, Cheyne G A 1972 Plasma biochemistry in relation to oedema of pregnancy. Journal of Obstetrics and Gynaecology of the British Commonwealth 79: 769–776

Rosenbaum A L, Churchill J A, Shakhasashiri Z A, Moody R L 1969 Neuropsychologic outcome of children whose mothers had proteinuria during pregnancy. Obstetrics and Gynecology 33: 118–123

Rudolph J E, Scwihizir R T, Barius S A 1979 Pregnancy in renal transplant patients: A review. Transplantation 27: 26–29

Schewitz L J, Friedman E A, Pollak V E 1965 Bleeding after renal biopsy in pregnancy. Obstetrics and Gynecology 26: 285–304

Segonds A, Luradour N, Suc J M, Orfila C 1979 Postpartum hemolytic uremic syndrome: a study of three cases with a review of the literature. Clinical Nephrology 12: 229–242

Sims E A H 1961 Serial studies of renal function in pregnancy complicated by diabetes mellitus. Diabetes 10: 190–195

Smith K, McClure Browne J C, Shackman R, Wrong O M 1965 Acute renal failure of obstetric origin. An analysis of 70 patients. Lancet 2: 351–354

Strauch B S, Hayslett J P 1974 Kidney disease and pregnancy. British Medical Journal 4: 578–582

Studd J W 1973 The origin and effects of proteinuria in pregnancy. Journal of Obstetrics and Gynaecology of the British Commonwealth 80: 872–883

Sun N C J, Johnson W J, Sung D T W, Woods J E 1975 Idiopathic postpartum renal failure. Review and case report of a successful renal transplantation. Mayo Clin Proc 50: 395–398

Tenney B, Dandrow R V 1961 Clinical study of hypertensive disease in pregnancy. American Journal of Obstetrics and Gynecology 81: 8–15

Weber F L, Snodgrass P J, Powell D E, Rao P, Hoffman S L, Brady P G 1979 Abnormalities of hepatic mitochondrial urea-cycle enzyme activities and hepatic ultrastructure in acute fatty liver of pregnancy. Journal of Laboratory and Clinical Medicine 94: 27–41

Webster J, Rees A J, Lewis P J, Hensby C N 1980 Prostacyclin deficiency in haemolytic uraemic syndrome. British Medical Journal 281: 271

Werko L, Bucht H 1956 Glomerular filtration rate and renal blood flow in patients with chronic diffuse glomerulonephritis during pregnancy. Acta Medica Scandinavica 153: 177–186

Williams G 1977 Renal disease in pregnancy. Journal of Clinical Pathology 29 (suppl) 10: 77–90

UK Transplant Service Annual Report 1980 pp 26–36

5. Diabetes mellitus and pregnancy

M. Ivo Drury John M. Stronge

HISTORICAL

In contrast with the general literature on diabetes mellitus, that of pregnancy in the diabetic woman is of recent origin. Bouchardat, a French physician, in his treatise on Diabéte Sucrè published in 1883, stated that the pregnant diabetic was unknown to him. In the Boston Medical and Surgical Journal of 1899, Taylor stated that the Boston Lying-In Hospital had cared for 10 000 obstetric cases during the preceding 25 years without finding a single case of diabetes mellitus. The occurrence of a reducing substance in the urine of pregnant women however, was well known, to the extent that Jaksch (1895) considered that the presence of glycosuria after the oral administration of 100 grammes of grape sugar might be regarded as a sign of pregnancy. In 1882, Van Noorden reported on a survey of 427 diabetic women and found that pregnancy had occured in only 5 per cent. The first case report on diabetes in pregnancy was that of Bennewitz, who in 1826 described a patient with intense thirst and polyuria in three successive pregnancies — 'The taste of the urine resembled beer but was much sweeter and it contained 2 ozs saccharine matter per lb'. In 1882, Matthews Duncan, a name familiar to obstetricians for his description of a particular method of placental delivery, presented a paper entitled 'On Puerperal Diabetes' to the London Obstetrical Society. He stated 'Of diabetes in pregnancy and parturition our knowledge is scanty in the extreme. Obstetrical works generally make no reference to the subject. Apart from Bennewitz's and my own cases, none has been published and no general account of this terrible disease is to be found in the whole history of midwifery.' He reported that, including three cases of his own, 'all of which I have any knowledge' — this made a total of 22 pregnancies in 16 women. In these pregnancies 47 per cent of the infants died, four women died in coma or collapsed within a few days of delivery and seven others died within two years. In 1907, Eshner, reviewed the cases published before that date and recorded eight pregnancies in known diabetics and 27 others in whom diabetes was diagnosed during pregnancy; 28 infants were lost and 19 mothers died at varying periods after delivery. It is not surprising that Eshner should teach that: 'A diabetic woman should not marry, or, if married, she should not become pregnant'. The classical paper of that era was that of J. Whitridge Williams, Professor of Obstetrics at Johns Hopkins, published in 1909. His was the first attempt to classify the glycosurias of pregnancy, and he wrote that 'A positive Fehling's test during pregnancy does not necessarily indicate the existence of diabetes, but is usually due to lactosuria or to transient alimentary or recurrent glycosuria.' He reviewed the literature on diabetes in pregnancy and added five cases; omitting 15 doubtful cases, there were 64 pregnancies in 43 women. The fetal loss was 50 per cent, and 13 of the 43 mothers died during labour or the puerperium. In the nine cases in which pregnancy occurred in known diabetics, there were five maternal deaths.

This gloomy position continued until 1922, when Banting & Best revolutionised the outlook for diabetics with their discovery of insulin. The fertility of diabetics, hitherto impaired by their disease, was restored to normal, so that the rare and difficult problem of pregnancy in the diabetic became at the same time more common and more manageable. With increasing experience of the problem there was a remarkable reduction in maternal mortality and at present, given reasonable co-operation by the patient, a maternal death is exceptional. Fetal survival figures have also improved, but are still far from satisfactory.

In 1950 at the 12th British Congress of Obstetrics and Gynaecology, Peel & Oakley stated that 'the risk of intrauterine death of the fetus rises gradually from the 32nd to the 49th week; after 36 weeks the risk of intrauterine death exceeds the risk of neonatal death. Therefore, our view is that 36 weeks is the optimum date for termination, in the absence of special indications for earlier or later interference.' Fouracre Barns questioned this, and quoted from his own experience of patients divided into two groups according to time of delivery. He found that the fetal loss was the same for the two groups and concluded that early termination merely 'changed the death bed of the fetus, whilst subjecting the mother to greater risks incurred by interference.' Drury (1961) suggested that a compromise seemed best and recommended delivery at 37 weeks. Our current management programme includes delivery at term and is based on the experience of one of the authors (M.I.D.) with 825 pregnancies (845 infants) in 434 clinical diabetics in the three Dublin Maternity Hospitals, National Maternity (1951–1981), Coombe Lying-In (1954–1981) and Rotunda (1979–1981).

The pregnancies were consecutive and no pregnancy was terminated. No maternal deaths have occurred and the perinatal loss was 7.8 per cent (Tables 5.1 and 5.2).

Table 5.1 Dublin 1951–1981. 825 pregnancies (845 infants) in 434 clinical diabetics. National Maternity Hospital (1951–1981): Coombe (1954–1981): Rotunda (1979-1981).

Fetus dead on referral	10
Delivered elsewhere (S.B.)	1
Spontaneous abortion	69
Viable infants	765
No MATERNAL DEATH	

Table 5.2 Dublin 1951–1981

765 Viable I.D.M.	
Intrauterine deaths	28
Neonatal Deaths	32
Live born	705
	765
Perinatal Loss = 7.8%	

Since 1975, 262 viable infants have been delivered. Eleven intrauterine deaths occurred but no neonatal deaths — a perinatal loss of 4.2 per cent. Since 1979, 109 viable infants have been delivered and three intrauterine deaths occurred but no neonatal deaths — a perinatal loss of 2.7 per cent. The Caesarean section rate was 25 per cent. This continued improvement is, we believe, attributable to a policy of strict control of diabetes mellitus.

PHYSIOLOGY

In normal pregnancy metabolic adaptations occur in the mother to provide for the nutrition of the fetus whose primary fuel is glucose received by facilitated diffusion across the placenta. Amino acids, of which alanine is the most important are actively transported across the placenta. As a result the fasting blood glucose and the fasting amino acids are low in pregnant women. There is a corresponding reduction in the level of fasting insulin. Since this low level of insulin occurs in association with normal levels of glucagon and growth hormone the metabolic mode is ketogenic. The maternal need of alternative fuels is met by increasing levels of free fatty acids and of ketones. Thus, the metabolism in normal pregnancy is reminiscent of a starvation state.

In early pregnancy, carbohydrate tolerance improves due to the increasing levels of oestradiol and progesterone which diminish gluconeogenesis and facilitate glycogen deposition. Later on, however, there is an increased output of the insulin antagonists, human placental lactogen and cortisol. This is counter-balanced by an increase in the output of insulin from the beta cell of the pancreas.

The modification of carbohydrate metabolism which is a feature of normal pregnancy has important diagnostic and therapeutic implications. Thus the standard criteria for abnormality in the oral glucose tolerance test are not applicable in pregnancy. Furthermore levels of blood glucose which are acceptable indices of good diabetic control in normal circumstances are not so in pregnancy. This can readily be appreciated by noting that in normal women the fasting blood glucose is much lower in the pregnant than in the non-pregnant state. Specific criteria for pregnancy were laid down by O'Sullivan and Mahan (1964) as follows viz.

In performing the oral glucose tolerance test 100 grammes of glucose is administered and the blood samples are taken fasting and at one, two and three hours after the draught. The maximum permitted glucose values in mmol/l at these times are:

(venous whole blood — true glucose method)

Fasting (mmol/l)	1 hour	2 hour	3 hour
5	9.2	8	7

If *any two* of these values are equalled or exceeded the oral glucose tolerance test is abnormal.

GESTATIONAL DIABETES MELLITUS

In normal women the need for extra insulin during pregnancy is well within the reserve capacity of the beta cell. If, however, this reserve is diminished, carbohydrate tolerance becomes impaired. As the demand for insulin is greatest in late pregnancy impairment is most likely at that stage. The degree of impairment is variable and in most cases is detectable only by an oral glucose tolerance test, but in a few it is florid and substantial doses of insulin may be required. In at least 95 per cent of cases, carbohydrate tolerance returns to normal after delivery (Table 5.3) and this may occur even if a large dose of insulin was required during pregnancy.

Table 5.3   Gestational diabetes mellitus — return to normal after puerperium. Age 30, 2^{+0}, Glycosuria, Family history of diabetes mellitus.

BG (mmol/l)	Fasting	1 hour	2 hour	3 hour
At 36 weeks	9.6	11.5	10.0	9.6
After puerperium	4.1	7.8	6.7	5.6

Diagnosis of gestational diabetes

Recognition of gestational diabetes demands a high index of suspicion based on the following clues:

1. A family history of diabetes — especially in first degree relatives.
2. 'Significant' glycosuria.
3. A history of unexplained perinatal death especially fetal death, of a large-for-dates infant, or of a malformed infant.
4. Gross obesity.
5. Development of macrosomia or of unexplained hydramnios.

Glycosuria is common because at least 15 per cent of pregnant women have a temporary lowering of the renal threshold for glucose. The specificity of glycosuria can be increased by defining 'significant' glycosuria as that which occurs in a second fasting specimen. The patient is instructed to void on waking. A little later, whilst still fasting, a second specimen is voided and tested. In normal pregnant women the fasting blood glucose is so low that glycosuria at that time is very unlikely to be due to lowering of the threshold. Conversely glucose in such a specimen is more likely to be meaningful.

Although the presence of a single clue to gestational diabetes is less reliable, (Table 5.4) it should not be ignored (Drury & Timoney, 1970).

With careful history taking many patients will come under suspicion at an early stage in pregnancy when an abnormal glucose tolerance test is unlikely. The definitive glucose tolerance test is postponed but, to avoid a catastrophe, all suspect cases should have a fasting blood glucose measurements and postprandial blood glucose at fortnightly intervals. This practice eliminates wasteful use of the glucose tolerance test whilst ensuring that deterioration in tolerance is not missed by deferring that test. If the fasting blood glucose exceeds 5 mmol/l or the postprandial level exceed 6.5 at any time, the glucose tolerance test is done forthwith. It must be emphasised however that a normal oral glucose tolerance test before the 39th week does *not* necessarily exclude the diagnosis. In such cases the test should be repeated at 39 weeks when the definitive judgement is made. A normal glucose tolerance test at that stage excludes the diagnosis. When the glucose tolerance test becomes positive the patient is asked to attend for monitoring of blood glucose. In the great majority of patients with impaired tolerance minor adjustments of carbohydrate intake restore the blood glucose to normal. In those who are overweight, calorie intake lshould be limited to avoid undue weight gain. Over-enthusiastic attempts at weight control should be avoided as prolonged maternal ketonaemia may be harmful to the fetus. If dietary measures do not maintain the fasting blood glucose at about 5 mmol/l and the postprandial level at

Table 5.4   Investigations for gestational diabetes mellitus. 772 mothers studied.

Indication for Oral Glucose Tolerance Test	Number of women	Gestational Diabetes Mellitus
Glycosuria (G)	488	72 (15%)
G and suggestive obstetrical history (OH)	64	35 (55%)
G and family history of diabetes (FH)	78	26 (33%)
G + OH + FH	11	6 (54%)
OH	79	15 (18%)
FH	42	2 (5%)
OH and FH	9	6 (66%)
Angina Pectoris	1	1
	772	163 (21%)

If more than one clue is present, abnormal carbohydrate tolerance is much more likely to be found.

Table 5.5   Gestational diabetes mellitus requiring insulin when pregnant.

Maturity (weeks)	Post-prandial Blood Glucose mmol/l
17	5.8
20	13.2
	14.0
27 Insulin	8.1
33 increasing	5.8
38 to 60 units daily	5.9

The oral glucose tolerance test was normal after the puerperium

about 6.5 mmol/l the use of insulin should be considered. Occasional patients will need daily doses of 40 units or more and in spite of this may return to normal after delivery (Table 5.5).

Management of gestational diabetes

Perinatal mortality is not increased in recognised cases of gestational diabetes. If insulin has been required or if complications (e.g. hydramnios, macrosomia, pre-eclampsia) arise, management should be as defined for clinical diabetes (vide infra). In the great majority spontaneous labour is awaited.

If insulin has been used it should be phased out quickly after delivery. If the blood glucose then rises it is reintroduced but a further attempt at withdrawal may be made after the puerperium. If insulin is required after the puerperium the patient is not a gestational but a clinical diabetic in whom the diagnosis came to light during pregnancy.

Excepting those few cases who need insulin, all others should have an oral glucose tolerance test after the puerperium. The criteria for assessment of the test at this stage are those of the *non-pregnant* state. If this test is abnormal the patient is classified as a clinical diabetic; if negative the correct designation is gestational diabetes. It should be clear from the foregoing that the status of the patient in whom impaired carbohydrate tolerance develops during pregnancy can only be defined after the puerperium.

Clinical diabetics are referred to the diabetic clinic for continuing supervision. A significant number of gestational diabetics become clinical with the passage of time. The significance of pruritus vulvae and of thirst, polyuria and weight loss should be explained, so that diagnosis will not be delayed. If family planning is necessary, oral contraceptives should be avoided. The importance of weight control and the necessity to report early, if pregnant, should be stressed.

Infants of mothers with gestational diabetes
Perinatal mortality is not increased in established cases of gestational diabetes (Drury & Timoney 1970). There is a small but definite increase in the incidence of macrosomia. This tendency may be minimised by introducing insulin if blood glucose levels exceed the ideal range already defined. We do not consider that the routine use of insulin is justified.

In any unexplained fetal or neonatal death the possibility of unrecognised gestational diabetes should be considered and at autopsy special attention should be paid to the histology of the pancreas and gonad. In the absence of rhesus incompatibility, beta cell hyperplasia is compelling evidence of gestational diabetes as is the presence of increased interstitial tissue in the testis or of luteinisation of the theca interna of the ovary. Such findings override a normal oral glucose tolerance test because this test may rapidly return to normal after delivery. Occasionally the measurement of Haemoglobin A_1 (Hb A_1) may provide the necessary evidence. If gestational diabetes is suspected and corroborative evidence is unavailable, e.g. because of maceration in the fetus, the patient should be under close supervision in a subsequent pregnancy.

CLINICAL DIABETES MELLITUS

Before the introduction of insulin in 1922, pregnancy was rare and often lethal for mother and fetus. With the availability of insulin the pregnant woman with diabetes became more common and with increasing experience and knowledge the maternal risk has virtually disappeared. Perinatal loss is still significant although it is now very low in specialised centres. The outcome of pregnancy is determined by:

1. Patient compliance.
2. Strict control of the diabetes.
3. Commitment of the special team.

These factors are closely linked in that strict control of the diabetes is only possible if the patient cooperates fully with a physician who understands the nuances of insulin manipulation which are required. The physician and obstetrician members of the team should see all patients together at joint outpatient sessions and should be available for consultation on a 24-hour basis.

Classification of diabetes mellitus (Table 5.6)
Priscilla White (1971) introduced a classification system by which cases are graded according to the duration of diabetes, the age of the patient and the presence of diabetic complications. This classification should permit comparison between results from various centres. Regrettably many published series fail to distinguish between Class A clinical diabetes and gestational diabetes. This misleads by inflating the series

Table 5.6   Classification of White (1971).

A	Abnormal oral glucose tolerance test (after the puerperium)
B	Onset of diabetes over 20 *and* duration less than 10 years
C	Onset of diabetes between 10 and 19 *or* duration 10 to 19 years
D	Onset of diabetes before 10 or duration more than 20 years or with minimal vascular disease
F	Renal disease (proteinuria in excess of 100 mg/dl)
H	Ischaemic heart disease
R	Proliferative retinopathy
T	Renal transplant

size and by weighting favourably the fetal survival figures since gestational diabetes carries such a small fetal risk (Drury, 1980).

White's classification, although valuable, is based on the prepregnant state and does not include other significant risk factors, e.g. maternal age, parity, distance of domicile from hospital, social or personal inadequacy, presence of associated disease, and late referral. Neither does it take into account significant prognostic factors arising during pregnancy, e.g. macrosomia, hydramnios, hypertension with proteinuria, and fetal growth retardation. In our view therefore the White classification is only one aspect of the overall evaluation by which the timing and mode of delivery are decided.

General problems

The care of the pregnant diabetic is beset by problems which are common to all cases:

1. In the second half of pregnancy an increase in insulin requirement occurs in most cases so that frequent adjustments are necessary.
2. As strict control of the diabetes is vital, hypoglycaemic episodes are frequent.
3. As the renal threshold for glucose may be lowered, urine tests may be misleading.
4. Polyhydramnios (4 per cent) and preclampsia (12 per cent) are more common in diabetics.
5. As pre-term delivery will be required in a number of cases, neonatal morbidity is common.
6. Congenital malformations are increased threefold in infants of diabetic mothers.

An approach to management

In our view the management is primarily clinical and demands an obsessional commitment from the medical team. The number of personnel should be small to ensure continuity of care. A team with appropriate skill and experience can only be provided in special centres to which all cases in the region should be referred.

Prospective parents should be seen before conception if at all possible so that the partners may meet the physician, obstetrician and nurse, in the setting where the patient will attend. At this visit methods of family planning are discussed and the system of management during pregnancy is explained. This interview provides the opportunity for explanation and encouragement. The importance of strict control of the diabetes at the time of conception and throughout pregnancy is stressed.

Antenatal care

We advise patients to report at the special joint clinic as soon as pregnancy is suspected. Arrangements are made for blood glucose profiles at weekly intervals. The required samples should be taken a day or two before the visit to the clinic so that the results are available to the clinicians when the patient attends. The patient may attend at the hospital for blood tests but ideally the samples should be collected at home during the course of a normal working day, by arrangement with the district nurse or family practitioner. Many of our patients (or their spouses) have been taught to take blood — an ideal solution because samples can be collected at odd times, e.g. in the small hours if nocturnal hypoglycaemia is suspected. In the early stages a brief stay in hospital may be desirable especially if the patient is new to the service. This provides an opportunity to meet members of the team, to become familiar with the ward and to improve control of the diabetes. Apart from this initial admission which is by no means invariable we do not recommend hospitalisation unless problems arise. Routine admission in the last few weeks is an expensive and unnecessary luxury and ignores the consequences of separating a mother from her spouse and family.

Control of diabetes — assessment and attainment

The most important single determinant of success is strict control of the diabetes defined as a fasting blood glucose of about 5 mmol/l with postprandial values of about 7 mmol/l. The degree of control should be constantly monitored by a combination of methods viz. urinalysis, home monitoring of blood glucose, blood glucose profiles, glycolysated haemoglobin (Hb A_1 or Hb A_1C).

URINALYSIS

Urine testing is a poor guide because the absence of glycosuria merely means that the blood glucose is less than 10 mmol/l but may still be at an unacceptably high level. On the other hand patients may be misled by heavy glycosuria which is really due to lowering of the renal threshold.

HOME MONITORING OF BLOOD GLUCOSE

Blood glucose can be measured at home with special strips which may be read with the eye or on a home monitor. This is an ideal approach provided that the patient has been well instructed so that she performs the test properly and understands how to adjust the dose of insulin in the light of the result.

BLOOD GLUCOSE PROFILES

In all cases (even if home monitors are used) a blood glucose profile should be available at each clinic visit. The minimum requirement is a fasting and a postprandial blood glucose test but we recommend four tests, i.e. fasting: noon: afternoon: late night.

GLYCOLYSATED HAEMOGLOBIN (Hb A_1 OR A_1C)

The percentage of haemoglobin which is glycolysated correlates well with the mean of the blood glucose levels over the preceding four weeks. Thus Hb A_1 levels reflect overall control and correlate with blood glucose profiles. If however the Hb A_1 is abnormally high in the face of normal blood glucose profiles the patient should be admitted for multiple analyses of blood glucose using an indwelling venous cannula. Phases of poor control may be detected in this way.

Achieving control of diabetes

In all patients, a special diet is required to provide for the special needs of pregnancy and to restrict weight gain to a maximum of 12 kg. Because pregnancy is a ketogenic state, the allowance of carbohydrate should be generous — at least 200 g, forming about 50 per cent of the total calorie allowance. In the presence of heavy glycosuria due to a low renal threshold more carbohydrate may be needed to avoid maternal ketonaemia, in the interest of the fetus. The allowance of protein is about 1.3 g/kg body weight and the remainder is made up of fat. In the overweight, enthusiastic attempts at weight reduction should be avoided lest significant ketonaemia should develop. The aim should be the modest one of limiting weight gain to the ideal. Sodium should not be restricted and diuretics should not be used even if water retention and pre-eclampsia develop.

We do not recommend oral hypoglycaemics in any woman who might conceive. If a woman on oral agents conceives and is referred to us, we immediately change her to insulin.

Insulin

In a few patients the desired control may be achieved with insulin once a day. Most patients require twice daily injections of a mixture combining a quick acting insulin (e.g. Actrapid M.C. or Velosulin) and one of intermediate duration (e.g. Semitard or Insulatard). The modern 'non-immunogenic' preparations may be advantageous.

The extent to which insulin requirement changes as pregnancy advances varies from patient to patient and on the same patient may vary from pregnancy to pregnancy. It is not our experience that a falling insulin requirement in the last few weeks indicates failing placental function.

Restricting the blood glucose within the defined range may lead to hypoglycaemic episodes. These may be profound because the normal physiological response to hypoglycaemia is blunted during pregnancy. At least one member of the household (or a neighbour) should be familiar with the manifestations of hypoglycaemia and the administration of glucagon. Anxiety has been expressed that severe hypoglycaemia may be harmful to the fetus. We doubt this as one of the authors (M.I.D.) has seen 100 patients who were in hypoglycaemic coma at least once during pregnancy; in four of these the infant did not survive but in no case was the death related in time to the episode of coma. Maternal hypoglycaemia is not associated with congenital malformations.

By contrast maternal ketoacidosis is often lethal to the fetus and in our series 11 intrauterine deaths occurred *during* 14 such episodes. Diabetic ketoacidosis is so serious that prevention is vital. Patients should be instructed to report immediately if they begin to vomit as a delay of a few hours may be crucial.

Complications of diabetes mellitus

Hypoglycaemia and ketoacidosis have already been discussed. Vascular complications of diabetes may contribute to perinatal mortality and morbidity as malformations seem to be more common in White's Classes D and F (Tables 5.6 and 5.9). The most readily identifiable are retinopathy and nephropathy.

RETINOPATHY

Fundoscopy should be performed at first visit and repeated frequently. Background retinopathy is of little significance but observation is important as proliferative changes may appear, albeit rarely. New lesions commonly arise during pregnancy but usually regress after delivery. If proliferative changes exist or develop (Class R) meticulous observation is needed. Light coagulation may be required but this is exceptional. In general, pregnancy does not have a deleterious effect and indeed strict control of DM may be beneficial not only in the short term but in demonstrating to the patient that she is capable of maintaining high standards.

NEPHROPATHY

Even in Class F cases the success rate for pregnancy is high and there is no evidence that pregnancy has any permanent effect on the course of nephropathy (see Ch. 4, p. 78). Meticulous control of diabetes may have long-term benefits.

Complications of pregnancy

URINARY TRACT INFECTIONS

Asymptomatic bacteriuria and symptomatic infections are common and should be treated promptly and intensively because the associated vomiting may lead to ketoacidosis.

PRE-ECLAMPSIA

Pre-eclampsia, defined as the onset during pregnancy of hypertension (or its worsening) and proteinuria, is in our experience ten times more frequent in diabetic than in non-diabetic primigravidae. It is often acute in onset and rapidly progressive, demanding early delivery and thereby contributing to perinatal morbidity and mortality. In multigravidae pre-eclampsia is less common and less florid and expectant treatment may be possible. Nevertheless it is wise to deliver such cases at 38 weeks.

HYDRAMNIOS

Hydramnios is uncommon in well controlled patients, and when it arises a fetal anomaly should be suspected. Ultrasonography in late pregnancy should exclude anencephaly, spina bifida and hydrocephaly. Significant hydramnios in the absence of a fetal anomaly is an indication for admission to improve control of the diabetes.

MACROSOMIA (over 4000 g)

The obstetrician should record regularly his clinical assessment of fetal size and weight. Macrosomia is an indication for more intensive control of the diabetes, if necessary by admission. Regrettably, macrosomia occasionally occurs in spite of impeccable control; the beta cells of the fetus may be stimulated by substances other than glucose, e.g. aminoacids. Alternatively, factors other than fetal hyperinsulinism may cause macrosomia. A surprising result of our policy of late delivery has been a reduction in the incidence of macrosomia.

Assessment of fetal wellbeing

The mystery of late intrauterine death, for so long a feature of pregnancy in diabetics, has conditioned thinking and management for decades. The minds of many have been exercised in considering whether such deaths were due to hypoglycaemia, cardiac arrhythmia, or acid-base changes in the fetus. In turn great importance has been attached to procedures believed to be valuable in predicting fetal death.

OESTRIOL MEASUREMENTS

The value of oestriol measurements as an index of fetal wellbeing is doubtful. Diurnal variations are considerable but this deficiency can be minimised by using an oestriol/creatinine ratio. Whilst an increasing ratio is comforting, a falling ratio does not necessarily mean that fetal death is imminent. Distler et al (1978) have evaluated the realiability of unconjugated plasma oestriols.

This measurement has the advantage that it is not influenced by alterations in maternal renal function which is important as Class F cases are those in whom anxiety is most likely. We rarely estimate oestriol levels but if retardation of fetal growth is suspected serial measurements may provide reassuring evidence of wellbeing.

ANTEPARTUM CARDIOTOCOGRAPHY (CTG)

There is a substantial risk of false positive and a slight risk of false negative results in stress and non-stress CTG. We reserve this study for occasional cases e.g. when the mother reports a reduction in fetal movements. We suspect that undue dependence on CTG contributes to the unacceptably high rate of Caesarean section reported from many centres.

ULTRASONOGRAPHY

Ultrasound is helpful in assessing gestational age. If maturity is in doubt, measurement of the crown-rump length in the first trimester and of the biparietal diameter in the second trimester is carried out. Wladimiroff et al (1978) suggested that calculation of the head-chest ratio helps in the detection of macrosomia. In our view, clinical assessment is reliable, provided it is made weekly by the same experienced observer, who should record his estimation of fetal weight especially in the last weeks. Preoccupation with biochemical and biophysical assessment of the fetus should not take the emphasis away from control of the diabetes. Given optimum control, the use of fetal monitoring should be of the same order of frequency as in non-diabetic women.

Timing of delivery

The policy of pre-term delivery stemmed from the fear of intra-uterine death. Prior to 1973 this practice resulted in 17 neonatal deaths from hyaline membrane disease. The introduction of the lecithin-sphingomyelin (LS) ratio in 1973 made possible the prediction of fetal lung maturity and since then death from respiratory distress has become very rare (Drury et al, 1977). Gabbe et al (1977) confirm our view that an LS ratio of two or more virtually guarantees lung maturity. They reported hyaline membrane disease in 3 per cent of infants of diabetic mothers when the LS ratio was two or more, an incidence similar to that in infants of normal mothers. In contrast Cruz et al (1976) reported that nine of 150 infants of diabetic mothers developed hyaline membrane disease in spite of an LS ratio in excess of two. Our preference for vaginal delivery may be an important factor in this context, as respiratory distress syndrome is more likely following delivery by Caesarean section. Ambiguities of the LS ratio sparked off a search for more reliable indicators of lung maturity, e.g. specific phospholipid fractions such as phosphatidylglycerol (see Ch. 3, p. 64 and Ch. 6, p. 131).

Occasionally, complications force delivery in the face of an unfavourable LS ratio. In such cases a short sharp course of prednisolone orally may accelerate the production of surfactant. If steroids are used there will be a transitory increase in insulin requirement. We rarely use steroids and prefer to deliver quickly if the fetus is in jeopardy (see Ch. 6, p. 132).

We now deliver uncomplicated well controlled patients at term and reserve the LS ratio for patients whose maturity is uncertain and especially if delivery by Caesarean section is planned. Strict control of the diabetes has given us the confidence to go to full term and cease the routine use of the LS ratio. During the years 1975 to 1978 our patients were delivered at 38 weeks; in 1979 at 39 weeks and since 1980 at 40 weeks. Delivery at full term has the following advantages:

1. Spontaneous labour is frequent (20 per cent); induction is more often successful and the Caesarean section rate is lower.
2. Lung maturity is assured and neonatal morbidity is less.

Mode of delivery

Diabetes is not a reason for elective Caesarean section and should be reserved for obstetrical indications, e.g. hypertension with proteinuria, malpresentation; previous Caesarean section. We have always believed that vaginal delivery is best (Drury, 1961). Brudenell (1978) agrees that 'the ideal way to deliver the baby of a diabetic mother would be for her to go into labour spontaneously at term and be delivered normally by the vaginal route'. However he considers that this ideal cannot be attained because 'even with close control occasional late intrauterine deaths may occur and the baby may still be larger than average so that the risk of difficult delivery still exists although to a much lesser degree than formerly'. We share these anxieties but our results overall justify our policy of allowing well controlled uncomplicated cases to go to full term. Since January 1979, 57 women have been delivered at 39 weeks or later (28 at 40 weeks or later) without loss. During the same period in 11 Class F.R. patients (Table 5.6) one was delivered at 39 weeks and four at 40 weeks all without loss. With fastidious control of the diabetes late intra-uterine death is rare and the timing of delivery should be an individual decision in each pateint. Like all mothers the diabetic woman aspires to spontaneous labour and delivery with its inherent advantages, notably the virtual elimination of neonatal morbidity.

Induction of labour should not be performed unless there is a reasonable prospect of a vaginal delivery. Vaginal suppositories of Prostaglandin E_2 may be helpful in ripening the cervix. We reserve electronic fetal monitoring for patients in whom fetal distress is expected e.g. liquor is reduced or meconium is passed. We agree with Havercamp et al (1979) that the routine use of electronic fetal monitoring significantly increases the Caesarean section rate without any demonstrable reduction in perinatal mortality. O'Driscoll et al (1977) in a prospective study of 1000 consecutive primigravidae concluded that 'clear liquor early in labour virtually ensures the birth of a healthy infant, provided that the duration of labour is limited and delivery is effected without trauma, and conversely meconium — or no liquor — marks the fetus who may suffer death or brain damage during normal labour'. The widespread use of electronic monitoring is based on the concept that in the diabetic the fetal risk is high. With meticulous control of the diabetes this is not so and in the last 60 patients under our care electronic monitoring was used in only two patients.

Control of diabetes in labour
On the morning of the planned induction insulin and breakfast are taken as usual. The forewaters are ruptured at noon and the patient returns to the antenatal ward to await labour. Meals and insulin are given as usual until labour begins. Two thirds of the patients start in labour within 20 hours of rupture of the forewaters. When spontaneous labour is established one litre of five per cent dextrose in water containing 12 units of quick acting insulin is infused over 8 hours. The blood glucose is estimated hourly on a monitor, and the dose of insulin is adjusted to maintain blood glucose values between 5 and 7 mmol/l. Hyperglycaemia should be avoided lest it cause hypoglycaemia in the newborn (Table 5.7).

Table 5.7   Labour at 38 weeks — usual meals and insulin.

Morning dose 28 units Retard and 4 units Neutral
blood glucose hourly during labour (mmol/l)
4.8 — 3.8 — 6.6 — 4.1 — 7

Table 5.8   Caesarean section at term Age 30 years Class B

5% Dextrose water with 12 units Acrapid per litre
Blood glucose at 15 minute intervals (mmol/l)
2.6 — 3.3 — 5.2 — 7.3 — 3.5 — 2.4 — 7.6

In the remaining third an oxytocin infusion is set up at 8.00 a.m. on the day after surgical induction. Insulin and breakfast are replaced by an intravenous infusion as detailed above. We expect a short duration of labour and if delivery is not imminent within eight hours Caesarean section is performed (Table 5.8). Brudenell (1978) considers that a diabetic may be allowed to labour for 12 hours but in our view this is too long. Our induction practice carries a small risk of fetal infection but this risk is outweighed by the fact that two-thirds of our patients do not require oxytocin infusion and our Caesarean section rate is 25 per cent. After delivery if the patient does not feel well the insulin infusion may be continued until normal eating is resumed at which stage twice daily insulin is reintroduced.

INFANTS OF DIABETIC MOTHERS

With strict control of the diabetes the classical ruddy, chubby, hirsute and large baby is rarely seen. Maternal hyperglycaemia causes neonatal morbidity by stimulating hyperinsulinism in the fetus which in turn increases fat deposition and may delay the formation of pulmonary surfactant.

The neonatal death rate has fallen dramatically. From 1951 to 1981 there were 32 neonatal deaths in 765 viable infants (4.1 per cent) but in the last six years no neonatal deaths have occurred in 262 viable infants. Late delivery has virtually eliminated the problem of respiratory distress in the newborn and the commonest cause of perinatal death is now congenital malformation.

Malformations

Significant malformations occur in about 4 per cent of infants of diabetic mothers. As a similar excess does not occur in infants of diabetic fathers the intra-uterine milieu is likely to be the operative factor. Miller (1979) has shown a correlation between the occurrence of malformations and high Hb A_1 levels in early pregnancy. Strict control of diabetes prior to the time of conception is an ideal worth pursuing. The spectrum of malformations is wide but cardiac anomalies and neural tube defects are the most common. Long standing diabetics especially those with vascular disease are more likely to have malformed infants (Table 5.9).

Table 5.9 Malformations 1975–1980.

Maternal age	Parity	Class	Years of diabetes	Anomaly
28	1 + 1	B	3	Anencephaly
37	3 + 2	D	20	Holoprosencephaly
23	0 + 0	C	9	Iniencephaly
25	0 + 0	C	14	Cardiac
25	1 + 0	C	9	Cardiac
18	0 + 0	D	13	Cardiac
24	0 + 0	D	15	Cardiac

Perinatal morbidity

We define morbidity as the occurrence of any condition which necessitates the detention of the infant in the special care neonatal unit for longer than 36 hours. By this standard 48 (32 per cent) of 150 infants of diabetic mothers delivered consecutively at the National Maternity Hospital, Dublin, in the years 1975 to 1978 inclusive were morbid (Table 5.10).

Table 5.10 150 infants of diabetic mothers 1975–1978
National Maternity Hospital Dublin. Morbidity in 48 infants
(32%).

Jaundice (requiring phototherapy)	26
Respiratory Distress Syndrome	14
Malformations	12
Hypoglycaemia	4
Shoulder Dystocia	4
Septicaemia	2
Small for dates	2

In 16 of the infants more than one condition was present.

Planned delivery was postponed to 39 weeks gestation in 1979 and to 40 weeks in 1980. Of 62 infants delivered at the National Maternity Hospital since 1979, 12 (19 per cent) were morbid, but of 17 delivered after spontaneous labour none were morbid. We conclude that spontaneous labour after 38 weeks is ideal for the infant. One of the benefits of delaying induction is that 20 per cent have a spontaneous onset of labour.

Because of other complications, premature delivery is indicated or occurs spontaneously, and here the infant will usually experience problems, e.g. respiratory distress syndrome, hypoglycaemia, hypocalcaemia, hyperbilirubinaemia, hyperviscosity, macrosomia and trauma.

Respiratory distress syndrome

Delivery at full term almost eliminates respiratory distress syndrome. In the last 209 live-born infants delivered at the National Maternity, seven developed respiratory syndrome. Two of the seven were delivered at 34 weeks, three inhaled liquor or meconium, one had a spontaneous pneumomediastinum, and the remaining case followed delivery at 38 weeks despite a normal LS ratio.

Hypoglycaemia

If the maternal diabetes is not well controlled the fetus suffers hyperglycaemia which stimulates the beta cells of the fetal pancreas. The combination of substrate with excess insulin increases the deposition of glycogen and adipose tissue. After delivery the available substrate is much less but the excess of insulin continues and favours glycogen storage whilst inhibiting gluconeogenesis and lipolysis. The frequency of hypoglycaemia varies the definition used. We define hypoglycaemia as a blood glucose of less than 1.7 mmol/l. Symptoms include hypotonia, hypothermia, apnoea and convulsions. Pulsed doses of glucose should be avoided because they sustain the high output of insulin. Five per cent dextrose solution should be infused intravenously at a rate of 0.24 g/kg/hour.

Hypocalcaemia

Serum calcium levels of 1.65 mmol/l or less are found in 50 per cent of infants. This may be due to increased levels of calcitonin and of parathormone; hyperphosphataemia and hypomagnesaemia are often associated. Clinical manifestations include apnoea, neuromuscular irritability and convulsions.

Hyperbilirubinaemia

Jaundice occurs in 10 per cent of infants i.e., four times more frequently than in other hospital babies. Amongst those delivered electively, however late, the incidence is still high at 20 per cent. This does appear not to affect future development since prompt phototherapy prevents brain damage. However, the separation of mother and infant diminishes bonding and inhibits the institution of breast feeding which we encourage for all infants of diabetic mothers.

Hyperviscosity

At the National Maternity whole blood viscosity, measured at a low shear rate in umbilical cord blood was found to be significantly increased in 20 infants of diabetic mothers (Foley et al, 1981). Hyperviscosity correlated with macrosomia, suggesting a relationship with control of the diabetes. Packed cell volume and whole blood viscosity were closely correlated suggesting that the increased viscosity is secondary to polycythaemia. Increased viscosity could not be related to any particular symptoms in the neonate. Hyperviscosity might be a factor in unexplained intrauterine death. The work of Stuart et al (1980) in measuring fetal blood flow may be applicable in this context.

Macrosomia and birth trauma

Forceps delivery in our series is the same as that for the hospital as a whole — 5 per cent. Shoulder dystocia is a problem and may result in fracture of clavicles and even death. At the National Maternity Hospital between 1975 and 1978, 42 of 150 liveborn infants weighed more than 4000 grammes (28 per cent). In this group there were 13 cases of shoulder dystocia (8.5 per cent) and in four the clavicle was fractured. In the period 1979 to 1981, four of 62 liveborn infants weighed 4000 grames or more and there were two cases of shoulder dystocia (3.2 per cent). This change reflects the contribution of strict control of the diabetes to diminishing the incidence of macrosomia. Nevertheless it is of paramount importance that a senior obstetrician be present at all deliveries in case shoulder dystocia should occur.

SUMMARY

1. The physiological adaptation of normal pregnancy creates a demand for extra insulin. In a small number of women an inadequate islet reserve results in abnormal carbohydrate tolerance. If this gestational diabetes mellitus is not recognised perinatal death may result. In the great majority of patients carbohydrate tolerance returns to normal immediately after delivery.

2. Pregnancy in the clinical diabetic is not a hazard for the mother. Perinatal mortality in centres which specialise in this problem is now less than 5 per cent. Strict control of the diabetes is the key to a successful outcome. Well controlled uncomplicated cases should be delivered vaginally at term.

REFERENCES

Barnes-Fouracre H U 1950 Discussion on management of pregnancy in diabetics. Transactions of the 12th Congress of Obstetrics & Gynaecology 12: 169

Bennewitz H G 1826 Osann's 12ter Jahresberichte der koniglichen poliklinischen Institutes der Universitat zu Berlin. G Remier 12: 23

Bourchardat A 1851 Du diabéte sucré ou glycosurie, son traitement hygiénique. Bailliére, Paris, p 70

Brudenell J M 1978 Delivering the baby of the diabetic mother. Journal of The Royal Society of Medicine 71: 207–211

Cruz A C, Bubi W C, Birk S A, Spellacy W N 1976 Respiratory distress syndrome with mature lecithin/sphynogomyelin ratios: diabetes mellitus and low apgar scores. American Journal of Obstetrics and Gynecology 126: 78–82

Distler W, Gabbe S G, Freeman R K 1978 Oestriol in pregnancy unconjugated and total plasma oestriol levels in comparison to 24 oestriol and creatinine excretion in the management of diabetic pregnancies. American Journal of Obstetrics and Gynecology 130: 424–431

Drury M I 1961 Diabetes mellitus complicating pregnancy — first Grave's lecture. Journal of Medical Science 10: 425–453

Drury M I, Timoney F J 1970 Latent diabetes in pregnancy. Journal of Obstetrics and Gynecology of the British Commonwealth 77: 24–28

Drury M I, Greene A T, Stronge J M 1977 Pregnancy complicated by clinical diabetes mellitus — a study of 600 pregnancies. Obstetrics and Gynecology 49: 519–522

Drury M I 1980 Diabetes and pregnancy: a plea for uniform data reporting. Diabetes Care 3:6: 705

Duncan J M 1882 On puerperal diabetes. Transactions of the London Obstetrical Society 24: 256–285

Eshner A A 1907 The relations between diabetes mellitus and pregnancy: with report of a case of diabetes mellitus in which glycosuria disappeared with inception of pregnancy and relapsed after delivery. American Journal of Medical Sciences 134: 375–379

Foley M E, Collins R, Stronge J M, Drury M I, MacDonald D 1981 Blood viscosity in umbilical cord blood from infants of diabetic mothers. Journal of Obstetrics. (In Press)

Gabbe S G, Lowensohn R I, Westman J U, Freeman R K, Goebelsmann U 1975 Lecithin/sphyngomyelin ratio in pregnancy complicated by diabetes. American Journal of Obstetrics and Gynecology 128: 757–760

Havercamp A D, Orleans M, Langendoerfer S, McFee J, Murphy J, Thompson H 1979 Controlled trial of the differential effects of intrapartum fetal monitoring. American Journal of Obstetrics and Gynecology 134: 399–412

Von Jaksch R V 1885 Uber Acetonurie und Diaceturie. A Hirschwald, Berlin, p 84

Miller E H, Hare J W, Cloherty J P, Dunn P J, Soeldner J S, Kitzmiller J S 1979 Major congenital anomalies and elevated Hb A_1C in early weeks of diabetic pregnancy. Diabetes 28: 347

Mintz D, Skyler J S, Chez R A 1978 Diabetes mellitus and pregnancy. Diabetes Care 1: 49–63

O'Driscoll K, Coughlan M, Fenton V, Skelly M 1977 Active management of labour: care of the fetus. British Medical Journal 2: 1451–1453

O'Sullivan J B, Mahan C H 1964 Criteria for the OGTT in pregnancy. Diabetes 13: 278–285

Peel J H, Oakley W G 1950 Management of pregnancy in diabetics. Transactions of the 12th Congress of Obstetrics & Gynaecology 12: 161

Stuart B, Drumm J, Fitzgerald D E, Duignan N 1980 Fetal blood velocity wave forms in normal pregnancy. British Journal of Obstetrics and Gynaecology 78: 780–785

Taylor F W 1899 Diabetes mellitus and pregnancy. Boston Medical and Surgical Journal 160: 205–207

Van Noorden C H 1882 Die zuckerkrankheit. Berlin, p 88–94

White P 1971 Pregnancy and diabetes Joslin's diabetes mellitus. Lea and Febiger, Boston, p 588

Whitridge Williams J 1909 Clinical significance of glycosuria in pregnant women. American Journal of Medical Sciences 137:1: 1–26

Wladimiroff J W, Bloemsa C A, Wallenburg H C S 1978 Ultrasonic diagnosis of the large for dates infant. Obstetrics and Gynecology 52: 285–287

Perinatal medicine

6. The care of the low birthweight infant

A. Lucas   Cliff Roberton

A human being is more likely to die on the first day of his life than any other day — except the last one! Approximately 40 per cent of all children who die between the moment of birth and their 15th birthday do so during the first week of life (Table 6.1). In an attempt to reduce mortality major advances have been made in the intensive care of the critically ill low birthweight infant during the last decade and those of interest to the obstetrician will be reviewed in this chapter.

However not all neonatology is intensive care, and a major neonatal challenge is how, and with what to nourish the ill low birthweight baby. The pre-eminence of human milk as food for human babies is once more established. Even in the full-term neonate, breast feeding is a complex biological activity involving not only the transfer of a highly evolved food from mother to infant, but also protection of the neonate against infection, modification of neonatal gut flora and mother infant bonding. Several new concepts relating to normal infant feeding will be considered in this chapter together with the special problems of feeding low birth-weight infants.

Table 6.1 Causes of death in childhood in England and Wales in 1968 and 1978.

	1968	1978
Total live births	814519	597533
Total deaths < 15 yrs	20217	11312
Deaths 1–14 yrs	5247	3531
Deaths 1/12–12/12	4847	2819
Late neonatal deaths (7–28 days)		
Malformation	627	442
Pneumonia	234	70
Anoxia, RDS, immaturity	121	113
Others	561	320
TOTAL	1443	945
Early neonatal deaths		
Anoxia, hypoxia including RDS	2437	Anoxia etc. 450 RDS 793
Immaturity	1715	500
Malformation	1359	1035
Birth injury etc.	1153	421
Pneumonia	220	70
Haemolytic disease	238	33
Others	1650	931
TOTAL	8682	4233

Data for 1968 from HMSO (1970) for 1978 from HMSO (1980)

The last quinquennium has also seen an explosion of data on the serious long term deleterious effects of mother child separation in the early neonatal period (see Ch. 7). Allowing maximum mother–child contact even when the infant is of low birthweight is a major challenge for those responsible for establishing clinical and nursing practices in maternity hospitals, and the Cambridge routines designed to promote this contact will be described.

CARE OF INFANTS ON POSTNATAL WARDS

The importance of close contact between a mother and her newborn infant is clearly outlined in Chapter 7.

Fortunately, most maternity hospitals now have 'rooming-in' on the postnatal wards, and the normal infants are with their mothers for the majority of the day. Even in hospitals with 'rooming-in', however, large numbers of babies are routinely admitted to the neonatal unit. The national figures for neonatal unit admissions are shown in Table 6.2, and although a downward trend is evident in nearly all regions in

Table 6.2 Admissions to Special Care Units after birth as a percentage of all livebirths in each region of England and Wales.

Region	1974	1975	1976	1977	1978	1979
Northern	21.4	21.1	22.5*	21.8	21.5	19.3
Yorkshire	22.3	22.6	23.2*	23.1	21.5	19.0
Trent	15.7	17.1	17.7	19.0*	17.2	14.7
East Anglia	27.0*	23.5	21.9	20.2	18.4	17.2
NW Thames	18.9	20.5	22.2	23.0*	22.2	19.2
NE Thames	18.5	17.4	20.7*	19.6	16.8	15.0
SE Thames	16.3	18.6	19.7	21.9*	17.9	17.4
SW Thames	16.3	19.2	18.8	20.0*	17.3	15.8
Wessex	14.5	16.6	16.0	16.8*	16.0	12.7
Oxford	21.0*	18.7	17.2	16.7	13.5	12.8
South Western	13.5	13.6	14.4	15.4*	15.1	13.9
West Midlands	14.8	15.4	16.1	17.9*	16.6	17.0
Mersey	21.4	22.6	19.2	23.3*	20.6	17.0
North Western	16.3	17.0	19.4*	18.8	16.6	14.8

Source: Unpublished DHSS data for livebirths delivered in NHS hospitals and for Special Care Unit deaths and discharges each year.

* Year admission rate peaked in each region

the last two years, the admission of approximately 17 per cent of all infants is unnecessary. Furthermore in many hospitals, as many as 40 per cent of all live births are separated from their mothers. Since the prematurity rate (i.e. babies less than 2.50 kg) remains constant in the United Kingdom at around 6.5 per cent the vast majority of infants admitted to neonatal units must be mature, and are usually admitted because of an abnormal delivery or brief delay in starting to breathe — although by five to ten minutes of age they were pink and lusty with no respiratory compromise. There are various spurious reasons given for high admission rates to neonatal units:

1. To reduce the neonatal mortality: neonatal mortality is primarily due to mal-formation, *severe* birth asphyxia or problems of very low birthweight (VLBW)

infants; it will not therefore, be reduced by admitting healthy, unasphyxiated infants weighing more than 1.80 to 2.00 kg to the neonatal unit.

2. The Sheldon report recommended that all infants weighing less than 2.50 kg, plus breech, forceps and Caesarean section deliveries should be admitted. In the face of a rising forceps and Caesarean section rate this is particularly absurd, since the object of surgical or instrumental intervention is to keep the baby in good condition, and to prevent asphyxia and morbidity. If such infants are asymptomatic immediately after delivery they do not require admission.

3. Because neonatal units are safer than postnatal wards, and no one is on duty in the postnatal ward who can be trusted with the babies. This is totally incorrect microbiologically, and nonsense from a nursing point of view. Those who make this statement must be unaware of the scant attention which is given, particularly at night, to large healthy infants in neonatal units, by nurses who are rushed off their feet caring for critically ill infants on ventilators. On the postnatal ward the same large infant receives uninterrupted special care from one devoted nurse — his mother.

4. To keep bed occupancy high on the neonatal unit to justify the nursing establishment and placate administrators — hardly credible but true!

We have found that most infants over 2.5 kg can be managed on a postnatal ward with their mothers with the greatest of ease, total safety, and without any special medical or nursing provision being made (Table 6.3) (Whitby et al, 1982).

Table 6.3   Inborn admission to Cambridge SCBU 1979–1980.

Birthweight	Number delivered	Number admitted	per cent
< 1.50 kg	120	120	100%
1.5–2.0	171	136	80%
2.0–2.5	380	85	22%
2.5	7695	163	2.1%
Total	8366	504	6%

However, many maternity hospitals find problems caring for healthy asymptomatic infants 1.80 to 2.50 kg on a postnatal ward. In Cambridge we have arranged for all infants of this birthweight who are healthy to be concentrated on one postnatal ward which also takes routine postnatal cases. Rooming-in is the rule for all infants. No extra nursing staff are allocated to the ward, though at night we ensure that a trained nurse is always in charge. The only routines expected of the nursing staff are the ability to do Dextrostix six- to eight-hourly, give tube feeds, and supervise photo-therapy. This ward enabled us to nurse most 1.80 to 2.50 kg infants with their mothers throughout the puerperium. Furthermore, many of the infants of this weight who require admission to the neonatal unit for some neonatal illness can be transferred to the postnatal ward to be with their mothers prior to discharge. Of 256 surviving infants of this birth weight born in the Cambridge Maternity Hospital during a thirteen month period 233 (90 per cent) went home with their mothers (Table 6.4). The details of the care these infants received on the postnatal ward over a thirteen month period is given in Table 6.5.

Contrary to popular belief, this type of ward is extremely easy to establish and run,

Table 6.4   Outcome of infants 1.8–2.50 kg Born in Cambridge March 1979–March 1980 inclusive.

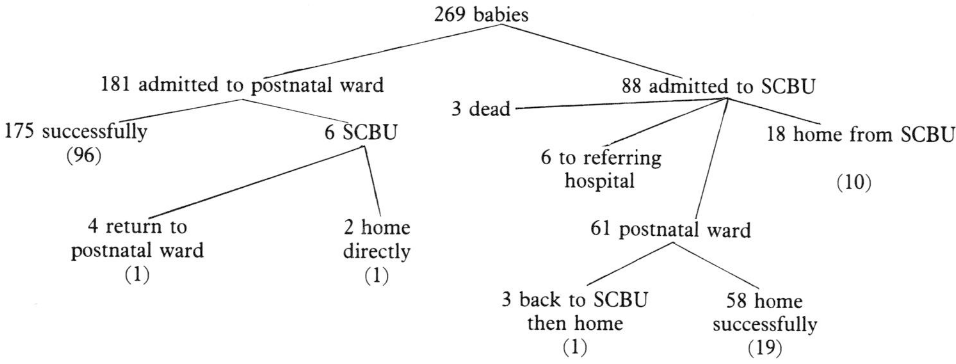

Of 256 'Cambridge Babies' who survived 233 (90%) went home with their mother and of these 128 (55%) were making some attempt to breast feed.

The figures in brackets refer to the number of babies breast feeding on discharge.

and although some extra support is required from the neonatal medical staff, it is undoubtedly popular with the mothers and nursing staff, who, after being initially wary about the additional responsibility are now enthusiastic supporters of such a system.

As a result of these arrangements, only 6 per cent of infants born in the Cambridge Maternity Hospital need admission to the special care baby unit (Table 6.3), a considerable difference from the data in Table 6.2.

EFFECTIVENESS OF NEONATAL INTENSIVE CARE

On neonatal mortality

Some of the fall in neonatal mortality in the United Kingdom which has occurred during the past decade (Table 6.1, 6.6) reflects improvements in socio-economic conditions and the fall in the birth rate, and although there are dissenting voices (e.g. Jones et al, 1976) most workers recognise the important role that neonatal intensive care has played in this reduction, particularly in infants weighing less than 2.0 kg (Stewart et al, 1978; Borkowff et al, 1979).

Normally formed infants weighing more than 2.0 kg at birth should rarely if ever die. Birth trauma has, or should have disappeared (Chamberlain et al, 1975); intrapartum asphyxia is now recognisable in the early stages thereby reducing the number of infants delivered in terminal apnoea. Inhalation pneumonia, and surfactant deficient respiratory distress syndrome (RDS) in infants over 2.0 kg should be rarely, if ever fatal; severe early onset sepsis due to the group B streptococci (GBS) and other organisms is recognisable and treatable (p. 140), and rhesus haemolytic disease is now rare (Table 6.1).

For normally formed infants weighing 1.5 to 2.0 kg, neonatal death should also be rare. In Cambridge we have a 3.5 per cent mortality at this birth weight, and most of those have lethal malformations. Similar figures are reported elsewhere for the UK (Mutch et al, 1981), and the USA (Wung et al, 1979). Sadly, the mortality in other

Table 6.5   Data of infants 1.80–2.50 kg born in Cambridge Maternity Hospital March 1979–March 1980.

	Never admitted to special care baby unit	Admitted at birth to SCBU then transferred to the post-natal ward	Always on SCBU
Number	175	58	27
Mean birthweight	2.27 kg	2.12 kg	1.97 kg
Mean gestation	36.5	35	32.4
Diagnosis on SCBU			
RDS		14	10
Transient tachypnoea		12	8
Normal prem.		17	4
Mild Birth Asphyxia		5	—
Normal small for dates		4	—
Malformation		1	3 (2)★
Others		5	2 (1)★
Transfer to P.N.W.			
Weight		2.05 kg	
Age		3.4 days	
Problems on P.N.W.			
Tube feeding	33	33	
Jaundice	39	12	
Phototherapy	16	9	
Dextrostix	167	7	
Low values	5	—	
Conjunctivitis	16	—	
Skin infections	2		
Transient tachypnoea	2		
Malformations	6	1	
Antiobiotic (i.m. oral or topical)	6	3	
Duration of stay on P.N.W.	8.7 days	9 days	
Discharge			
Mean age	8.3 days	13.7 days	22.7 days
Mean weight	2.28 kg	2.18 kg	2.16 kg
Feeding			
Breast	96	19	10
Bottle	75	35	8

Readmissions		
3. Bronchiolitis	4. Bronchiolitis	1 Bronchiolitis
2. Bronchitis		1 URTI (2 admissions)
2. Hernias	1. Failure to thrive (× 4)	1 Apnoea with feed
2. Pyloric stenosis	2. Hernias	
	1. Squint	
2. Fracture femur (1 ? NAD)	1. Pyloric stenosis, bronchiolitis (2 admissions)	
1. D & V	1. Disseminated BCG-osis	
1. Adenovirus pneumonia (died)	3. D & V	
1. Myocarditis (died)	1. Balanitis, skull fracture (2 admissions)	
1. Congenital Rubella with Patent Ductus	1. Dislocated hip	
	1. SIDS	

★ Figures in parenthesis = deaths

Table 6.6   Neonatal mortality/1000 live births by birthweight in England and Wales.

Birthweight (g)	1968	1973	1978
< 1000	812 (1795)	808 (1228)	754 (1031)
1001–1500	451 (1701)	408 (1220)	291 (886)
1501–2000	140 (1356)	128 (985)	86 (618)
2001–2500	33 (1280)	31 (961)	20 (542)
> 2500	5.2 (3999)	4.9 (3134)	3.7 (2044)
TOTAL	12.4 (10125)	11.9 (7528)	8.7 (5186)

Figures in brackets — absolute numbers of deaths Pharaoh P.O.D. (Pers. Comm).

Table 6.7   Mortality rates by birthweight in different centres including malformations.

Location	Reference	% mortality 500–1000g birthweight	% mortality 1000–1500g birthweight
University College Hospital	Stewart and Reynolds, 1979	52%	17%
University of Florida 1977–1978	Nelson et al, 1979	61%*	17%
Hammersmith Hospital 1976–mid 1979	Jones et al, 1979a	74%	24%
Kings College Hospital 1976–mid 1979	Gamus et al, 1979	68%	15%
Vermont 1976–1978	Philip, 1979	57%	16%
Cambridge 1977–1980	(unpublished)	51%	17%
Boston 1975–1978	Brown and Taeusch, 1979	56%†	17%
Cleveland 1976	Fanaroff and Merkatz, 1977	45%	16%
Toronto 1976–1978	Milligan and Shennan, 1980	—	11%
Milwaukee 1973–1975§	Borkowff et al, 1979	83%	3.2%
Melbourne 1977–1978	Yu and Hollingsworth, 1979	40%	

* All infants < 1.00 kg
† Infants 700–999g
§ Excluding malformations.

studies, including the national data is two to three times higher (Congdon & Lealman, 1980; Steiner et al, 1980) (Table 6.6).

At lower birthweights, the reported results are surprisingly consistent with a mortality around 15 to 17 per cent for infants between 1.0 and 1.50 kg, and about 50 per cent in infants less than 1.0 kg (Table 6.7); again, the United Kingdom national figures as shown in Table 6.6 are disappointing.

As more results appropriately broken down are published, it is becoming apparent that above a birthweight of 1.25 kg neonatal mortality should be rare. Since 1.25 kg represents a gestation of approximately 29 weeks, the implication is clear; provided a normally formed infant is delivered beyond 29 completed weeks of gestation neonatal death should be a rarity, and should one occur the events surrounding the death should be subjected to detailed scrutiny.

On handicap rate in low birthweight survivors

The outcome for LBW survivors has steadily improved from that reported in the 1950s and early 1960s (Drillien, 1965, 1967; Davies & Tizard, 1975) though current evidence suggests that the handicap rate has levelled out (Stewart et al, 1978; Jones et al, 1979; Stanley & Hobbs, 1980; Dale & Stanley, 1980; Stewart et al, 1981).

Results from units offering vastly differing standards of neonatal intensive care (Hommers & Kendall, 1976; Stewart et al, 1978; Kumar et al, 1980; Jones et al, 1979; Steiner et al, 1980) report strikingly similar handicap rates. About 5 to 8 per cent survivors weighing 1.0 to 1.5 kg at birth have a severe handicap, with a similar percentage suffering a mild handicap. This incidence is approximately doubled in survivors who weighed less than 1.0 kg.

This suggests that the major impact of neonatal intensive care over the last two decades has been to save lives rather than reduce even further the number of handicapped VLBW surviving infants.

On handicap rate in full-term infants

It is crucial to realise that the majority of perinatally acquired handicap occurs in term infants, usually as a result of perinatal asphyxia, trauma or infection (Hagberg et al, 1975; Brimblecombe et al, 1978). Recent evidence suggests that with improvements in perinatal facilities, the absolute amount of handicap generated in term infants is however falling, compared with the static handicap rate of VLBW infants (Dale & Stanley, 1980).

INFANT FEEDING

Recent concepts

Mammalian milks vary greatly in their composition, and milk composition is related to each species' needs, yet only in recent years have some of the specific adaptations of human milk to human infants' nutritional needs become appreciated. Furthermore, milk contains non-nutritional factors such as hormones and prostaglandins (vide infra) which may modulate neonatal physiology. In addition, feeding may induce adaptive changes in the neonate's gastrointestinal tract, and his metabolism which equip him for extrauterine nutrition, and may exert long term effects on the metabolic handling of nutrient substrates in later life (Kramer, 1980).

AMINO ACIDS

Cystine is a non-essential amino-acid for adults since it is synthesised from methionine along the sulphur amino-acid pathway which involves the hepatic enzyme cystathionase. However since cystathionase activity only develops postnatally in man (Sturman et al, 1970; Gaull et al, 1978) cysteine is an essential amino-acid for the human neonate. Human milk contains abundant cystine and indeed has the lowest methionine to cystine ratio amongst all sources of animal protein. In contrast, cows' milk contains a substantially greater methionine to cystine ratio and is therefore theoretically inappropriate for human infants (György, 1971).

Taurine, another sulphur amino-acid is present in breast milk, and is particularly abundant in the milk of the cat: kittens are exquisitely sensitive to dietary taurine deficiency which causes retinal degeneration and blindness (Hayes et al, 1975). Taurine may also be important to the developing central nervous system (Sturman & Gaull, 1975). There is a high concentration of taurine in the free amino-acid pool in human milk (Rassin et al, 1977) whereas in cows' milk it is substantially lower. Gaull et al (1977) showed a progressive fall in plasma and urine taurine concentration in preterm infants fed on synthetic cows milk based formulae. At present, however, no syndrome due to taurine deficiency has been identified in either term or preterm infants.

CHANGES IN BREAST MILK COMPOSITION

There has been recent speculation that the longitudinal changes known to occur in human milk content might be adapted to the infant's changing requirements. Thus the higher milk sodium content in early lactation (Pittard & Clark, 1977; Lucas et al, 1978) might compensate for the reduced ability of the human infants kidney to conserve salt in early postnatal life. Furthermore the significant postnatal fall in milk protein (Lonnerdal et al, 1976) could relate to the neonate's decreasing protein need for growth. Another intriguing yet unproven possibility, is that longitudinal changes in milk fatty acids might be correlated with the neonates changing needs for substrates for central nervous system development (Hall & Oxberry, 1977; Crawford et al, 1976): thus the long chain polyunsaturated fatty acids (LCP) content of milk falls as grey matter development decelerates (LCP is particularly incorporated into brain cells) and the milk saturated fatty acid content rises as the infants glial cells begin to produce myelin which incorporates large quantities of such fatty acids.

ANTIBACTERIAL ASPECTS OF BREAST MILK

Human milk contains a wide variety of factors and mechanisms with antibacterial powers in the neonatal gut. These factors together with their speculated mode of action are listed in Table 6.8. The importance of most of these factors has yet to be

Table 6.8   Factors in human milk and their roles in the neonatal gut.

Protective factor	Speculated role
Macrophages	Phagocytosis, co-operation with lymphocytes
Lymphocytes	
B cells	Production of immunoglobulins especially IgA
T cells	? lymphokines e.g. transmission tuberculin sensitivity
	IgA (and lesser amounts IgG and IgM): dimeric IgA attached to secretory piece resists digestion in the gut.
Trypsin inhibitor	Present in early lactation: further reduces digestion of immunoglobulins in early postnatal life.
Complement	Activated C3: Opsonic, chemotactic, anaphylotoxic
Lysozyme	cleaves peptidoglycans in bacterial cell walls
Lactoferrin B 12 binding protein Folate binding protein	inhibit bacterial growth by chelating respectively iron, B12 and folate thus depriving gut bacteria of these growth factors
Antistaphylococcal factor	A fatty acid, thermostable and antistaphylococcal
Lactoperoxidase system:	A peroxidase which together with hydrogen peroxide and thiocyanate forms an enzyme and substrate system for killing catalase negative bacteria
Interferon and perhaps other antiviral factors	antiviral
Bifidus factor	encourages the growth of harmless lactobacilli in the guts of breast fed infants reducing the potentially pathogenic E. coli population

(reviewed by Reiter 1978)

established in vivo, but collectively they must account for the anti-infective effect of breast feeding which is supported by considerable epidemiological evidence (Gerrard, 1974; Cunningham, 1977).

HORMONES AND PROSTAGLANDINS IN BREAST MILK

In recent years steroids, thyroxine, gonadotrophins, LHRH, TRH, erythropoietin, melatonin, prolactin (Sack, 1980) epidermal growth factor (Starkey & Orth, 1977), TSH and ACTH (Kodovsky et al. 1980) and prostaglandins (Lucas & Mitchell, 1980) have been found in breast milk. The concentration of some of these factors may be much greater in milk than in the maternal circulation; the concentration of prostaglandins E and F is 100 times higher in human milk than in maternal plasma. The possibility that these hormones may stimulate adaptations to extrauterine life is an exciting area for further study.

PHYSIOLOGICAL RESPONSE TO FEEDING

Feeding has multiple physiological effects on newborn infants including dynamic changes in intermediary metabolism and hormone release, changes in respiratory pattern (Wilkinson, 1979) and changes in regional cerebral blood flow (Yao et al, 1971; Dear, 1980), and sleep state (Murlin et al, 1925). These normal effects may be of even greater importance — or possibly even deleterious, when feeding preterm infants. In the immediate postnatal period, feeding may stimulate some of the adaptive physiological changes which permit the infant to switch from intravenous nutrition via the placenta to intermittent feeding and fasting, and metabolic independence (vide infra).

FEEDING PRETERM INFANTS

Sick preterm infants, particularly those with respiratory distress cannot tolerate enteral feeding during the first two to four days of life (see p. 135). The short term vulnerability of the unfed preterm infant has been recognised for many years. At 1.0 kg the infant's estimated survival time in the totally starved state (based on energy reserves) is about 4.5 days, and at 2 kg 12 days (Heird & Anderson, 1977). If, therefore, very low birthweight infants with RDS cannot tolerate enteral feeds within two to four days of birth they need intravenous nutrition.

ADAPTATION TO EXTRAUTERINE FEEDING

Following preterm birth an infant is deprived of the mode of nutrition for which he is adapted — namely parenteral nutrition via the placenta. In addition, the loss of maternal regulation of fetal metabolism, and control of circulating substrates occurs at a time when the gut and liver, together with their enzyme systems, are functionally immature (Smith, 1976). Nevertheless, even the most premature of infants may seem to be able to adapt to enteral feeding as much as fourteen weeks 'too soon' in biological terms. This ability suggests that there is a triggering mechanism which stimulates the necessary postnatal changes in the gut and in intermediary metabolism. That feeding itself might be the trigger, is suggested by the fact that feeding piglets within the first 24 hours of life stimulates structural and enzymic changes in the digestive tract not seen in unfed animals (Widdowson et al, 1976; Stoddard & Widdowson, 1976) and by the animal studies of Asplund (1972) and Gentz et al (1971) who demonstrated that feeding after birth stimulated key adaptive changes in intermediary metabolism.

A possible mechanism for these feeding induced events after birth is now emerging. Following the onset of enteral feeding in both term and preterm infants there are dramatic increases in the levels of many gastro-intestinal tract hormones including gastrin, enteroglucagon, gastric inhibitory polypeptide (GIP), pancreatic polypeptide (PP), motilin and neurotensin; in some cases, the hormone elevation far exceeds that found in healthy adults undergoing maximal gut hormonal stimulation (Lucas et al, 1980 a–c, 1981). Extrapolating from knowledge of the function of these hormones in animals and adults it is likely that they stimulate many of the adaptive events which equip the newborn infant for extrauterine nutrition. These studies also raise the possibility that it may be possible to devise feeding regimes for preterm infants which will stimulate optimally these postnatal adaptations.

THE DIETARY NEEDS OF PRETERM INFANTS

The optimal dietary requirements for preterm infants are unknown and must be based on reasonable assumptions. One such 'reasonable assumption' has been put forward by the American Academy of Paediatrics who contend that 'the optimal diet for the low birthweight infant may be defined as one that supports a rate of growth approximating to that of the third trimester of intrauterine life without imposing stress on the developing metabolic or excretory systems'. One short-coming of this prescription is that although *intrauterine* growth retardation carries recognised risks for the future development of the child, no such convincing data exists for the infant who exhibits growth retardation postnatally. In other words, the optimal postnatal growth rate for low birthweight infants has yet to be defined. Paediatricians are concerned nevertheless, by the fact that the preterm infant's poor postnatal growth is occurring at a time when his brain is undergoing a critical growth phase (Dobbing, 1974), and is perhaps especially vulnerable to the effects of suboptimal nutrition. Although this concept is supported by epidemiological evidence, for example from postnatally starved full term infants in third world (Evans et al, 1980) the quantitative relationship between postnatal growth and neurological vulnerability in low birth-weight infants is unknown. Furthermore, there are dangers in imposing a nutritional overload on the immature metabolic and excretory system; for example the neurologi-cally damaging effects of certain hyperaminoacidaemias (Menkes et al, 1972; Gold-man et al, 1974) induced by dietary protein overloading in the neonatal period.

If, despite the foregoing discussion, the American Academy of Paediatrics assump-tion about desirable growth rates is accepted, then it becomes possible to perform a theoretical calculation of the dietary needs of the low birthweight infant. Such a computation may be based on a combination of two types of information:

1. A knowledge of the average body composition of the fetus at each gestational age or weight group (which may be obtained by analysis from abortuses or stillborn infants).
2. Metabolic balance studies to determine absorption and retention of each dietary component.

Based on such considerations there is an increasing awareness that human milk designed evolutionarily for full-term infants may not meet the special requirements of the low birthweight neonate.

Protein. Protein intake is a critical variable in determining growth rate. Milk protein in different mammals relates clearly to growth: for example mature human milk contains 0.9 g per cent of protein, and the infant doubles in birthweight in 180 days, whereas corresponding figures for the sheep are 5.5 g per cent and 10 days (Visser, 1979). Human milk given at 150 ml/kg/day provides only around 1.5 g per kg per day of protein, yet Senterre (1979) has estimated on the basis of balance studies on infants weighing 1.48 to 2.18 kg that as much as 3.5 to 4 g protein/kg/day may be optimal, and within the renal capacity for acid and solute excretion.

Protein quality may also be of considerable importance in view of the low birthweight infant's limited capacity to convert methionine to cystine and cystine to taurine and catabolise tyrosine which is abundant in casein rich milks such as cows milk (Gaull et al, 1977; Rassin et al, 1977). Such considerations are pertinent to the detailed design of special preterm infant formulae. The risks of iatrogenic brain damage from hyperaminoacidaemias (Menkes et al, 1972; Goldman et al, 1974) must be weighed against the possible advantages of 'optimal' growth.

Fat. This is the principle source of calories in human milk. The preterm infant may, however, malabsorb this dietary component, and several groups have recommended feeding medium chain triglycerides which are better absorbed (Roy et al, 1975), may spare dietary nitrogen (Tautibhedhyangkul & Hashim, 1975) and may enhance dietary calcium and magnesium absorption (Tautibhedhyangkul & Hashim, 1978). Nevertheless, the metabolic handling by low birthweight infants of unphysiological amounts of dietary medium chain triglycerides needs further investigation.

Fat quality also deserves consideration. It has been speculated that fatty acid substrates needed by low birthweight infants may differ according to the stage of neurological development (Hall & Oxberry, 1977). The composition of myelin, a tissue with a remarkably low turnover rate, may be influenced greatly by the spectrum of fats in the diet (Sinclair & Crawford, 1972), and possible neurological and developmental consequences of this have received little attention.

Carbohydrate. The digestive capacities of the preterm infant's gut may need to be taken into account in planning carbohydrate intakes. Pancreatic amylase secretion is so poor, even in term infants during the first two months of life, that starches cannot be regarded as a useful source of carbohydrate (Husband et al, 1970). Most disaccharides however are well digested. Maltase and sucrase develop early (sixth to eighth month of gestation), but lactase normally develops at term. Nevertheless lactase activity increases rapidly in preterm infants after birth (Boellner et al, 1965) and in our experience, by the time they are taking full feeds, even the very high lactose content of breast milk (7 g per 100 ml) is tolerated. If the maximum lactose intake is exceeded (Aurichio et al, 1965) then diarrhoea and metabolic acidosis ensues, but there are theoretical advantages in keeping lactose intake as high as possible as fermentation of undigested lactose in the large bowel favours a low pH and the growth of lactobacilli which inhibits that of potentially pathogenic E. coli (Bullen & Nillis, 1971). If another source of carbohydrate is substituted for lactose, a short chain saccharide is probably preferable to a monosaccharide such as glucose, since the later will increase the feed osmolality and consequent osmotic water shifts across the gut could play a role in the genesis of necrotising enterocolitis (NEC). Maltodextrins have been used successfully for some years in infant formulae, but there is now interest in another medium chain glucose polymer, Polycose which has been studied in adults, and an initial trial in low birthweight neonates has been encouraging (Brans, 1980).

Minerals. Balance studies indicate that human milk and standard cows' milk formulae supply considerably less calcium than is required for optimal skeletal mineralisation (Shaw, 1976). In utero, the net amount of calcium transferred daily to the fetus is around 130 to 155 mg/kg of fetus per day whereas premature infants receive only 100 mg/kg enterally, and with a 30 per cent absorption from artificial formulae, such infants may only receive 20 per cent of their requirement (Tsang, 1980). Phosphate supply is probably equally limiting for skeletal mineralisation. After birth, blood calcium falls and there is a subsequent rise in parathormone and 1.25 dihydroxyvitamin D (Tsang, 1980) presumably in an attempt to increase calcium and phosphate absorption from the gut. Recent studies suggest that administering additional oral calcium and phosphate may prevent postnatal bone mineralisation defects (Tsang, 1980). Nevertheless frank symptomatic rickets, as opposed to radiological or biological changes of rickets in preterm infants fed on breast milk is uncommon. Possibly the future use of growth promoting diets for preterm infants may enhance calcium and phosphate needs to the point where frank symptomatic rickets develops.

The work of Dauncy et al (1977) suggests that other minerals such as copper and zinc may need to be supplemented in the diet of preterm infants. The requirement for other trace elements such as selenium is more controversial.

Low birthweight infants are especially susceptible to iron deficiency because of their smaller iron stores at birth and the rapid increase in red cell mass as erythropoietin rises after about six weeks of age. Lundstrom et al (1978) have demonstrated that low birthweight infants receiving no supplemental iron may develop iron deficiency by three months of age. However the right time to start supplementary iron is disputed. Free iron in the gut may encourage bacterial overgrowth (hence protective role of lactoferrin). Our policy is to start iron supplementation at six weeks of postnatal age.

Vitamins. Little is known about vitamin requirements of preterm infants. It is likely that the fast growing infant will need supplementary vitamin C and folate.

Recent work by Lakdawala and Widdowson has shown that 0.8 μg of water soluble vitamin D sulphate is present per 100 ml of human milk. This approximates to the daily requirement of vitamin D and may explain why healthy, full-term, breast-fed infants do not develop rickets. The amount of vitamin D required by the rapidly growing preterm infant with steatorrhoea and defective calcium and phosphate absorption (see above) is uncertain, but to prevent the appearance of biochemical and radiological changes of rickets we supplement infants less than 1.50 kg with 1500 units of vitamin D daily.

A large literature exists on the possible beneficial effects of the antoxidant vitamin E in the prevention of anaemia (Chadd & Fraser, 1970) but the value of this vitamin in protecting against the toxic effects of oxygen such as retrolental fibroplasia and bronchopulmonary dysplasia (Ehrenkranz et al, 1979; Johnson et al, 1974) is being evaluated. Recently Hittner et al (1981) have produced convincing evidence that high doses of vitamin E have a protective effect against retrolental fibroplasia. These workers used doses of vitamin E that were around 140 times the amount that would be received by infants fed on mature expressed breast milk: clearly further work is needed to examine the possible toxic effects of such a practice.

Caloric intake. For practical purposes most low birthweight infants achieve satisfactory weight gain with diets supplying 110 to 150 kcals/kg/day. (Human milk contains 65 to 70 kcals per 100 ml.) Some groups have recommended high caloric feeding, but Drew et al (1979) could find no difference in growth rate in infants 1.50 kg or less on 80 kcal/100 ml compared with 65 kcal/per 100 ml feedings.

METHOD OF FEEDING

Infants below 34 weeks' gestation are usually unable to suck efficiently, and even if they appear to do so, the risk of aspiration makes oral feeding unacceptable. If enteral rather than i.v. feeding is chosen it may be given via an orogastric or nasogastric tube or by the transpyloric route (nasoduodenal or nasojejunal). Feeds may be given hourly or two-hourly as a bolus or as a continuous infusion.

The extent to which these 'unphysiological' modes of feeding affect postnatal adaptation, gut hormone release, gut function and metabolism is an interesting area for study. Intravenous feeding precludes the potentially important effects on gut hormone release of food in the gut lumen (Lucas et al, 1980 a–c; Lucas, 1981) and eliminating sucking may remove the 'cephalic' or 'anticipatory' phase of digestion; transpyloric feeding also bypasses the gastric phase. Bolus feeds are arguably more physiological than continuous feeds and possibly phasic stimulation of the gut might result in greater peak levels of released hormones. Indeed unpublished studies (Aynsley-Green & Sibley) suggest that infants regain their birth weight faster on bolus intragastic feeding compared with continuous feeding by this route. The risks of aspiration and apnoea on bolus feeds must however, be considered.

Transpyloric versus intragastric feeding

Transpyloric feeding (given by continuous infusion) has received considerable attention in recent years. Earlier literature reports a wide variety of possible harmful side-effects such as intestinal perforation, NEC (which may have been related to the leaching of PVC plasticisers from the tubing), intussusception, renal perforation, decreased fat absorption, diarrhoea and alteration of intestinal flora (Schreiner, 1980). Others have emphasised the safety of this procedure (Rhea et al, 1975). Three controlled studies have been performed comparing continuous transpyloric with bolus nasogastric feeds (Wells & Zachman, 1975; Pereira & Lemos, 1976; Uauy et al, 1975). Two of these are only in abstract form. One study showed no difference between the groups and the other two showed increased weight gain and caloric intake on transpyloric feeds. The evidence in favour of transpyloric feeding is therefore scanty. We use it only for selected infants who fail to tolerate intragastric feeds.

Total parenteral nutrition (TPN)

The value of routine parenteral nutrition in very low birthweight infants has not yet been established. Yu et al (1979) reported that a TPN fed group of infants did no better in terms of postnatal weight loss than a milk fed group in the first week of life, though they subsequently gained their birthweight faster. Gibbs (1980) reported that TPN fed infants remained growth retarded (especially in length) and their weight gains did not differ from enterally fed infants.

TPN is however of undoubted value in the management of certain groups of sick infants such as those undergoing gut surgery, or infants with NEC (see p. 143) TPN should only be performed in centres where nursing staff are experienced in its use and where laboratory facilities are available for the essential metabolic monitoring of intravenously fed infants.

At a time when the National Health Service is struggling to meet financial demands it should be recognised that compared with enteral nutrition TPN is expensive and labour intensive.

Several regimes for TPN in low birthweight infants have been proposed (Yu et al, 1979; Kerner & Sunshine, 1979). In essence, most regimes aim to meet the nutritional requirements of preterm infants as discussed above, using a combination of glucose, amino-acid solutions, fat emulsion, electrolytes, trace elements and vitamins. These are infused either into an umbilical arterial catheter (if one is present for blood gas monitoring), a long central venous line or a peripheral vein. Monitoring should include (certainly in the first week) daily blood electrolytes, bilirubin, haemoglobin, acid-base status, and a check for turbidity (hyperlipidaemia) and at least weekly blood samples taken for liver function, plasma proteins and blood culture.

Recognised complications related to central catheters include bacteraemia, fungaemia, superior vena cava thrombosis, perforation of central veins, pleural effusion, haemorrhage and pulmonary emboli. (Kerner & Sunshine, 1979). Fewer complications of this nature are seen with peripheral venous lines (Gibbs, 1980), but the use of hyperosmolar infusions, in our experience substantially reduces the life span of peripheral infusion sites.

Metabolic complications include azotaemia, hyperaminoacidaemias, hypoamino-acidaemias, hyperammonaemia, hepatocellular damage, cholestasis, hyperglycaemia, glycosuria and electrolyte and acid base disturbances. In addition, lipid infusions, particularly if given in bolus fashion rather than spread out over 24 hours may result in altered pulmonary function, displacement of albumin bound free fatty acids, liver damage, coagulation disorders, interference with biochemical tests (e.g. spurious hyponatraemia) and fat emboli (Kerner & Sunshine, 1979). There is also the possibility that such infusions could change the lipid configuration of myelin. Aminoacid solutions used in clinical practice in most centres have been designed for adult use, and in the near future solutions designed specifically for paediatric patients may become available.

Although *total* parenteral nutrition has multiple complications, and, we believe has few neonatal applications other than for gastro-intestinal failure, we have found supplementary nutrition by the intravenous route to be clinically useful. Many small sick infants will tolerate 1 to 2 ml of breast milk per hour enterally, but full enteral nutrition is impossible. Supplementation with an infusion through a peripheral vein of a Vamin-Glucose-Electrolyte-Vitamin solution made up of 25 per cent vamin glucose, and 75 per cent 10 per cent dextrose in 0.18 per cent saline with added electrolytes and vitamins has few if any of the hazards associated with TPN. Such a solution containing 460 kcal/litre given at 100 to 120 ml/kg/24 hours gives the infant an adequate supply of nitrogen, and considerably increases his caloric intake when enteral feeding is restricted.

MILK FOR PRETERM INFANTS

In the British Isles, in recent years, there has been a major, though by no means universal swing away from the use of cows' milk formulae towards the use of breast milk for feeding high risk low birthweight neonates. Currently cited advantages of human milk include the greater absorbability of fat, relatively low renal solute load, specific protein composition with a high content of cystine and taurine and probable protective effects against infection and NEC (Fomon et al, 1977).

As discussed above, human milk is unlikely to meet all the calculated nutritional needs of preterm infants, but these deficits can to some extent be offset by the greater fluid intake of 220 to 250 ml/kg appropriate for preterm infants once they are well. However it remains to be established whether very preterm infants fed on breast milk will suffer any long-term morbidity as a result of their apparently suboptimal dietary intake. Infants fed on human milk may be fed milk from a milk bank or their own mothers expressed milk.

HUMAN MILK BANKS

There has recently been a resurgence of human milk banks. Most of the banks in this country are run on goodwill, minimal funds, minimal equipment and minimal staffing, and yet there is now increasing awareness that for donor milk to be used optimally, the scientific and organisational aspects of milk banking must be taken seriously. Paediatricians are now finding themselves grappling with the problems that the dairy industry had to solve decades ago. A donated sample of milk, before reaching a recipient infant might (typically) be collected in a breast shield (and contaminated with skin organisms), stored in the home freezer or refrigerator, transported, thawed if frozen, pooled, pasteurised, cooled, frozen, thawed, issued for use but still stored for several hours at 4°C while portions are instilled down a nasogastric tube. Such handling may substantially change the character of the original biological secretion. Bacteriological contamination may include potential pathogens (Lucas & Roberts, 1977); these workers also raise the possibility that bacterial enzymes secreted into milk could damage milk quality and bacterial toxins might accumulate. Freezing and thawing possibly (Gibbs et al, 1978), and heat treatment definitely damages many of the anti-infective factors in milk. Evans et al (1978) showed that accurate pasteurisation for 30 minutes at 62.5°C produced a loss of 23.7 per cent of the lysozyme, 56.8 per cent of the lactoferrin, 34 per cent of the IgG but no loss of IgA; whereas after inaccurate pasteurisation for the same period (73°C) only minimal quantities of these constituents remained intact. Fat absorption is also reduced when milk is pasteurised (Williamson et al, 1978). Once pasteurised or frozen, milk may not protect against NEC (Kliegman et al, 1979a). For these reasons some units recommend the use of raw milk (Carroll et al, 1979), but others are concerned about its bacteriological safety (Baum, 1979). Another pitfall in the use of human milk is that significant milk calories can be lost if milk is allowed to stick to feeding utensils, giving sets and feeding tubing (Lucas, unpublished). Perhaps of more concern is that the milk donated to milk banks is often so called drip breast milk (DBM) — that is the milk that drips from the opposite breast during feeding; this occurs in about 20 per cent of lactating mothers (Gibbs et al, 1978). This milk can be collected conveniently into a shell, but its use creates problems since the composition is unlike breast milk (Lucas et al, 1978); in particular it has a low fat and therefore low caloric content. The fat content of DBM falls progressively during lactation, and after three months of lactation DBM may only have 1 g/100 ml of fat compared with 4 g/100 ml in expressed milk. The possible deleterious effects of such a low fat and therefore coloric intake need further assessment by long term clinical trials.

MOTHERS OWN 'PRETERM' MILK

Compared with the infant fed on banked human milk, a low birthweight neonate receiving his own mothers milk has a significantly different diet. Not only is this milk expressed (rather than drip), but most units would accept that it can be given raw in this situation, and thus have its protective factors preserved intact. Of current interest are the fascinating studies of Atkinson et al (1978, 1980) who have shown the milk of mothers who deliver preterm infants may have a higher nitrogen and electrolyte content, and therefore be more 'adapted' to their infant's needs. The extent of the adaptation needs further work.

SPECIAL PREMATURE FORMULAE

Over the next few years an increasing number of infant formulae will be on the market specially designed for the calculated needs of low birthweight infants. At the same time, those committed to human milk banking will be looking at ways of separating and reconstituting human milk to provide custom-built human milk formulae (Lucas et al, 1980d). Whether these formulae will prove to be better than the infants own mothers 'preterm milk' will be an important area for investigation.

CARE OF THE CRITICALLY ILL VLBW INFANT

In this section we will review the management of ill infants concentrating on infants with respiratory distress syndrome (RDS) but also discussing three other important conditions, group B streptococcal (GBS) sepsis, necrotising enterocolitis (NEC) and intraventricular haemorrhage (IVH).

Respiratory distress syndrome in the low birthweight infant

The treatment of this condition is now so good that death from RDS alone is now a rarity (Table 6.9). The overall mortality is about 10 per cent (Table 6.10) the majority of the deaths occurring in infants weighing less than 1.25 kg at birth, either from IVH or the complications of long-term artificial ventilation.

Table 6.9 Causes of death in infants with RDS (Cambridge 1975–1979) inborn and outborn.

RDS + IVH	39
RDS + Acute air leak	5
RDS + Bronchopulmonary dysplasia	6
RDS + Infection	7
RDS + Asphyxial brain damage	4
RDS + Necrotizing enterocolitis	2
RDS + Massive pulmonary haemorrhage	1
RDS Solo	8

Table 6.10   Cambridge Maternity Hospital (inborn) 1975–1980.

Birthweight	Total number of infants with RDS	Total deaths in infants with RDS	Number of infants ventilated for RDS	Number of deaths in ventilated infants
<1.0 kg	36	20* (56%)	32	19* (59%)
1.0–1.5 kg	129	32† (25%)	91	32† (35%)
1.5–2.0 kg	141	5 (3.5%)	44	5 (11%)
2.0–2.5 kg	102	2§ (2.5%)	16	2§
>2.5 kg	144	1 (1%)	10	1
TOTAL	552	60 (11%)	148	48 (31%)

* Including 5 postneonatal deaths
† Including 5 postneonatal deaths
§ Including 1 postneonatal death.

Surfactant

Much of the improvement in the prognosis for infants with RDS has arisen from a better understanding of surfactant physiology.

The composition of surfactant is shown in Table 6.11. Dipalmitoyl lecithin (DPL),

Table 6.11   Composition of surfactant.

Protein 10% w/w	Lipid 90%
Lipids % w/w total lipid	
Phosphatidylcholine	72.6%
Phosphatidylglycerol	4.5%
Phosphatidylinositol	4.5%
Phosphatidylethanolamine	4.1%
Cholesterol	3.2%
Triacylglycerol	4.6%
Unesterified Fatty Acids	2.6%
Sphingomyelin	2.1%
Lysophosphatidylcholine	0.2%
Others	1.6%

although the major constituent needs the presence of the other compounds, in particular phosphatidylglycerol (PG) to be an effective surface tension lowering agent.

The amount of surfactant present in an infants lung is assessed by measuring the lecithin–sphyngomyelin ratio (LS ratio) on the liquor antenatally or on gastric or pharyngeal aspirate obtained postnatally. Other techniques for measuring surfactant are reviewed by O'Brien & Cefalo (1980). Infants with an LS ratio of less than 1.5:1 have a 70 per cent incidence of RDS; those with an LS ratio between 1.5:1 and 2:1 have a 40 per cent incidence, whereas in those with LS ratios greater than 2:1, RDS is uncommon unless the mother is a diabetic (Harvey et al, 1975). RDS with a mature LS ratio in infants of diabetic mothers is due to an isolated deficiency of PG (Cunningham et al, 1978) (see Ch. 3, p. 64).

It is now apparent that PG should be measured when analysing liquor antenatally. If PG is present, RDS is extremely unlikely (Golde & Moseley, 1980) even with an LS ratio less than 2:1 (Whittle et al, 1981).

SURFACTANT SYNTHESIS AND RELEASE
Surfactant is synthesised in the type 2 pneumonocytes by the choline incorporation pathway. This pathway is rapidly inhibited by pH values below 7.2 (Fig. 6.1) (Merritt

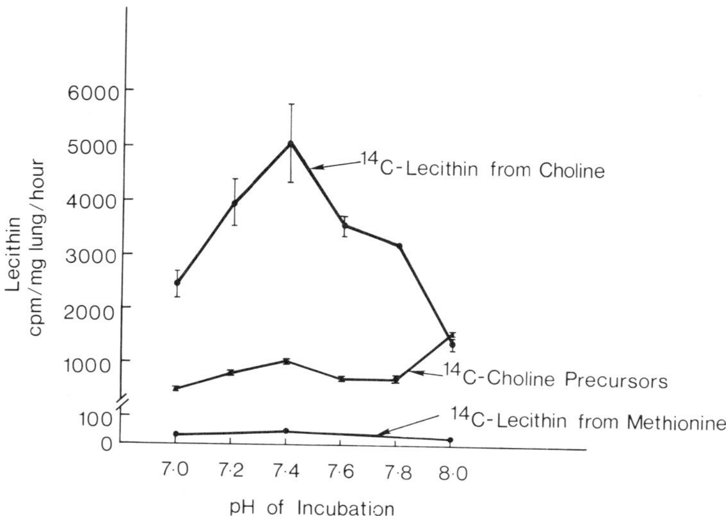

Fig. 6.1 Rate of incorporation of ^{14}C into lecithin in monkey lung slices (Data of Merritt & Farrell, 1976).

& Farrell, 1976). Hypothermia also inhibits surfactant synthesis (Gluck et al, 1972). Surfactant is released from the pneumonocytes in part by adequate but not excessive alveolar expansion (Lawson et al, 1979) and in part by prostaglandin activity plus cholinergic and beta adrenergic stimulation (Oyarzun & Clements, 1977, 1978).

The production of surfactant in the human fetal lung increases at 30 to 34 weeks gestation, and will not occur in the absence of corticosteroids (Gross, 1979; Torday, 1980). Thyroxine is also required (Cunningham et al, 1980) and hypothyroid human neonates probably have an increased incidence of RDS (Fisch et al, 1975; Schönberger et al, 1981). Drugs which induce surfactant production include opiates (Glass et al, 1971), aminophylline (Sevanian et al, 1979, Hadjigeorgiou et al, 1979) the betamimetics (Kanjanapone et al, 1980) and biosolvon (Lorenz et al, 1974). Surfactant synthesis is inhibited by insulin (Gross, 1979; Neufeld et al, 1979).

Although glucocorticoids have been widely used to induce surfactant synthesis in the human fetus (Liggins & Howie, 1972; Howie & Liggins, 1977; Caspi et al, 1976; Dluholucky et al, 1976; Block et al, 1976; Thornfeldt et al, 1978; Morrison et al, 1978; Taeusch et al, 1979; Ballard et al, 1979; Papageorgiou et al, 1979; Young et al, 1980; Schutte et al, 1980), we believe that the reports require careful evaluation because:

1. The mothers, and therefore their babies are given other drugs including betamimetics (Caspi et al, 1976; Howie & Liggins, 1977. Ballard et al, 1979) which influence surfactant synthesis and release (Oyarzun & Clements, 1977; Kanjanapone et al, 1980).
2. Steroids have deleterious effects: an increased risk of infection for the mother and baby (Taeusch et al, 1979; Johnson & Schneider, 1978; Young et al, 1980), and adrenal suppression (Taeusch et al, 1978), hypoglycaemia (Papageorgiou et al, 1979) and hypercholesterolaemia (Andersen & Friis-Hansen, 1978) in the infants. Fatal pulmonary oedema is reported in women given steroids plus the

betamimetics required to delay delivery long enough for the steroids to induce surfactant (Jacobs et al, 1980) and peptic ulceration may also occur in glucocorticoid treated women (Semchyschyn, 1981).

The majority of the above trials including Liggins & Howie (1977) excluded women who were *not* in labour, and there is little evidence that steroids work in such patients. Furthermore, in women requiring premature delivery before the onset of labour, pre-eclampsia, glucose intolerance, or renal disease are contraindications to steroid administration.

The only benefit from antenatal steroids seems to accrue in male infants (Ballard et al, 1980) between 30 and 32 weeks' gestation and 1.00 to 1.50 kg who deliver between 24 hours and seven days after receiving steroids.

In 1975 to 1978 in over 15 000 deliveries in Cambridge, 114 women delivered at 30 to 32 weeks gestation, but only 22 would have qualified for antenatal steroids. All 22 women delivered healthy infants; 13 developed RDS, but in only three was it severe enough to require intermittent positive pressure ventilation (IPPV). No infant died. For these reasons we see little point in administering steroids generally to women in premature labour even between 30 to 32 weeks gestation. There is even less reason to give steroids to women over 32 weeks gestation where the incidence and mortality of RDS is even lower. Other studies have reached the same conclusion (Depp et al, 1980). Studies must now concentrate on gestations less than 30 weeks where there is a striking dearth of data, except for the small numbers of Liggins & Howie (1977) and Ballard et al (1979).

Delivering premature infants
Milder asphyxia than that which causes brain damage in *term* infants will damage the *preterm* infant's lungs (Cruz et al, 1976; Brumley & Crenshaw, 1980); furthermore, asphyxiated preterm infants are more likely to die from RDS (Roberton & Tizard, 1975), and more likely to develop an IVH. Intrapartum asphyxia is one of the major determinants of whether or not low birthweight survivors have subsequent neurological handicap.

Women in labour at short gestation must therefore have intrapartum fetal monitoring (Bowes et al, 1980; Zanini et al, 1980), and if signs of fetal distress develop the infant should be delivered immediately by Caesarean section if necessary.

The perinatal paediatrician's aphorism to his perinatal obstetric colleague must be 'give me a premature baby in good condition, and I'll give you a neurologically intact survivor'.

THE PREMATURE BREECH
There is compelling evidence that vaginal breech delivery increases the mortality in infants less than 1.50 kg (Bowes et al, 1977; Stewart, 1977; Goldenberg & Nelson, 1977; Duenhoelter et al, 1979; Bowes et al, 1979; Smith et al, 1980), and also increases handicap (Ingemarsson et al, 1978). There are dissenting voices (Woods, 1979) and Caesarean section carries a morbidity for the mother. Therefore, whether Caesarean section is preferable in breech presentation must depend on how much maternal morbidity is acceptable in all mothers so delivered in order to prevent death or damage in a proportion of the infants and that is something which cannot be

decided by a randomised controlled trial. We believe that such infants should be delivered by Caesarean section.

CAESAREAN SECTION AND RDS

The classical papers on this topic have little data at gestations less than 32 weeks (Butler & Alberman, 1969; Usher et al, 1971). In Cambridge (Table 6.12) Caesarean section at these gestations, does *not* increase morbidity or mortality from RDS and is not only safe for the premature breech, but is used to effect safe delivery of the premature infant and prevent fetal or maternal morbidity in such conditions as severe pre-eclampsia or abruptio placentae.

Table 6.12A Outcome of infants 28–31/52 delivered at Cambridge Maternity Hospital 1975–1979 (malformations excluded).

Delivery	Total	RDS	RDS + IPPV	Deaths
Caesarean section	76	61	44	11
Vaginal	72	47	26	12

Table 6.12B Indications for Caesarean section and outcome.

Indication	Total	RDS	RDS + IPPV	Deaths
Severe pre-eclampsia	26	21	18	4
Breech (in labour)	12	9	5	1
Placenta praevia-labour or bleeding	10	8	5	2
Abruptio placenta	5	5	4	1
Severe growth retardation	4	1	–	–
Prolonged membrane rupture and pyrexia	4	2	2	–
Cord prolapse	3	3	1	1
Fetal distress in labour	3	3	3	2
Chornic renal disease	3	2	1	–
Miscellaneous	5	4	4	–

Management of RDS

The overall management of RDS is to keep the infant alive until he resynthesises his own surfactant. However in the future it may be possible to administer a surfactant to the infant. Fujiwara et al (1980) gave bovine surfactant to neonates and demonstrated improved oxygenation, although the installation of 10 ml of a fluid containing animal protein into a neonate's lung is not a technique to be undertaken lightly. The synthetic, non-protein containing surfactant used by Morley et al (1981) is preferable. They showed a significantly lower mortality in premature infants receiving a single puff of 25 mg of synthetic surfactant containing 70 per cent DPL and 30 per cent PG. Treated babies still developed RDS, but it was less severe.

Control of body temperature in infants with RDS

Babies who get cold die more often (Silverman & Blanc, 1957) as do babies who get too hot (Yashiro et al, 1973). The modern practice of nursing sick VLBW infants under overhead radiant heaters to improve access is not without risk. Burns and

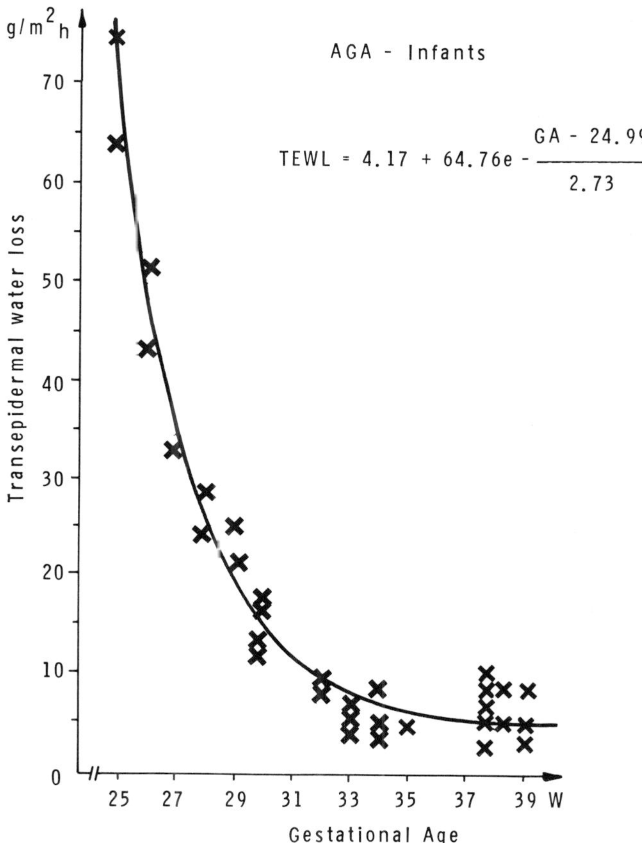

Fig. 6.2 Trans-epidermal water loss at different gestations. A 1.0 kg infant has a surface area of 0.1 m²
and a 3.5 kg infant a surface area of 0.2 m². (Data of Hammarlund & Sedin, 1979).

severe hyperthermia have been reported (Fleischman, 1977; Committee on environmental hazards, 1978) but the major hazard of these devices is a great increase in the transepidermal fluid loss creating major problems with fluid balance.

The VLBW infant does not loose much water from sweating, but probably as a result of defective skin keratinisation, his transepidermal fluid loss even when nursed in incubators may exceed 100 ml/kg/24 hours (Fig. 6.2) (Hammarlund & Sedin, 1979; Rutter & Hull, 1979). The amount lost may increase by a further 50 to 60 per cent if the relative humidity falls from 60 to 20 per cent, and be even greater under radiant heaters (Bell et al, 1980).

The high insensible water losses have surprisingly few effects on metabolic rate and oxygen consumption (Okken et al, 1979) so long as the infant's body temperature under a radiant heater or in a incubator with a heat shield in situ is kept at 36.5°C (Yeh et al, 1979; Bell et al, 1980; Marks et al, 1980). The vast increase, however, in insensible water loss, particularly under radiant heaters makes the management of fluid and electrolyte balance difficult with the constant risk of severe dehydration and hyperosmolarity.

Feeding
To the older observations of Dunn (1963) that infants with RDS have a paralytic ileus and of Wharton & Bower (1965) that feeding causes aspiration, have been added the newer observations that passing naso-gastric tubes is a noxious stimulus causing hypoxia; once in situ the tube causes airway obstruction and increases the work of breathing (Stocks, 1980), and putting even small quantities of fluid into the stomach lowers the PaO_2 (Wilkinson & Yu, 1974), and the functional residual capacity (FRC). (Pitcher-Wilmott et al, 1979). It is not surprising that such infants may develop NEC (p. 143) or become apnoeic and regurgitate (Herbst et al, 1979). Feeds should therefore be given with great care to infants with RDS, and are probably contraindicated initially in infants receiving more than 60 per cent oxygen, CPAP or IPPV.

Fluid and electrolyte balance
In his classic paper Usher (1963) recommended that infants with RDS should receive 65 ml/kg of intravenous glucose-bicarbonate solution per 24 hours. Over the subsequent 10 years this volume increased to 150 ml/kg/24 hours and beyond for various reasons:

1. The high fluid intakes needed to prevent dehydration under radiant heaters tended to be given indiscriminately to all small infants.
2. Jaundice caused brain damage and was aggravated by dehydration (Wennberg et al, 1966). 150 to 170 ml/kg of milk was given to infants feeding orally, particularly if they were small for dates, in an attempt to prevent hypoglycaemia and jaundice (Smallpiece & Davies, 1964); similar volumes were then given intravenously.
3. Infusing sufficient fluid to achieve a urine osmolarity less than 200 mosmol/kg

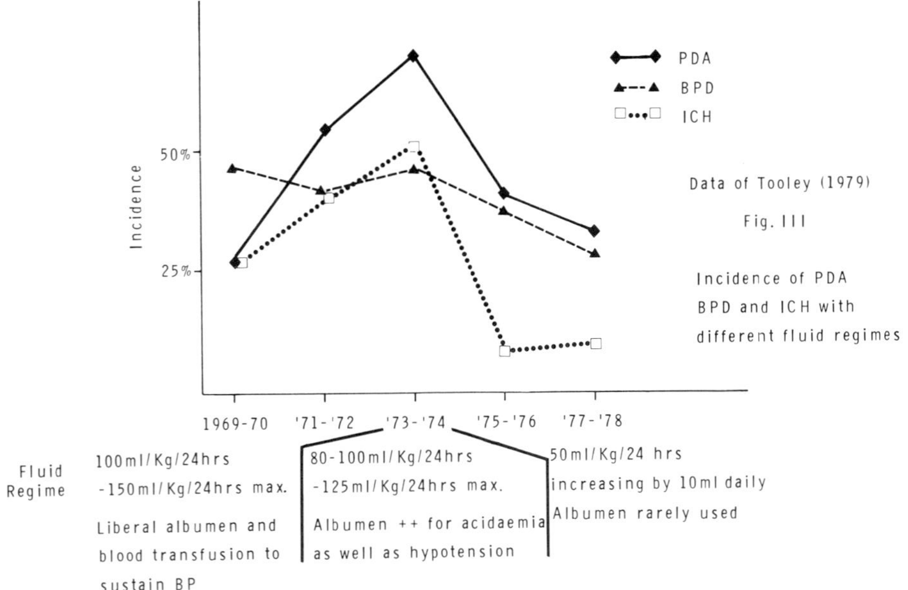

Fig. 6.3   Incidence of PDA, BPD and ICH with different fluid regimes. (Data redrawn from Tooley, 1979.)

(Jones et al, 1976) while theoretically appealing is, unjustified in sick infants with compromised renal function, and results in fluid overload.
4. Large quantities of intravenous crystalloid, plasma and blood have been administered to counteract hypotension in the neonate.

This excessive fluid intake has increased four serious illnesses, patent ductus arteriosus (PDA), NEC, IVH, and bronchopulmonary dysplasia (BPD) (Tooley, 1979; Brown, 1979; Bell et al, 1978). Other factors were probably involved in this increase, but, as Figure 6.3 shows, reduction in fluid intake was followed by a lower incidence of the condition.

We believe, therefore, that Usher's (1963) original recommendation is correct for sick VLBW infants less than 48 hours old. Adjustments can then be made in the light of biochemical and clinical assessment of the infant. An intake of 20 to 30 ml/kg/24 hours maybe adequate for an infant with inappropriate ADH production, whereas small infants under radiant heat sources may require 250 to 300 ml/kg/24 hours.

Acid base homeostasis
The fact that excessive use of bicarbonate can be damaging (Simmons et al, 1974, Wigglesworth et al, 1976) should not obscure the fact that profound metabolic acidaemia is equally damaging to the central nervous system (Dawes et al, 1964), cardiovascular function (Beirholm et al, 1975), and surfactant synthesis (Merritt & Farrell, 1976). Every effort, including infusion of base, should be made to keep the infants pH greater than 7.25. In many cases, inadequate oxygenation, hypotension or sepsis are responsible for acidaemia and prevention of these will prevent metabolic acidaemia.

Blood pressure and blood volume
Infants with RDS have a lower blood pressure than healthy infants at the same gestation (Neligan & Smith, 1960; Broughton-Pipkin & Smales, 1977). Infants with systolic blood pressures less than 40 mmHg have a poorer prognosis (Hall & Oliver, 1971; Alden et al, 1972), are more likely to have a metabolic acidaemia and poor renal function (Lay et al, 1980), and if the hypotension is not quickly corrected, the incidence of IVH is increased (Fujimura et al, 1979). We aim therefore to detect and correct hypotension and anaemia as soon after birth as possible, and use plasma or blood transfusion to keep the blood pressure greater than 35 to 40 mmHg and the haematorcrit greater than 40 per cent.

Ventilatory assistance

CPAP. Continuous positive airways pressure has been with us for 10 years (Gregory et al, 1971). Controlled trials have failed to show a large increase in survival rate in infants receiving CPAP particularly in those less than 1.50 kg, but early application CPAP shortens the course of the disease, the duration of oxygen therapy and reduces the intensity of any subsequent ventilator therapy (Rhodes & Hall, 1973; Durbin et al, 1976; Mockrin & Bancalari, 1975; Belenky et al, 1976).

IPPV. Studies in the late 1960s and early 1970s (Smith et al, 1972; Herman & Reynolds, 1973) showed that a pressure limited, flow generator type of ventilator set at rates of 20 to 40 min, inspiratory to expiratory ratios of 1.5:1, 2:1 and even 3:1, plus positive and expiratory pressure (PEEP) of 3 to 5 cm H_2O was the most effective way of oxygenating infants. Recently, fast ventilator rates are again being used (Bland et al, 1977), supporting some of the older literature (Owen-Thomas et al, 1968).

Drug therapy

Antibiotics. Because of the problems with Group B streptococcal sepsis (p. 140) most neonatologists routinely administer penicillin prophylactically to all infants with signs of RDS.

Tolazoline. This combines alpha-adrenergic blocking actions with a histaminic effect, and dilates the muscular pulmonary arteries (Lock et al, 1979a), probably by the histaminic actions (Goetzman & Milstein, 1979). It has been used in severely hypoxic infants with RDS with a large right to left shunt sustained by high pulmonary artery pressures (Goetzman et al, 1976; Mackintosh & Walters, 1979; Stevens et al, 1980). About half the infants with RDS receiving Tolazoline show no PaO_2 response and a further 25 per cent have a small rise in PaO_2 which is probably within the variation expected from other changes in therapy. However in 25 per cent of infants, usually less than 24 hours of age, there is brisk improvement in PaO_2 over one to two hours (Fig. 6.4).

Curare. Pancuronium has recently been introduced into ventilator care in the neonate. Striking improvements in an infant's oxygenation may be seen following curarisation, particularly in those who are breathing out of phase with the ventilator (Henry et al,

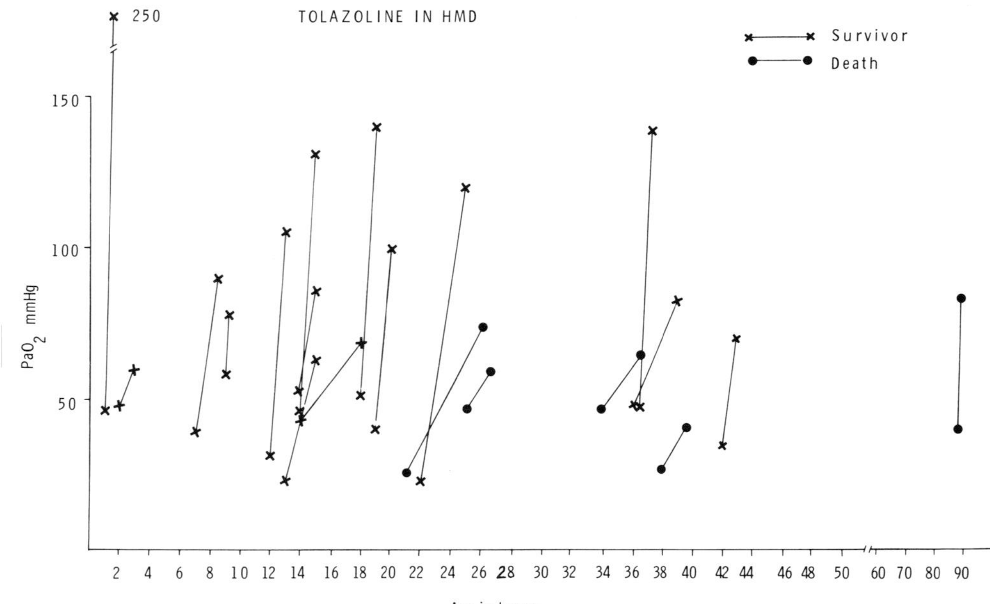

Fig. 6.4   Increase in arterial PO_2 in infants receiving Tolazoline. The first dot is the PaO_2 immediately preceeding the Tolazoline and the second dot is the PaO_2 when the next sample was taken.

1979; Crone & Favorito, 1980). In addition curarised infants have a lower incidence of pulmonary barotrauma (p 140) probably due to the lower peak inspiratory pressures which can be used (Stark et al, 1979; Pollitzer et al, 1981).

Monitoring infants with RDS

All sick neonates should have their e.c.g. monitored continuously, and their blood pressure, temperature and respiration monitored frequently.

BLOOD GAS MONITORING

In the last few years it has become possible to record continuously an infants PaO_2 using umbilical artery catheters which have a miniturised PaO_2 cell built into their tip. Not only is hypoxia rapidly detected with such catheters, but hyperoxaemia with the risk of retrolental fibroplasia (RLF) can be avoided. The catheters have a sampling lumen to allow blood to be withdrawn for pH, $PaCO_2$ and other chemical and haematological measurements, and should be inserted into all infants requiring more than 40 per cent oxygen (Conway et al, 1976; Pollitzer et al, 1980).

The use of these catheters has highlighted the deleterious effect of handling sick infants (Fig. 6.5). All nursing procedures cause falls in PaO_2 (Speidel, 1978), and aspirating an endotracheal tube or puncturing a peripheral artery can cause marked and prolonged hypoxaemia. This inaccuracy of PaO_2 measurements obtained by direct arterial puncture casts serious doubt over the safety of this technique for preventing hyperoxaemia or RLF. In the absence of a continuous PaO_2 catheter, an ordinary umbilical catheter should be inserted, and blood gases measured at least three- to four-hourly.

An apparatus for continuous transcutaneous PO_2 ($TcPO_2$) measurement is now available. Its accuracy and value in experienced hands is established (Huch et al,

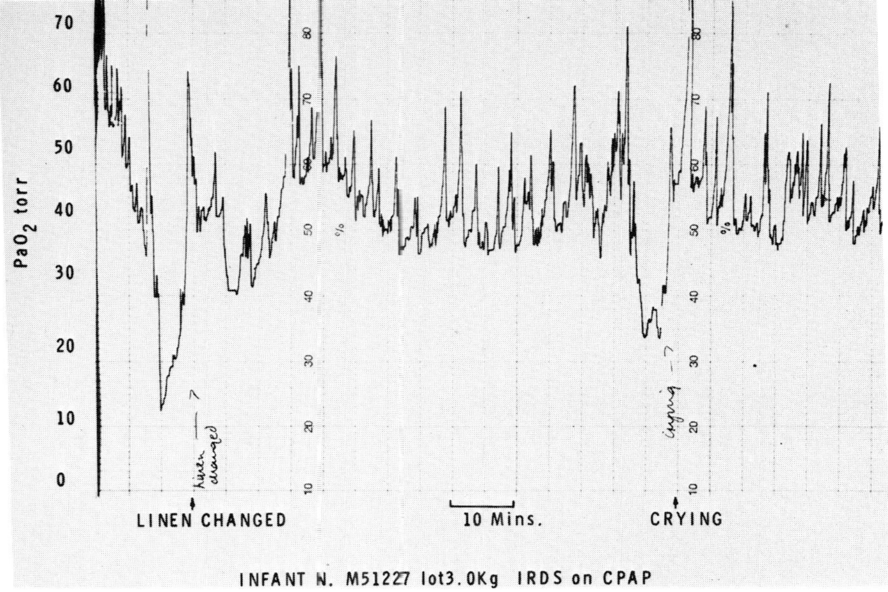

Fig. 6.5   Spontaneous swings in PaO_2 (recorded by Searle Polarographic Catheter) in an infant with RDS on CPAP.

1976; LeSouef et al, 1978; Peabody et al, 1978a). However the device may underestimate hyperoxaemia particularly during hypotension, shock, or Tolazoline infusion (LeSouef et al, 1978; Peabody et al, 1978b; Buntain et al, 1979), exposing the infant to risk of RLF.

Complications of RDS

PATENT DUCTUS ARTERIOSUS

The ductus is less sensitive to the oxygen stimulus to closure in premature infants (McMurphy et al, 1972), and this problem may be aggravated by pulmonary disease such as RDS causing hypoxaemia, and by the excessive use of intravenous fluids (see p. 136).

In infants with RDS, PDA usually presents at the end of the first week of life with bounding pulses, a loud systolic murmur and pulmonary crepitations; chest X-ray shows cardiomegaly and a peri-hilar haze. The $PaCO_2$ rises and more vigorous ventilation is required to control the blood gases.

Treatment. Since fluid overload may cause PDA, it is reasonable to restrict fluid to a 100 ml/kg/24 hours, and give frusemide, but Digoxin is unlikely to help (Berman et al, 1978).

If all these measures fail, since prostaglandins keep the ductus patent (Coceani et al, 1978), and infants with PDA have a higher prostaglandin levels than those without (Lucas & Mitchell, 1978) a prostaglandin synthetase inhibitor such as indomethacin can be given. About 50 to 75 per cent of PDA are reported to close following indomethacin (McCarthy et al, 1978; Halliday et al, 1979), and this matches our own experience. If after two repeat courses of indomethacin, the ductus has not closed it should be ligated since this can now be done with minimal morbidity (Merritt et al, 1978; Cotton et al, 1978).

AIR LEAKS

Spontaneous pneumothorax and pneumomediastinum have long been recognised as complications of RDS, but the incidence rises to 30 to 40 per cent in infants with RDS on IPPV (Yu et al, 1975; Ogata et al, 1976; Madansky et al, 1979). The development of a pneumothorax doubles the mortality from RDS (Ogata et al, 1976; Madansky et al, 1979) (Table 6.13) and considerably increases the incidence of IVH (Dykes et al, 1980; Lipscombe et al, 1981).

BRONCHOPULMONARY DYSPLASIA (BPD)

This chronic lung fibrosis develops in infants with severe RDS who receive long-term positive pressure ventilation. Factors involved are oxygen toxicity, infection, retention of secretions behind an indwelling endotracheal tube, over-hydration with or without a PDA (Brown, 1979; Tooley, 1979), but most important of all is air leaks from high pressure IPPV (Reynolds & Taghizadeh, 1974; Berg et al, 1975; Stahlman et al, 1979; Table 6.13). Almost all the reported cases of BPD occur in infants who have been exposed to peak inflating pressures exceeding 30 cm H_2O (Roberton, 1976).

Table 6.13   Cambridge Maternity Hospital 1975–1978. Intensity of treatment of RDS as the air leak developed.

Type of Therapy:	No ventilatory assistance:		CPAP		IPPV (<25 cms H_2O)		IPPV (25–30 cms H_2O)		IPPV (>30 cms H_2O)	
	Air leak	No air leak	Air leak	No air leak	Air leak	No air leak	Air leak	No air leak	Air leak	No air leak
Number of Infants:	7	179	5	21	6 (2)★	15	9 (4)★	9	22 (10)★	20
Number developing Bronchopulmonary Dysplasia:	–	–	–	–	1	–	–	–	6	1
Deaths:	–	–	3	–	2 (α)	–	2	3	15 (β)	10

(α) Including the one with Bronchopulmonary dysplasia (BPD)
(β) Including three with BPD
★   Figures in brackets: infants with just pulmonary interstitial emphysema.

The treatment of BPD is to keep the ventilator pressures as low as possible, to close a patent ductus if present, and to give diuretics (Shannon, 1979).

ACUTE GROUP B STREPTOCOCCAL SEPSIS IN THE NEONATE

It has recently become apparent that infants dying early in life with what was diagnosed as RDS were infected (Jeffrey et al, 1977; Menke et al, 1979). Post mortem studies demonstrated atelectasis with atypical hyaline membranes (Ablow et al, 1976), which could lead an inexperienced pathologist to diagnose RDS in the absence of positive bacteriology.

The role of GBS in this syndrome has become frighteningly apparent; in the USA it causes one neonatal death per one thousand live births (Howard & McCracken, 1974). As more blood cultures are taken from acutely ill infants immediately after birth other organisms are being found to cause an identical illness including group D (Headings et al, 1978) and G streptococci (Nieberg, 1979), pneumococci (Bortolussi, et al, 1977), Strep. viridans (Jeffrey et al, 1977), haemophilus species (Bale & Watkins, 1978; Lilien et al, 1978), and other Gram negative organisms including, in our experience, salmonella heidelberg, bacillus cereus, and anaerobes.

Over 25 per cent of healthy women may carry GBS in the vagina as an apparently non-pathogenic commensal (Beachler et al, 1979; Siegel et al, 1980) though most studies, including those in the United Kingdom, report carrier rates of 5 to 10 per cent (Schauf & Hlaing, 1976). A much smaller number of women carry other potentially pathogenic organisms. 50 per cent of infants born through a colonised birth canal become colonised themselves (Reid, 1975; Anthony et al, 1979; Yow et al, 1980), but serious disease develops in less than 5 per cent of them (Embil et al, 1978; Anthony & Okada, 1977). The infants most likely to develop acute neonatal GBS sepsis are born to heavily colonised mothers (Anthony et al, 1979), with no IgG anti-bodies against the organism (Baker & Casper, 1976; Vogel et al, 1980) who have premature onset of labour, or premature rupture of the membranes (Pasnick et al, 1980; Gerard et al, 1979).

In some units there is a high nosocomial colonisation rate within the nursery, but this form of transmission is unlikely to cause the severe early onset form of GBS sepsis (Aber et al, 1976).

Neonatal signs and diagnosis
It is not possible to differentiate GBS sepsis from RDS at a stage in the illness early enough to give antibiotics only to infants with GBS. However compared to infants with RDS, those with GBS sepsis tend to be more mature, become apnoeic earlier, have lower blood pressures, are easier to ventilate, have different X-ray pictures (Ablow et al, 1976; Menke et al, 1979), and abnormal white blood cell counts (Manroe et al, 1977; Boyle et al, 1978).

Diagnosis can be confirmed by identifying Gram positive cocci in gastric aspirate (Yeung & Tam, 1972), pharyngeal aspirate (Slack & Mayon-White, 1978) and ear swabs (Scanlon, 1971), or by the demonstration of GBS antigen by countercurrent immunoelectrophoresis on serum, c.s.f. or concentrated urine (Baker et al, 1980; Bromberger et al, 1980). Nevertheless the absence of these findings does not exclude

GBS disease, and in some patients RDS and GBS sepsis can co-exist (Jacob et al, 1980).

Antenatal prevention
The eradication of the organism from the vagina by oral antibiotic therapy was not possible in one study (Gardner et al, 1979) and in another the women recolonised between treatment and eventual delivery (Hall et al, 1976). However, Yow et al (1979) showed that giving 500 mg of ampicillin i.v. six-hourly during labour to carrier mothers eliminated the GBS colonisation in the neonate, and Merenstein et al (1980) showed that oral penicillin, or erythromycin given to the mother from 38 weeks gestation until delivery prevented infant colonisation. The logistics of swabbing all women at 38 weeks are colossal, but, perhaps by selecting a high risk group (Pasnick et al, 1980) it will be possible to considerably reduce the number of infants colonised, thereby reducing the number of neonatal infections.

Prevention of GBS sepsis in the neonate
Universal institution of good umbilical cord care may help to reduce infant colonisation (Wald et al, 1977). Giving penicillin to all infants has been suggested (Steigman et al, 1978; Lloyd et al, 1979), but one controlled trial has shown no benefit from this routine (Ramamurthy, et al, 1979) and the very much larger study (Siegel et al, 1980) while showing a reduced colonisation and symptomatic infection rate with GBS in treated infants, demonstrated increasing problems with penicillin-resistant organisms in the nursery during the study, and concluded that routine penicillin proplylaxis was unjustifiable. We believe that the safest approach is to give penicillin to all dyspnoeic newborn infants immediately the respiratory illness is recognised (Cowan et al, 1979). We take cultures from all such infants, irrespective of gestation, chest X-ray or clinical findings, and start them 50 000 units/kg/bd. If there is anything to suggest heavy GBS infection (e.g. positive Gram stains or countercurrent immunoelectrophoresis of other suggestive clinical features), we would double the penicillin dose and add gentamycin which acts synergistically with penicillin against GBS (Schauf et al, 1976) and increases the anti-bacterial spectrum in case another organism is present. If the cultures are negative 48 hours later the antibiotics can be stopped.

NECROTISING ENTEROCOLITIS

This condition has emerged during the last decade, and now affects approximately 5 per cent of all infants less than 2.0 kg, with the incidence increasing to 25 per cent in some series (Book et al, 1976b; Stoll et al, 1980; Ryder et al, 1980).

Aetiology
Many factors have been implicated, and these are summarised in Figure 6.6. Most cases are multifactorial, but in a few infants, a single agent may predominate.

Gut hypoperfusion may be due to serious illness, birth asphyxia, hypoxia, hypotension, heart failure from a PDA or hyperviscosity (Kitterman, 1975; Ryder et al, 1980; Hakanson & Oh, 1977; Santulli et al, 1975; Bunton et al, 1978) or venous

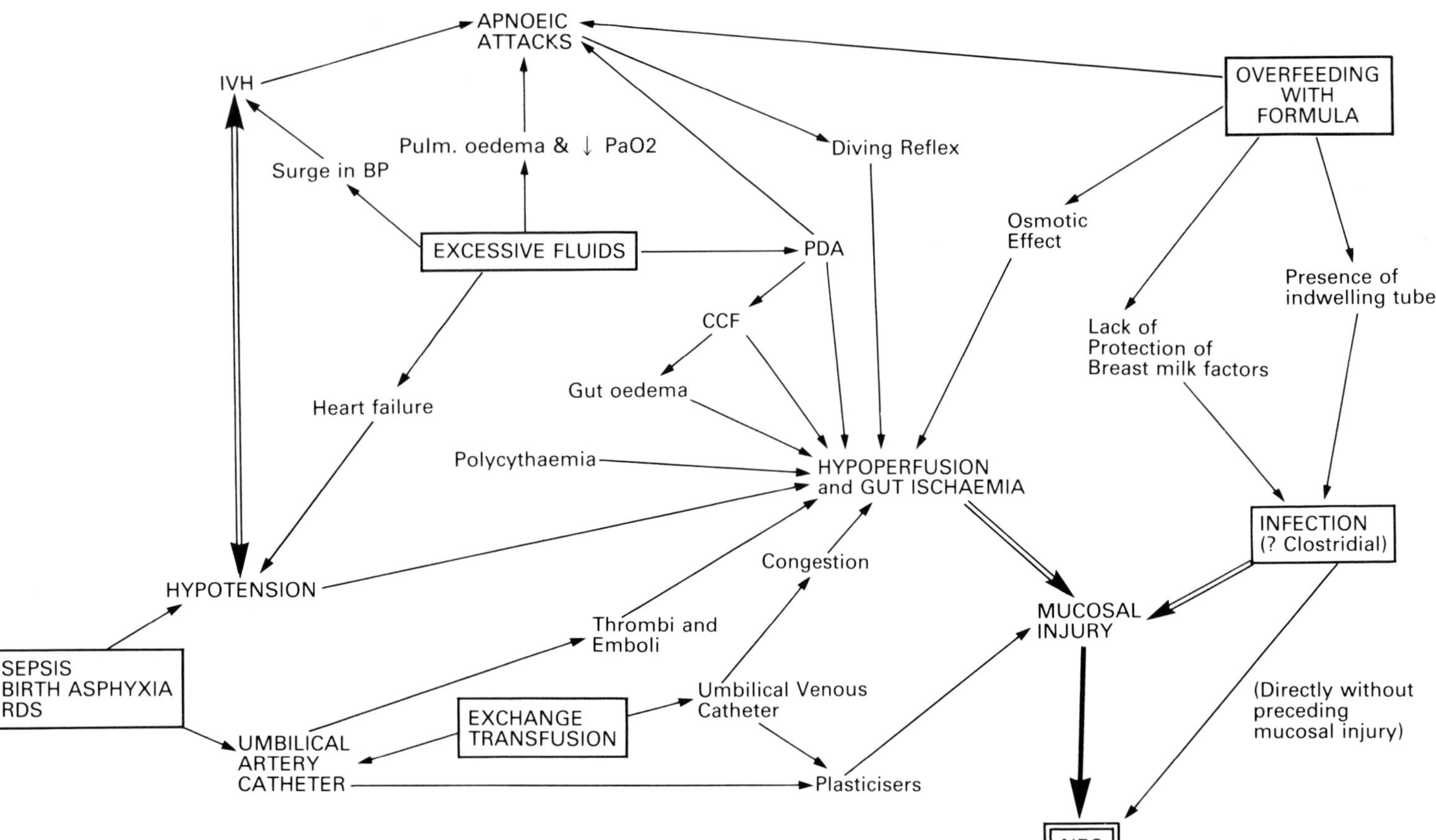

Fig. 6.6   Aetiological factors in NEC. Major factors are enclosed in dark boxes.

stasis from an indwelling umbilical catheter (Orme & Eades, 1968; Touloukian et al, 1973).

The umbilical artery catheter has been much maligned as a cause of intestinal ischaemia (Bunton et al, 1978; Livaditis, 1974) either by causing obstruction simply by its presence in the aorta, or by causing thrombi. These thrombi can then propagate along the aorta and its branches or disseminate emboli. More recent studies have not implicated umbilical artery catheterization (Stoll et al, 1980; Ryder et al, 1980).

Infection is suggested by the fact that a positive blood culture is often found in NEC, and many cases occur in clusters (Book et al, 1977; Powell et al, 1980; Howard et al, 1977). The organisms implicated include clostridium butyricum (Howard et al, 1977), Clostridium perfringens (welchii) (Kosloske et al, 1978; Kliegman et al, 1979b), klebsiella (Frantz et al, 1975; Ryder et al, 1980), E. coli (Speer et al, 1976) and Enterobacter cloacae (Powell et al, 1980). In other studies, even of epidemics, no pathogens (Book et al, 1977; Guinan et al, 1979), or a variety of pathogens have been isolated (Kosloske & Ulrich, 1980). Many of these organisms are found in asymptomatic infants (Kindley et al, 1977; Smith et al, 1980) suggesting that the gut mucosa needs to be damaged by hypoxia before normally commensal organisms become invasive.

A third aetiological factor is fluid intake (Bell et al, 1979). This may cause NEC by generating gut oedema or by the high fluid intake causing PDA (Brown, 1979), chronic lung diease or IVH leading to the episodes of apnoea, hypoxia, hypotension which precede NEC.

Finally, over-vigorous infant feeding, in particular the use of partially digested milks containing 650 mos mol/litre (Book et al, 1975), or concentrated formula with more than 20 kcal/once (Frantz et al, 1975) have been blamed (Goldman, 1980; Ryder et al, 1980). In units where a major effort is made to delay feeding sick infants, and when starting it, to do so very gradually, the incidence of NEC has fallen (Brown & Sweet, 1978).

Diagnosis

The infant presents with abdominal distension, bilious vomiting, and the passage of bloody stool (Kosloske, 1979; Ryder et al, 1980) and may have other signs of disseminated sepsis, with apnoea, temperature instability and lethargy. He often has an ileus, and may develop signs of peritonitis.

In the early stages, abdominal X-ray will show abnormalities of gut gas pattern, and some gut wall thickening (Kogutt, 1979). Subsequently intramural gas bubbles appear, and may extend into the biliary tree (Daneman et al, 1978); ascites may develop. Perforation may occur at any stage, and infants with NEC should have daily X-rays to exclude the presence of free intraperitoneal air.

Prevention

There is a lower incidence of NEC in infants who have previously received antibiotics for various reasons (Guinan et al, 1979; Ryder et al, 1980). However although some studies show that oral administration of aminoglycosides reduces the incidence of NEC in at risk infants (Egan et al, 1976; Grylack & Scanlon, 1978) others do not (Boyle et al, 1978; Rowley & Dahlenburg, 1978).

The widespread administration of aminoglycoside antibiotics is fraught with microbiological hazards (McCracken & Eitzman, 1978); and there can be no justification for this routine except as an adjunct to barrier nursing techniques during a nursery epidemic (Book et al, 1977; Powell et al, 1980).

One intriguing observation is the possibility that one can predict the development of NEC by testing the infants stools for lactose (Book et al, 1976).

Treatment

MEDICAL

The infant's stomach should be aspirated regularly, oral feeds discontinued and the infant fed intravenously for seven to 10 days (Torma et al, 1973; Frantz et al, 1975; Kosloske, 1979) using a long line (Shaw, 1973). Umbilical venous and arterial catheters should be removed, and a peripheral intravenous infusion set up for a seven to 10 days course of antibiotics, usually penicillin or cloxacillin plus gentamicin. We are impressed that since we have used intravenous metronidazole as well, our results have improved. Oral antibiotics are unnecessary (Hansen et al, 1980).

Frequent albumin, plasma or blood transfusions are indicated together with the routine supportive therapy for any sick hypotensive neonate; arterial blood must be used for blood gas analysis, since in hypotensive underperfused infants $TcPO_2$ may seriously underestimate PaO_2 (see above).

SURGICAL

Pneumatosis alone is not an indication for laparotomy particularly if it seems to be the benign form of NEC (Santulli et al, 1975; Leonidas & Hall, 1976). The main indication for surgery is perforation-indicated by free intra-abdominal air, or failure to improve after seven days of conventional treatment. The presence of a discoloured peritoneal exudate with organisms present on Gram stain may indicate those infants likely to require surgery (Kosloske & Lilly, 1978).

SEQUELAE

Up to 25 per cent of infants who survive without laparotomy may develop stenosis of the segment of bowel involved. Four to six weeks after the initial illness, these infants present with signs of intestinal obstruction. Barium studies will confirm the stenosis, and resection of the affected segment is required (Bell et al, 1978; Schwartz et al, 1980).

RESULTS

The mortality from NEC is about 25 per cent. Bell et al (1978) reported that nine out of 36 infants died, but five of these deaths were from associated chronic lung disease. No medically treated cases of NEC died, but of nine patients requiring laparotomy, four died of NEC and three of chronic lung disease.

INTRAVENTRICULAR HAEMORRHAGE

This condition is the cause of most deaths in neonates weighing less than 1.50 kg, and is particularly common in infants suffering from severe RDS (Table 6.9; Dykes et al, 1980).

Anatomy

The haemorrhage arises from the germinal layer which contains large, irregular thin walled vessels not identifiable as arterioles, venules or capillaries, and lies between the caudate nucleus and the ependyma in the floor of the lateral ventricle. The haemorrhage may localise there (a sub-ependymal haemorrhage, or germinal layer haemorrhage (GLH), or rupture into the c.s.f. and spread throughout the ventricules, or extend into the adjacent cortex.

Pathogenesis

In post mortem experiments on human neonatal brains, Hambleton & Wigglesworth (1976) following arterial injection showed that GLH and IVH arose from disruption of the germinal layer capillary network, and they postulated that IVH was due to surges in arterial blood pressure, a view supported by the animal data (Goddard et al, 1980; Reynolds et al, 1979).

In the human neonate the cerebral blood flow (CBF) autoregulates with blood pressure changes (Cowan, 1979), but raising the $PaCO_2$ increases CBF both in healthy (Leahy et al, 1980; Milligan, 1980), and sick neonates (Cooke et al, 1979). Furthermore, Lou et al (1979) showed that in mildly asphyxiated babies CBF was pressure passive and moderate increases in blood pressure caused a doubling or trebling of the infants CBF.

A reduced blood pressure when CBF is pressure passive may well cause ischaemia in the sub-ependymal layer, and Fujimura et al (1979) showed that low birthweight infants who subsequently developed IVH were hypotensive initially.

On the basis of these findings Pape & Wigglesworth (1979) have promulgated a theory to account for the development of IVH (Fig. 6.7). Anything that causes a major increase in CBF, increasing $PaCO_2$, increasing BP or both, can cause a GLH which may rupture out of a previously normal germinal layer and cause an IVH. In view of the data of Fujimura et al (1979) factors such as periods of hypotension which

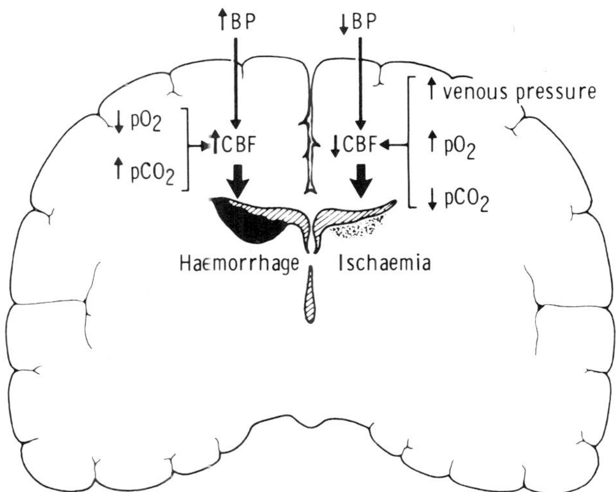

Fig. 6.7 Factors involved in causing either ischaemia, or hyperperfusion and haemorrhage in VLBW infants. (From Pape & Wigglesworth, 1979.)

render the subependymal layer ischaemic make the blood vessels, already fragile because of their anomalous configuration even more susceptible to such surges in CBF.

Incidence and sequelae

In the last few years, the use of CAT scanners (Krishnamoorthy et al, 1977; Papile et al, 1978a; Lee et al, 1979), and small portable real time ultrasound scanners (Pape et al, 1979; Graziani et al, 1980; Allen et al, 1980) have shown that GLH and IVH occur in up to 50 per cent of all infants weighing 1.00 to 1.50 kg at birth, and are even more common in infants weighing less than 1.00 kg (Papile et al, 1978a) and those on IPPV (Lee et al, 1979). Many of these haemorrhages are asymptomatic.

The implications of these findings are still being evaluated. Some of the survivors have resolution of the CAT scan changes (Papile et al, 1978a) and are making apparently normal developmental progress (Goldstein et al, 1976; Krishnamoorthy et al, 1979). Other infants may develop hydrocephalus within one to two weeks of birth, but there seems to be little point in doing serial lumbar punctures until there is ultrasound evidence of ventricular dilatation (Goldstein et al, 1976; Papile et al, 1980; Mantovani et al, 1980).

Up to 50 per cent of infants in whom serial LPs do not control the hydrocephalus and a c.s.f. shunting procedure is required may be handicapped (Chaplin et al, 1980).

REFERENCES

Aber R C, Allen N, Howell J T, Wilkenson H W, Facklam P R 1976 Nosocomial transmission of group B streptococci. Pediatrics 58: 356–353

Ablow R C, Driscoll S G, Effman E L, Jolles C J, Uauy R, Warshaw J B 1976 A comparison of early onset group B streptococcal neonatal infection and the respiratory distress syndrome of the newborn. New England Journal of Medicine 294: 65–70

Alden E R, Mandelkorn T, Woodrum D E, Wennberg R P, Parks C R, Hodson W A 1972 Morbidity and mortality of infants weighing less than 1000 grams on an intensive care nursery. Pediatrics 50: 40–49

Allen W C, Roveto C A, Sawyer L R, Courtney S E, 1980 Sector scan ultrasound imaging through the anterior fontanelle. American Journal of Diseases of Children 134: 1028–131

Andersen G E, Friis-Hansen B 1978 Hypercholesterolaemia in the newborn: Occurrence after antepartum treatment with betamethasone-phenobarbitone-ritodrine for the prevention of respiratory distress syndrome. Pediatrics 62: 8–12

Anthony B F, Okada D M 1977 The emergence of group B streptococcal infections of the newborn infant. Annual Review of Medicine 28: 355–369

Anthony B F, Okada D M, Hobel C J 1979. Epidemiology of the group B streptococcus: Maternal and nosocomial sources for infant acquisitions. Journal of Pediatrics 95: 431–436

Asplund K, 1972 Effects of postnatal feeding on the functional maturation of pancreatic islet cells of neonatal rats. Diabetologia 8: 153–159

Atkinson S A, Bryan M H, Anderson G H 1978 Human milk: Difference in nitrogen concentration in milk from mothers of term and premature infants. Journal of Pediatrics 93: 67–69

Atkinson S A, Radde I C, Chance G W, Bryan M H, Anderson G H 1980 Macromineral content of milk obtained during early lactation from mothers of premature infants. Early Human Development 4: 5–14

Aurichio S, Rubino A, Murset G 1965 Intestinal glycosidase activities in the human embryo, fetus and newborn. Pediatrics 35: 944–954

Baker C J, Casper D L 1976 Correlation of maternal antibody deficiency with susceptibility to neonatal group B streptococcal infection. New England Journal of Medicine 294: 753–756

Baker C J, Webb B J, Jackson C V, Edwards M S 1980 Countercurrent immunoelectrophoresis in the evaluation of infants with group B streptococcal disease. Pediatrics 65: 1110–1114

Bale J F, Watkins M 1978 Fulminant neonatal haemophilus influenza pneumonia and sepsis. Journal of Pediatrics 92: 233–234

Ballard R A, Ballard P L, Granberg J P, Sniderman E 1979 Prenatal administration of betamethasone for prevention of respiratory distress syndrome. Journal of Pediatrics 94: 97–101

Ballard P L, Ballard R A, Granberg J P, Sniderman S, Gluckman P D, Kaplan S, Grumbach M M 1980
  Fetal sex and prenatal betamethasone therapy. Journal of Pediatrics 97: 451–454
Baum J D 1979 Raw breast milk for babies in neonatal units. Lancet ii: 898
Beachler C W, Baker C J, Kasper D L, Fleming D K, Webb B J, Yow M D 1979 Group B streptococcal
  colonization and antibody status in lower socioeconomic parturient women. American Journal of
  Obstetrics and Gynecology 133: 171–173
Beirholm E A, Grantham R N, O'Keefe D D, Laver M B, Doggett W M 1975 Effects of acid-base changes,
  hypoxia and catecholamines on ventricular function. American Journal of Physiology 228: 1555–1561
Belenky D A, Orr R J, Woodrum D E, Hodgson W A 1976 Is continuous transpulmonary pressure better
  than conventional respiratory management of hyaline membrane disease? A controlled study. Pediatrics
  58: 800–808
Bell E F, Oh W D 1979 Fluid and electrolyte balance in very low birthweight infants. Clinics in
  Perinatology 6: 139–150
Bell E F, Warburton D, Stonestreet B S, Oh W 1979 High volume fluid intake predisposes premature
  infants to necrotising enterocolitis. Lancet ii: 90
Bell E F, Weinstein M R, Oh W 1980 Heat balance in premature infants: Comparative effects of
  convectively heated incubator and radiant warmer, with and without a plastic heat shield. Journal of
  Pediatrics 96: 460–465
Bell M J, Ternberg J L, Feigin R D, Keating J P, Marshall R, Barton L, Brotherton T 1978 Neonatal
  necrotizing enterocolitis. Annals of Surgery 187: 1–7
Berg T J, Pagtakhan R D, Reed M H, Langston C, Chernick V 1975 Bronchopulmonary dysplasia and lung
  rupture in hyaline membrane disease. Influence of continuous distending pressure. Pediatrics 55: 51–54
Berman W, Dubynsky O, Whitman V, Friedman A, Maisels M J 1978 Digoxin therapy in low birthweight
  infants with patent ductus arteriosus. Journal of Pediatrics 93: 652–655
Bland R D, Kim M H, Light M J, Woodson J L 1977 High frequency mechanical ventilation of low
  birthweight infants with respiratory failure from hyaline membrane disease. Pediatric Research 1977
  11: 531 (Abstract)
Block M F, Kling O R, Crosby W M 1976 Antenatal glucocorticoid therapy for the prevention of
  respiratory distress syndrome in the premature infant. Obstetrics and Gynecology 50: 186–190
Boellner S W, Beard A G, Panos T C 1965 Impairment of intestinal hydrolysis of lactose in newborn
  infants. Pediatrics 36: 542–550
Book L S, Herbst J J, Atherton S O, Jung A L 1975 Necrotizing enterocolitis in low birthweight infants fed
  an elemental diet. Journal of Pediatrics 37: 602–605
Book L S, Herbst J J, Jung A L 1976 Carbohydrate malabsorption in necrotizing enterocolitis. Pediatrics
  57: 201–204
Book L S, Herbst J J, Jung A L 1976b Comparison of fast- and slow-feeding rate schedule to the
  development of necrotizing enterocolitis. Journal of Pediatrics 89: 463–466
Book L S, Overall J C, Herbst J J, Britt M R, Epstein B, Jung A L 1977 Clustering of necrotizing
  enterocolitis. New England Journal of Medicine 277: 984–988
Borkowff H J, Grausz J P, Delfs E 1979 The effect of a perinatal center on perinatal mortality. Obstetrics
  and Gynecology 53: 633–640
Bortolussi R, Thompson T R, Ferrieri P 1977 Early onset pneumococcal sepsis in newborn infants.
  Pediatrics 60: 352–355
Bowes W A 1977 Results of the intensive perinatal management of very low birthweight infants. In:
  Anderson A, Beard R H, Brudenell J E, Dunn P M (eds) Preterm labour. Royal College of
  Obstetricians and Gynaecologists. London p 331–355
Bowes W A, Gabbe S G, Bowes C 1980 Fetal heart rate monitoring in premature infants weighing 1500 g or
  less. American Journal of Obstetrics and Gynecology 137: 791–796
Bowes W A, Taylor E S, O'Brien N, Bowes C 1979 Breech delivery. Evaluation of the method of delivery
  on perinatal results and maternal morbidity. American Journal of Obstetrics and Gynecology
  135: 965–970
Boyle R, Nelson J S, Stonestreet B S, Peter G, Oh W 1978 Alteration in stool flora resulting from oral
  kanamycin prophylaxis of necrotizing enterocolitis. Journal of Pediatrics 93: 857–861
Boyle R J, Chandler B D, Stonestreet B S, Oh W 1978 Early identification of sepsis in infants with
  respiratory distress. Pediatrics 62: 744–750
Brans Y W 1980 Meeting carbohydrate needs. In: Sunshine P (ed) Feeding the neonate weighing less than
  1500 g. Nutrition and beyond. Proceedings of Ross conference No. 79. Ross Laboratories, Columbus
  Ohio, p 23
Brimblecombe F S W, Rubissow J, Edelsten A D, Jones J 1978 A review of infant handicap and neonatal
  mortality in relation to the use of a special care unit. In: Brimblecombe F S W, Richards M P M,
  Roberton N R C (eds) Separation and special care baby units. Spastic International Medical Publications
  with William Heinemann, London, p 69–81

Bromberger P I, Chandler B, Gezon H, Haddon J E 1980 Rapid detection of neonatal group B streptococcal infections by latex agglutination. Journal of Pediatrics 96: 104–106

Broughton-Pipkin F, Smales O R C 1977 A study of factors affecting blood pressure and angiotensin $\bar{n}$ in newborn infants. Journal of Pediatrics 91: 113–119

Brown E G, Sweet A Y 1978 Preventing necrotizing enterocolitis in neonates. Journal of the American Medical Association 1978 240: 2452–2454

Brown E R 1979 Increased risk of bronchopulmonary dysplasia in infants with patent ductus arteriosus. Journal of Pediatrics 95, 865–866

Brown E R, Taeusch H W 1979 Intensive care of the very low birthweight infant. Lancet ii: 326–363.

Brumley G W, Crenshaw C 1980 Fetal lamb lung phosphatidylcholine; response to asphyxia and recovery. Journal of Pediatrics 97: 631–634

Bullen C L, Nillis A T 1971 Resistance of the breast fed infant to gastroenteritis. British Medical Journal iii: 338–343

Buntain W L, Conner E, Emrico J, Cassidy G 1979 Transcutaneous oxygen measurements as an aid to fluid therapy in necrotizing enterocolitis. Journal of Pediatric Surgery 14: 728–731

Bunton G L, Durbin G M, McIntosh N, Shaw D G, Taghizadeh A, Reynolds E. O. R, Rivers R P A, Urman G 1977 Necrotizing enterocolitis. Controlled study of 3 years experience in a neonatal intensive care unit. Archives of Disease in Childhood 52: 772–777

Butler N R, Alberman E D 1969 Perinatal problems. The second report of the 1958 British Perinatal Mortality survey. Livingstone, Edinburgh, p 186, Table 10.2

Carroll L, Osman M, Davies D P, McNeish A S 1979 Bacteriological criteria for feeding raw breast milk to babies on neonatal units. Lancet ii: 732–733

Caspi E, Schreyer P, Weinraub Z, Reif R, Levi I, Mundel G 1976 Prevention of the respiratory distress syndrome in premature infants by antepartum glucocorticoid therapy. British Journal of Obstetrics and Gynaecology 83: 187–193

Chadd M A, Fraser A J 1970 A controlled trial of vitamin E therapy in infancy. International Journal of Vitamin and Nutrition Research 40: 610–615

Chamberlain R, Chamberlain G, Howlett B, Claireaux A 1975 British Births 1970, Volume I. The first week of life. Heinemann London, p 242

Chaplin E R, Goldstein G W, Myerberg D Z, Hunt J V, Tooley W H 1980 Posthaemorrhagic hydrocephalus in the preterm infant. Pediatrics 65: 901–909

Coceani F, Bishai I, White E, Bodache D, Obley P M 1978 Action of prostaglandins, endoperoxides and thromboxanes on the lamb ductus arteriosus. American Journal of Physiology 234: H117–H122

Committee on Environmental hazards 1978 Infant radiant warmers. Pediatrics 61: 133–114

Congdon P J, Lealman G T, 1980 Low birthweight infants in Bradford 1972–1979. British Medical Journal 281: 594–596

Conway M, Durbin G M, Ingram D, McIntosh N, Parker D, Reynolds E D R, Soulter L P 1976 Continuous monitoring of arterial oxygen tension using a catheter tip, polarographic electrode in infants. Pediatrics 57: 244–250

Cooke R W I, Gribbin B, Gunning A J, Pickering D 1978 Ligation of patent ductus arteriosus in the very low birthweight newborn infant. Archives of Disease in Childhood 53: 271–275

Cooke R W I, Rolfe P, Howat P 1979 Apparent cerebral blood flow in newborns with respiratory disease. Developmental Medicine and Child Neurology 21: 154–160

Cotton R B, Stahlman M T, Bender H W, Graham T P, Carterton W Z, Kovar I 1978 Randomised trial of early closure of symptomatic patent ductus arteriosus in small preterm infants. Journal of Pediatrics 93: 647–651

Cowan F 1979 Blood pressure and cerebral blood flow in the healthy neonate. Paper presented to the Paediatric Research Society. Manchester September 1979

Cowan J, Gordon H, Sanderson P J, Valman H B 1978 Group B streptococcal infection in a maternity unit. British Journal of Obstetrics and Gynaecology 85: 541–545

Crawford M A, Hall B M, Lawrance B M, Munhambo A 1976 Current medical research and opinion 4 supplement 1, p 33

Crone R K, Favorito J 1980 The effects of pancuronium bromide on infants with hyaline membrane disease. Journal of Pediatrics 97: 991–993

Cruz A C, Buhi W C, Birk S A, Spellacy W N 1976 Respiratory distress syndrome with mature lecithin/sphingomyelin ratios, diabetes mellitus, and low apgar scores. American Journal of Obstetrics and Gynecology 126: 78–82

Cunningham A S 1977 Morbidity in breast fed and artificially fed infants. Journal of Pediatrics 90: 726–729

Cunningham M D, Desai N S, Thompson S A, Greene J M 1978 Amniotic fluid phosphatidylglycerol in diabetic pregnancies. American Journal of Obstetrics and Gynecology 193: 719–724

Cunningham M D, Hollingsworth D R, Belin R P 1980 Impaired surfactant production in cretin lambs. Obstetrics and Gynecology 55: 439–443

Dale A, Stanley F J 1980 An epidemiological study of cerebral palsy in Western Australia 1965–75; Spastic cerebral palsy and perinatal factors. Developmental Medicine and Child Neurology 22: 13–24

Daneman A, Woodward S, de Silva M 1978 The radiology of neonatal necrotizing enterocolitis. Pediatric Radiology 7: 70–77

Dauncy M J, Shaw J C L, Urman J 1977 The absorption and retention of magnesium, zinc, and copper by low birthweight infants fed pasteurised human breast milk. Pediatric Research 11: 1033–1039

Davies P A, Tizard J P M 1975 Very low birthweight and subsequent neurological defect. Developmental Medicine and Child Neurology 17: 3–17

Dawes G S, Hibbard E, Windle W F 1964 The effect of alkali and glucose infusions on permanent brain damage in rhesus monkeys asphyxiated at birth. Journal of Pediatrics 65: 807–818

Dear P R F 1980 Effect of feeding on jugular venous blood flow in the normal newborn infant. Archives of Disease in Childhood 55: 365–370

Depp R, Boehm J J, Nosek J A, Dooley S L, Hobart J M 1980 Antenatal corticosteroids to prevent neonatal respiratory distress syndrome; risk versus benefit considerations. American Journal of Obstetrics and Gynecology 137: 338–349

Dluholucky S, Babic J, Taufer I 1976 Reduction in incidence and mortality of respiratory distress syndrome by administration of hydrocortisone to mother. Archives of Disease in Childhood 51: 420–423

Dobbing J 1974 Later development of the brain and its vulnerability. In: Davis J A, Dobbing J (eds) Scientific foundation of paediatrics. Heinemann, London, p 565–577

Drew J G, Johnstone R, Finocchiaro C, Taylor P S, Goldberg H J 1979 Effect of high energy feedings on low birthweight infants. Medical Journal of Australia i: 467–468

Drillien C M 1965 Possible causes of handicap in babies of low birthweight. Journal of Obstetrics and Gynaecology of the British Commonwealth 72: 993–997

Drillien C M 1967 The incidence of mental and physical handicap in school age children of very low birthweight. Pediatrics 39: 238–247

Dudrick S J, Wilmore D W, Vars H M 1967 Long term parenteral nutrition with growth in puppies and positive nitrogen balance in patients. Surgical Forum 18: 356–357

Duenhoelter J H, Wells C E, Reisch J S, Santos-Ramos R, Jimenez H H 1979 A paired controlled study of vaginal and abdominal delivery of the low birthweight breech fetus. Obstetrics and Gynecology 54: 310–313

Dunn P M 1963 Intestinal obstruction in the newborn with special reference to transient functional ileus associated with respiratory distress syndrome. Archives of Disease in Childhood 38: 459–467

Durbin G M, Hunter N J, McIntosh N, Reynolds E O R, Wimberley P D 1976 Controlled trial of continuous inflating pressure for hyaline membrane disease. Archives of Disease in Childhood 51: 163–169

Dykes F D, Lazzara A, Ashmann P, Blumenstein B, Schwartz J, Brann A W 1980 Intraventricular haemorrhage; A prospective evaluation of etiopathogenesis. Pediatrics 66: 42–49

Egan E A, Mantilla G, Nelson R M, Eitzman D V 1976 A prospective controlled trial of oral kanamycin in the prevention of neonatal necrotizing enterocolitis. Journal of Pediatrics 89: 467–470

Ehrenkranz R A, Ablow R C, Warshaw J B 1979 Prevention of bronchopulmonary dysplasia with vitamin E administration during the acute stages of respiratory distress syndrome. Journal of Pediatrics 95: 873–878

Elman R, Weiner D O 1939 Intravenous alimentation with special reference to protein (amino-acid) metabolism. Journal of the American Medical Association 112: 796–802

Embil J A, Belgaumkar T K, McDonald S W 1978 Group B beta haemolytic streptococci in an intramural neonatal population. Scandinavian Journal of Infectious Diseases 10: 50–52

Evans D, Bowie M D, Hansen J D L, Moodie A D, van der Spuy H I J 1980 Intellectual development and nutrition. Journal of Pediatrics 93: 358–363

Evans T J, Ryley H C, Neale L M 1978 Effect of storage and heat on antimicrobial proteins in human milk. Archives of Disease in Childhood 53: 239–241

Fanaroff A A, Merkatz I R 1977 Modern obstetrical management of the low birthweight infant. Clinics in Perinatology 4: 215–237

Fisch R O, Bilek M K, Miller L D, Engel R R 1975 Physical and mental status at 4 years of age of survivors of the respiratory distress syndrome. Journal of Pediatrics 86: 497–503

Fleischman A R 1977 Another potential hazard of radiant warmers. Journal of Pediatrics 91: 984

Fomon S J, Zeigler E E, Vazquez H D 1977 Human milk and the small premature infant. American Journal of Diseases in Childhood 131: 463–467

Frantz I D, L'Heureux P, Engel, Hunt C E 1975 Necrotizing enterocolitis. Journal of Pediatrics 86: 259–263

Fujimura M, Salisbury D M, Robinson R O, Howat P, Emerson P M, Keeling J W, Tizard J P M 1979

Clinical events relating to intraventricular haemorrhage in the newborn. Archives of Disease in Childhood 54: 409–414

Fujiwara T, Maeta H, Chida S, Morita T, Watabey Y, Abe T 1980 Artificial surfactant therapy in hyaline membrane disease. Lancet i: 55–59

Gardner S E, Yow M D, Leeds L J, Thompson P K, Mason C O, Clark D J 1979 Failure of penicillin to eradicate group B streptococcal colonization of the pregnant woman. American Journal of Obstetrics and Gynecology 135: 1062–1065

Gaull G E, Hommes F A, Roux J F 1978 Human biochemical development. In: Faulkner F, Tanner J M (eds) Human growth i: Plenum Press, New York, p 23

Gaull G E, Rassin D K, Raiha N C R, Heinonen K 1977 Milk protein quantity and availability in low birthweight infants. III effects of sulphur amino-acids in plasma and urine Journal of Pediatrics 90: 356–360

Gamsu H R, Light F, Potter A, Price J F 1979 Intensive care and the very low birthweight infant. Lancet ii: 737

Gentz J, Persson B, Kellum M, Bengtsson G, Thorell J 1971 Effect of feeding on intravenous glucose tolerance and insulin response in piglets during the first day of life. Life Sciences 10: 137–144

Gerard P, Verghote-D'Hulst M, Bachy A, Duhaut G 1979 Group B streptococcal colonization of pregnant women and their neonates. Acta Paediatrica Scandinavica 68: 819–823

Gerrard J 1974 Breast feeding: Second thoughts. Pediatrics 54: 757–769

Gibbs J A H 1980 'Routine' total and supplemental parenteral nutrition for the very low birthweight infant. In: Sunshine P (ed) Feeding the neonate less than 1500 g — Nutrition and beyond. Proceedings of 79th Ross Conference, Ross, Laboratories, Ross, Columbus, Ohio, p 66

Gibbs J H, Fisher C, Bhattacharya S, Goddard P, Baum J D 1978 Drip breast milk; its composition, collection and pasteurisation. Early Human Development 1: 227–245

Glass L, Rajegowda B D, Evans H E 1971 Absence of respiratory distress syndrome in premature infants of heroin addicted mothers. Lancet i: 685–686

Gluck L, Kulovich M V, Eidelman A I, Cordero L, Khazin A F, 1972 Biochemical development of surfactant activity in mammalian lung. IV pulmonary lecithin synthesis in the human fetus and newborn, and etiology of the respiratory distress syndrome. Pediatric Research 6: 82–99

Goddard D, Lewis R M, Alcala H, Zeller R S 1980 Intraventricular haemorrhage — an animal model. Biology of the Neonate 37: 39–52

Goddard J, Lewis R M, Armstrong D L, Zeller R S 1980 Moderate rapidly induced hypertension as a cause of intraventricular haemorrhage in the newborn beagle model. Journal of Pediatrics 96: 1057–1060

Goetzman B W, Milstein J M 1979 Pulmonary vasodilator action of Tolazoline. Pediatric Research 13: 942–944

Goetzman B W, Sunshine P, Johnson J D, Wennberg R P, Hackel A, Merton D F, Bartoletti A L, Silverman N H 1976 Neonatal hypoxia and pulmonary vasospasm: response to Tolazoline. Journal of Pediatrics 89: 617–621

Golde S H, Mosley G H 1980 A blind comparison of the lung phospholipid profile, fluorescence microviscometry and the lecithin sphingomyelin ratio. American Journal of Obstetrics and Gynecology 136: 222–227

Goldenberg R L, Nelson K G 1977 The premature breech. American Journal of Obstetrics and Gynecology 127: 240–244

Goldman H I 1980 Feeding and necrotizing enterocolitis. American Journal of Diseases in Children 134: 553–555

Goldman H I, Goldman J S, Kaufman I 1974 Late effects of early dietary protein intake on low birthweight infants. Journal of Pediatrics 85: 764–769

Goldstein G. W, Chaplin E R, Maitland J, Norman D 1976 Transient hydrocephalus in premature infants: treatment by lumbar punctures. Lancet i: 512–515

Graziani L, Dave R, Desai H, Branca P, Waldroup L, Goldberg B 1980 Ultrasound studies in preterm infants with hydrocephalus. Journal of Pediatrics 97: 624–630

Gregory G A, Kitterman J S, Phibbs R H, Tooley W H, Hamilton W K 1971 Treatment of idiopathic respiratory distress syndrome with continuous positive airway pressure. New England Journal of Medicine 284: 1333–1340

Gross I 1979 The hormonal regulation of fetal lung maturation. Clinics in Perinatology 6: 377–395

Grylack L J, Scanlon J W 1978 Oral gentamicin therapy in the prevention of neonatal necrotizing enterocolitis. American Journal of Diseases of Children 132: 1192–1194

Guinan M, Schaberg D, Bruhn F W, Richardson C J, Fox W W 1979 Epidemic occurrence of neonatal necrotizing enterocolitis. American Journal of Diseases of Children 133: 594–597

Gyorgy P 1971 Biochemical aspects of human milk. American Journal of Clinical Nutrition 24: 970–975

Hadjigeorgiou E, Kitsiou S, Psaroudakis A, Segos C, Nicolopoulos D, Kaskarelis D 1979 Antepartum aminophylline for prevention of the respiratory distress syndrome in premature infants. American Journal of Obstetrics and Gynecology 135: 257–260

Hagberg B, Hagberg G, Olow I 1975 The changing panorama of cerebral palsy in Sweden 1954–1970. Acta Paediatrica Scandinavica 64: 187–192

Hakanson D O, Oh W 1977 Necrotizing enterocolitis and hyperviscosity in the newborn infant. Journal Pediatrics 90: 458–461

Hall B M, Oxberry J M 1977 Comparative studies on milk lipids and neonatal brain development. In: Peaker M (ed) Comparative aspects of lactation. Academic Press, New York

Hall R T, Barnes W, Krishnan L, Harris D J, Rhodes P G, Fayez J, Miller G L 1976 Antibiotic treatment of parturient women colonised with Group B streptococci. American Journal of Obstetrics and Gynecology 124: 630–634

Hall R T, Oliver T K Jr 1971 Aortic blood pressure in infants admitted to a neonatal intensive care unit. American Journal of Diseases of Children 121: 145–147

Halliday H L, Hirata T, Brady J P 1979 Indomethacin therapy for large patent ductus arteriosus in the very low birthweight infant. Results and complications. Pediatrics 64: 154–159

Hambleton G, Wigglesworth J S 1976 Origin of intraventricular haemorrhage in the preterm infant. Archives of Disease in Childhood 51: 651–659

Hammarlund K, Sedin G 1979 Transepidermal water loss in newborn infants. Acta Paediatrica Scandinavica 68: 795–801

Hansen T N, Ritter D A, Speer M E, Kenny J D, Rudolph A J 1980 A randomized controlled study of oral gentamicin in the treatment of neonatal necrotizing enterocolitis. Journal of Pediatrics 97: 836–839

Harvey D R, Parkinson C E, Campbell S 1975 Risk of respiratory distress syndrome. Lancet i: 42

Hayes K C, Carey R E, Smidt S Y 1975 Retinal degeneration associated with taurine deficiency in the cat. Science 188: 949–951

Headings D L, Herrera A, Mazzi E, Bergman M A 1978 Fulminant neonatal septicaemia caused by streptococcus bovis. Journal of Pediatrics 92: 282–283

Henry G W, Stevens D C, Schreiner R L, Grosfeld J L, Ballantine T V N 1979 Respiratory paralysis to improve oxygenation and mortality in large newborn infants with respiratory distress. Journal of Pediatric Surgery 14: 761–766

Herbst J J, Minton S D, Book L S 1979 Gastroesophageal reflux causing respiratory distress and apnoea in newborn infants. Journal of Pediatrics 95: 763–768

Hittner H M, Godio L B, Rudolf A J, Adams J M, Carcia-Prats J A, Freidman Z, Kautz J A, Monaco W A 1981 Retrolental fibroplasia effect of vitamin E in a double-blind clinical study of preterm infants. N. Engl J Med 305: 1365–1371.

HMSO 1970 The Registrar Generals Statistical Survey of England and Wales for 1968. London HMSO 1970. Table 17

HMSO 1980 Mortality Statistics: childhood and maternity. Office of Population Censuses and Surveys, London HMSO 1980 Tables 13 and 16

Herman S, Reynolds E O R 1973 Methods for improving oxygenation in infants mechanically ventilated for severe hyaline membrane disease. Archives of Disease in Childhood 48: 612–617

Hommers M, Kendall A C 1976 The prognosis of the very low birthweight infant. Developmental Medicine and Child Neurology 18: 745–752

Howard F M, Flynn D M, Bradley J M, Noone P, Szavatkowski M 1977 Outbreak of necrotizing enterocolitis caused by Clostridium Butyricum. Lancet ii: 1099–1102

Howard J B, McCracken G H 1974 The spectrum of group B streptococcal infections. American Journal of Diseases of Children 128: 815–818

Howie R N, Liggins G C 1977 Clinical trial of antepartum betamethasone therapy for prevention of respiratory distress in preterm infants. In: Preterm labour. Anderson A B M, Beard R W, Brudenell J M, Dunn P M (eds) Royal College of Obstetricians, p 281–289

Huch R, Huch A, Albani M, Barviel M, Schulte F J, Wolf H, Rupprath B, Emmrich P, Stechele U, Duc G, Bucher H 1976 Transcutaneous PO_2 monitoring in routine management of infants and children with cardiorespiratory problems. Pediatrics 57: 681–690

Husband J, Husband P, Mallinson C N 1970 Gastric emptying of starch meals in the newborn. Lancet ii: 290–292

Ingemarsson I, Westgren M, Svenningsen N W 1978 Long term follow up of preterm infants in breech presentation delivered by caesarean section. Lancet ii: 172–175

Jacob J, Edwards D, Gluck L 1980 Early onset sepsis and pneumonia observed as respiratory distress syndrome. American Journal of Diseases of Children 134: 766–768

Jacobs M M, Knight A B, Arias F 1980 Maternal pulmonary edema resulting from betamimetic and glucocorticoid therapy. Obstetrics and Gynecology 56: 56–59

Jeffrey H, Mitchison R, Wigglesworth J S, Davies P A 1977 Early neonatal bacteraemia, comparisons of group B streptococcal, other Gram positive and Gram negative infections. Archives of Disease in Childhood 52: 683–686

Johnson L, Schaffer D, Rubinstein D, Crawford C S, Boggs T R 1974 The role of vitamin E in retrolental fibroplasia. Pediatric Research 10: 425 (Abstract)

Johnson T R, Schneider J 1978 Steroids in premature rupture of membranes. New England Journal of Medicine 298: 56–57

Jones R A K, Cummins M, Davies P A 1979a Intensive care and the very low birthweight infant. Lancet ii: 737–738

Jones R A K, Cummins M, Davies P A 1979b Infants of very low birthweight. A 15 year analysis. Lancet ii: 1332–1335

Jones R W A, Rochefort M J, Baum J D 1976 Increased insensible water loss in newborn infants nursed under radiant heaters. British Medical Journal ii: 1347–1350

Kanjanapone V, Hartig-Beecken I, Epstein M F 1980 Effect of Isoxuprine on fetal lung surfactant in rabbits. Pediatric Research 14: 278–281

Kerner J A, Sunshine P 1979 Parenteral alimentation. Seminars in Perinatology 3: 417–434

Kindley A D, Roberts P J, Tulloch W H 1977 Neonatal necrotizing enterocolitis. Lancet i: 649

Kitterman J A 1975. In: Moore T D (ed) Necrotizing enterocolitis in the newborn infant. Report of the 68th Ross Conference on Pediatric Research. Columbus Ohio, Ross Laboratories, p 38–41

Kliegman R M, Pittard W B, Fanaroff A A 1979a Necrotizing enterocolitis in neonates fed human milk. Journal of Pediatrics 95: 450–453

Kliegman R M, Fanaroff A A, Izant R, Speck W T 1979b Clostridia as pathogens in neonatal necrotizing enterocolitis. Journal of Pediatrics 95: 287–289

Kodovsky O, Vancher Y, Gasparo M 1980 TSH and ACTH are present in rats milk; they retain physiological activity when given perorally to sucking rats. Pediatric Research 14: 502 (Abstract)

Kogutt M S 1979 Necrotizing enterocolitis of infancy. Radiology 130: 367–370

Kosloske A M 1979 Necrotizing enterocolitis in the neonate. Surgery, Gynecology and Obstetrics 148: 259–269

Kosloske A M, Lilly J R 1978 Paracentesis and lavage for diagnosis of intestinal gangrene in neonatal necrotizing enterocolitis. Journal of Pediatric Surgery 13: 315–320

Kosloske A M, Ulrich J A 1980 A bacterological basis for the clinical presentations of necrotizing enterocolitis. Journal of Pediatric Surgery 15: 558–564

Kosloske A M, Ulrich J A, Hoffman H 1978 Fulminating necrotizing enterocolitis associated with clostridia. Lancet ii: 1014–1016

Kramer M S 1980 Do breast feeding and delayed solid protect against obesity. Pediatric Research 14: 503 (Abstract)

Krishnamoorthy K S, Fernandez R A, Momose K J, De Long G R, Moylan F M B, Todres I D, Shannon D C 1977 Evaluation of neonatal untracranial haemorrhage by computerized tomography. Pediatrics 59: 165–172

Krishnamoorthy K S, Shannon D C, De Long G R, Todres I D, Davis K R 1979 Neurological sequelae in the survivors of neonatal intraventricular haemorrhage. Pediatrics 64: 233–237

Kumar S P, Anday E K, Sacks L M, Ting R Y, Delivoria-Papadopoulos M 1980 Follow upstudies of very low birthweight infants (1250 grams or less) born and treated within a perinatal center. Pediatrics 66: 438–444

Lakdawala D R, Widdowson E M 1977 Vitamin D in human milk. Lancet i: 167–168

Lawson E E, Birdwell R L, Huang P S, Taeusch H W 1979 Augmentation of pulmonary surfactant secretion by lung expansion at birth. Pediatric Research 13: 611–614

Lay K S, Bancalari E, Malkus H, Baker R, Strauss J 1980 Acute effects of albumin infusion on blood volume and renal functions in premature infants with respiratory distress syndrome. Journal of Pediatrics 97: 619–623

Leahy F, Cates D, MacCallum M, Rigatto H 1980 Effect of CO_2 and 100% oxygen on cerebral blood flow in preterm infants. Journal of Applied Physiology 48: 468–472

Lee B C P, Grassi E, Schechner S, Auld P A M 1979 Neonatal intraventricular haemorrhage. A serial computed tomography study. Journal of Computer Assisted Tomography 3: 483–490

Leonidas J C, Hall R T 1976 Neonatal pneumatosis coli — a mild form of neonatal necrotizing enterocolitis. Journal of Pediatrics 89: 456–459

LeSouef P N, Morgan A K, Soutter L P, Reynolds E O R, Parker D 1978 Comparison of transcutaneous oxygen tension with arterial oxygen tension in newborn infants with severe respiratory illnesses. Pediatrics 62: 692–697

Liggins G C, Howie R N 1972 A controlled trial of antepartum glucocorticoid treatment for prevention of the respiratory distress syndrome in premature infants. Pediatrics 50: 515–525

Lilien L D, Yeh T F, Novak G M, Jacobs N M 1978 Early onset haemophilus sepsis in newborn infants. Clinical, roentgenographic and pathologic features. Pediatrics 62: 299–303

Lipscombe A P, Thorburn R, Reynolds E O R, Stewart A, Blackwell R J, Cusick G, Whitehead M 1981 Pneumothorax and cerebral haemorrhage in preterm infants. Lancet i: 414–416

Livaditis A, Wallgren G, Faxelius G 1974 Necrotizing enterocolitis after catheterization of the umbilical vessels. Acta Paediatrica Scandinavica 63: 277–282

Lloyd D J, Belgaumkar T K, Scott K E, Wort A J, Aterman K, Krause V W 1979 Prevention of group B beta haemolytic streptococcal septicaemia in low birthweight neonates by penicillin administered within two hours of birth. Lancet i: 713–715

Lock J E, Coceani F, Olley P M 1979a Direct and indirect pulmonary vascular effects of tolazline in the newborn lamb. Journal of Pediatrics 95 600–605

Lock J E, Olley P M, Coceani F, Swyer P R, Rowe R D 1979 Use of prostacyclin in presistent fetal circulation. Lancet i: 1343

Löfgren D, Henriksson P, Jacobson L, Johansson O 1979 Transcutaneous PO_2 monitoring in neonatal intensive care. Acta Paediatrica Scandinavica 67: 693–697

Lonnerdal B, Forsum E, Hambraeus L 1976 A longitudinal study of the protein, nitrogen and lactose contents of human milk from Swedish well nourished mothers. American Journal of Clinical Nutrition 29: 1127–1133

Lorenz U, Ruttgers H, Fox G, Kubli F 1974 Fetal pulmonary surfactant induction by bromhexine metabolite VIII. American Journal of Obstetrics and Gynecology 119: 1126–1128

Lou H C, Lassen N A, Friis-Hansen B 1979 Impaired autoregulation of cerebral blood flow in the distressed newborn infant. Journal of Pediatrics 94: 118–121

Lucas A, Adrian T E, Bloom S R, Aynsley-Green A 1980a Plasma pancreatic polypeptide in the human neonate. Acta Paediatrica Scandinavica 69: 211–214

Lucas A, Adrian T E, Christofides N, Bloom S R, Aynsley-Green A 1980b Plasma motilin, gastrin and enteroglucagon and feeding in the human newborn. Archives of Disease in Childhood 55: 673–677

Lucas A, Aynsley-Green A, Blackburn A M, Adrian T E, Bloom S R 1981 Plasma neurotensin in term and preterm infants. Acta Paediatrica Scandinavica 70: 201–206

Lucas A, Gibbs J A H, Baum J D 1978 The biology of drip breast milk. Early Human Development 2: 351–361

Lucas A, Lucas P J, Chavin S I, Lyster R L J, Baum J D 1980d Human milk formula. Early Human Development 4: 15–21

Lucas A, Mitchell M D 1978 Plasma prostaglandins in preterm neonates before and after treatment for patent ductus arteriosus. Lancet ii: 130–132

Lucas A, Mitchell M D 1980 Prostaglandins in human milk. Archives of Disease in Childhood 55: 950–952

Lucas A, Roberts C D 1977 Bacteriological quality control in human milk banking. British Medical Journal i: 80–82

Lucas A, Sarson D L, Bloom S R, Aynsley-Green A 1980b Developmental aspects of gastric inhibitory polypeptide (GIP) and its possible role in the enteroinsular axis in neonates. Acta Paediatrica Scandinavica 69: 321–325

Lucas W, Kirschbaum T, Assali N S 1966 Cephalic circulation and oxygen consumption before and after birth. American Journal of Physiology 210: 287–292

Lundstrom U, Siimes M A, Dallman P R 1978 At what age does iron supplementation become necessary in low birthweight infants? Journal of Pediatrics 91: 878–883

McCarthy J S, Zies L G, Gelband 1978 Age dependent closure of the patent ductus arteriosus by indomethacin. Pediatrics 62: 706–712

McCracken G H, Eitzman D V 1978 Necrotizing enterocolitis. American Journal of Diseases in Children 132: 1167–1168

McIntosh N, Walters R O 1979 Effect of Tolazoline in severe hyaline membrane disease. Archives of Disease in Childhood 54: 105–110

McMurphy D M, Heymann N A, Rudolph A M, Melman K L 1972 Developmental changes in constriction of the ductus arteriosus; responses to oxygen and vasoactive agents in the isolated ductus arteriosus of the fetal lamb. Pediatric Research 6: 231–238

Madansky D L, Lawson E E, Chernick V, Taeusch H W 1979 Pneumothorax and other forms of pulmonary air leak in newborns. American Review of Respiratory Disease 120: 729–737

Manroe B L, Rosenfield C R, Weinberg A G, Browne R 1977 The differential leucocyte count in the assessment and outcome of early-onset neonatal group B streptococcal disease. Journal of Pediatrics 91: 632–637

Mantovani J F, Pasternak J F, Mathew C P, Allan W C, Mills M T, Casper J, Volpe J J 1980 Failure of daily lumbar punctures to prevent the development of hydrocephalus following intraventricular haemorrhage. Journal of Pediatrics 97: 278–281

Marks K H, Gunther R C, Rossi J A, Maisels M J 1980 Oxygen consumption and insensible water loss in premature infants under radiant heaters. Pediatrics 66: 228–232

Menke J A, Giacoia G P, Jockin H 1979 Group B beta haemolytic streptococcal sepsis and the idiopathic respiratory distress syndrome. A comparison. Journal of Pediatrics 94: 467–471

Menkes J H, Welcher D W, Levi H S 1972 Elevated blood tyrosine and ultimate intelligence of prematures. Pediatrics 49: 218–224

Merenstein G B, Todd W A, Brown G, Yost C C, Luzier T 1980 Group B beta haemolytic streptococcus: randomized controlled treatment study at term. Obstetrics and Gynecology 55: 315–318

Merritt T A, Farrell P M 1976 Diminished pulmonary lecithin synthesis in acidosis. Experimental findings as related to the respiratory distress syndrome. Pediatrics 57: 32–40

Merritt T A, DiSessa T G, Feldman B H, Kirkpatrick S E, Gluck L, Friedman W F 1979 Closure of the patent ductus arteriosus with ligation and indomethacin. Journal of Pediatrics 93: 639–645

Milligan D W A 1980 Failure of autoregulation and intraventricular haemorrhage in preterm infants. Lancet i: 896–898

Milligan J E, Shennan A T 1980 Perinatal management and outcome in the infant weighing 1000–2000 G. American Journal of Obstetrics and Gynecology 136: 269–273

Mockrin L D, Bancalari E H 1975 Early versus delayed initiation of continuous negative pressure in infants with hyaline membrane disease. Journal of Pediatrics 87: 596–600

Morley C J, Bangham A D, Miller N, Davis J A 1981 Dry artificial lung surfactant and its effect on very premature babies. Lancet i: 64–68

Morrison J C, Whybrew W D, Bucovaz E T, Schneider J M 1978 Injection of corticorteroids into mother to prevent neonatal respiratory distress syndrome. American Journal of Obstetrics and Gynecology 131: 358–365

Murlin J R, Conklin R E, Marsh E M 1925. Energy metabolism of newborn babies. American Journal of Diseases of Children 55: 678–682

Mutch L M M, Brown N J, Speidel B D, Dunn P M 1981 Perinatal mortality and neonatal survival in Avon. 1976–79. British Medical Journal 282: 119–122

Neligan G A, Smith C A 1960 The blood pressure of newborn infants in asphyxial states and in hyaline membrane disease. Pediatrics 26: 735–744

Nelson R M, Resnick M B, Eitzman D V 1979 Intensive care and the very low birthweight infant. Lancet ii: 737

Neufeld N D, Sevanian A, Barrett C T, Kaplan S A 1979 Inhibition of surfactant production by insulin in fetal rabbit lung slices. Pediatric Research 13: 752–754

Nieburg P I 1979 Fatal group G streptococcal sepsis in a neonate. Scandinavian Journal of Infectious Diseases 11: 93–95

O'Brien W F, Cefalo R C 1980 Clinical applicability of amniotic fluid tests for fetal pulmonic maturity. American Journal of Obstetrics and Gynecology 136: 135–144

Ogata E D, Gregory G A, Kitterman J A, Phibbs R H, Tooley W H 1976 Pneumothorax in respiratory distress syndrome. Incidence and effect on vital signs, blood gases and pH. Pediatrics 58: 177–183

Okken A, Jonxis J H P, Rispens P, Zijlstra W G 1979 Insensible water loss and metabolic rate in low birthweight newborn infants. Pediatric Research 13: 1072–1075

Orme R, L'E, Eades S M 1968 Perforation of the bowel in the newborn and the complication of exchange transfusion. British Medical Journal iv: 349–351

Owen-Thomas J B, Ulan O A, Swyer P R 1968 The effect of varying respiratory gas flow rate on arterial oxygenation during IPPV in the respiratory distress syndrome. British Journal of Anaesthesia 40: 493–502

Oyarzun M J, Clements J A 1977 Ventilatory and cholinergic control of surfactant in the rabbit. Journal of Applied Physiology 43: 39–45

Oyarzun M J, Clements J A 1978 Control of lung surfactant by ventilation, adrenergic mediators and prostaglandins in the rabbit. American Review of Respiratory Disease 117: 879–891

Papageorgiou A N, Desgranges M F, Masson M, Colle E, Shatz R, Gelfand M M 1979 The antenatal use of betamethasone in the prevention of respiratory distress syndrome. A controlled double blind study. Pediatrics 63: 73–79

Pape K E, Blackwell R J, Cusick G, Sherwood A, Houang M T W, Thorburn R J, Reynolds E O R 1979 Ultrasound detection of brain damage in preterm infants. Lancet i: 1261–1264

Pape K E, Wigglesworth J S 1979 Haemorrhage and the perinatal brain. Spastics International Medical Publications. Wm Heinemann, London, p 53–54 and 144–145

Papile L A, Burstein J, Burstein R, Koffler H, Koops B 1978a Incidence and evolution of subependymal and intraventricular haemorrhage. A study of infants with birthweights less than 1500 gm. Journal of Pediatrics 92: 529–534

Papile L A, Burstein J, Burstein R, Koffler H, Koops B L, Johnson J D, 1980 Posthaemorrhagic hydrocephalus in low birthweight infants: Treatment by serial lumbar punctures. Journal of Pediatrics 97: 273–277

Pasnick M, Mead P B, Philip A G S 1980 Selective maternal culturing to identify group B streptococcal infection. American Journal of Obstetrics and Gynecology 138: 480–484

Peabody J L, Gregory G A, Willis M M, Tooley W H, 1978a Transcutaneous oxygen tension in sick infants. American Review of Respiratory Disease 118: 83–87

Peabody J L, Neese A L, Philip A G S, Lucey J F, Soyka L F 1978b Transcutaneous oxygen monitoring in aminophylline treated apnoeic infants. Pediatrics 62: 698–701

Pereira G R, Lemos J 1976 Comparative study between transpyloric (nasojejunal) and intermittent gavage feeding in small preterm infants. Pediatric Research 10: 358 (abstract)

Philip A G S 1979 Intensive care and the very low birthweight infant. Lancet ii: 255

Pitcher-Wilmott R, Shutack J G, Fox W W 1979 Decreased lung volume after nasogastric feeding of neonates recovering from respiratory disease. Journal of Pediatrics 95: 119–121

Pittard W B, Clark D A 1977 Cellular and electrolyte changes in human breast milk with lactation. Pediatric Research 11: 448 (abstract)

Pollitzer M, Reynolds E O R, Shaw D G, Thomas R 1981 Pancuronium during mechanical ventilation speeds recovery of lungs of infants with hyaline membrane disease. Lancet i: 346–348

Pollitzer M J, Soutter L P, Reynolds E O R 1980 Continuous monitoring of arterial oxygen tension in infants: Four years of experience with an intravascular oxygen electrode. Pediatrics 66: 31–36

Powell J, Bureau M A, Pare C, Gaildry M L, Cabana D, Patriquin H 1980 Necrotizing enterocolitis. American Journal of Diseases in Children 134: 1152–1154

Ramamurthy R S, Pyati S P, Pildes R S 1979 Penicillin prophylaxis for group B streptococcal infection. Lancet ii: 246–247

Rassin D K, Gaull G E, Heinonen K, Räihä N C R 1977 Milk protein quantity and quality in low birthweigh infants. II effects of aliphatic amino-acids in plasma and urine. Pediatrics 59: 407–422

Reid T M S 1975 Emergence of group B streptococci in obstetric and perinatal infections. British Medical Journal ii: 533–535

Reiter B 1978 Review of the progress of Dairy Science. Antimicrobial systems in milk. Journal of Dairy Science 45: 131–147

Reynolds E O R, Taghizadeh A 1974 Improved prognosis of infants mechanically ventilated for hyaline membrane disease. Archives of Disease in Childhood 49: 505–515

Reynolds M L, Evans C A N, Reynolds E O R, Saunders N R, Durbin G M, Wigglesworth J S 1979 Intracranial haemorrhage in the preterm sheep fetus. Early Human Development 3: 163–186

Rhea J W, Ahmad M S, Mange M S 1975 Nasojejunal (transpyloric) feeding. A commentary. Journal of Pediatrics 86: 451–452

Rhodes P G, Hall R T 1973 Continuous positive airway pressure delivered by face mask in infants with idiopathic respiratory distress syndrome. A controlled study. Pediatrics 52: 1–5

Richards M. P. M, Roberton N R C 1978 Admission and discharge policies for special care baby units. In: Brimblecombe F S W, Richards M P M, Roberton N R C (eds) Separation and special care baby units. Spastics International Medical Publications, with William Heinemann, London, p 82

Roberton N R C 1976 Respiratory disease in early life. In: Stretton T B (ed) Recent advances in respiratory medicine. Churchill Livingstone, Edinburgh, p 222

Roberton N R C, Tizard J P M 1975 Prognosis for infants with idiopathic respiratory distress syndrome. British Medical Journal iii: 271–274

Rowley M P, Dahlenburg G W 1978 Gentamicin in prophylaxis of neonatal necrotizing enterocolitis. Lancet ii: 532

Roy C C, Ste Marie M, Chartrand L, Weber R T A, Bard H, Doray B 1975 Correction of the malabsorption of the preterm infant with a medium chain triglyceride formula. Journal of Pediatrics 86: 446–450

Rutter N, Hull D 1979 Water loss from the skin of preterm babies. Archives of Disease in Childhood 54: 858–868

Ryder R W, Shelton J D, Guinan M E, and the Committee on Necrotizing Enterocolitis: Necrotizing enterocolitis a prospective multicenter investigation. American Journal of Epidemiology 112: 113–124

Sack J 1980 Hormones in milk: In Freier, S, Eidelman A I (eds). Human milk, its biological and social values, p 56–61

Santulli T V, Schullinger J N, Heird W C, Gongaware R D, Wigger J, Barlow B, Blanc N A, Berdon W E 1975 Acute necrotizing enterocolitis in infancy. A review of 64 cases. Pediatrics 55: 376–387

Scanlon J 1971 The early detection of neonatal sepsis by examination of liquid obtained from the external ear canal. Journal of Pediatrics 79: 247–249

Schauf V, Deveikis A, Riff L, Serota A 1976 Antibiotic killing kinetics of group B streptococci. Journal of Pediatrics 89: 194–198

Schauf V, Hlaing V 1976 Group B streptococcal colonization in pregnancy. Obstetrics and Gynecology 47: 719–721

Schönberger W, Grimm W, Emmrich P, Gempp W 1981 Reduction of mortality rate in premature infants by substitution of thyroid hormones. European Journal of Pediatrics 135: 245–253

Schreiner R L 1980 Continuous and bolus feeding techniques in the low birthweight infant. Benefits and complications. In: Sunshine P (ed) Feeding the neonate weighing less than 1500 g — Nutrition and beyond. Proceedings of the 79th Ross Conference on Pediatric Research. Ross Laboratories, Columbus Ohio, p 78

Schutte M F, Treffers P E, Koppe J G, Breur W 1980 The influence of betamethasone and orciprenaline on the incidence of respiratory distress syndrome in the newborn after preterm labour. British Journal of Obstetrics and Gynaecology 87: 127–131

Schwartz M Z, Richardson J, Hayden C K, Swischuk L E, Tyson K R T 1980 Intestinal stenosis following successful medical management of NEC. Journal of Pediatric Surgery 15: 890–897

Semchyshyn S 1981 Gastrointestinal haemorrhage in the puerperium of pre-eclamptic patients who received glucorticoid therapy. American Journal of Obstetrics and Gynecology 139: 217–218

Senterre J 1979. In: Visser H K A (ed) Nutrition and metabolism of the fetus and neonate. Nijhoff, The Hague, p 195

Sevanian A, Gilden C, Kaplan S A, Barrett C T 1979 Enhancement of fetal lung surfactant production by aminophylline. Pediatric Research 13: 1336–1340

Shannon D C 1979 Chronic complications of respiratory therapy in the newborn. In: Thebault D W, Gregory G A (eds) Neonatal pulmonary care. Addison-Wesley, Menlo Park, California, p 401–409

Shaw J C L 1973 Parenteral nutrition in the management of sick low birthweight infants. Pediatric Clinics of North America 20, 333–358

Shaw J C L 1976 Evidence for defective skeletal mineralisation in low birth weight infants: the absorption of calcium and fat; Pediatrics 57: 16–25

Siegel J D, McCracken G H, Threlkeld N, Milvenan B, Rosenfield C R 1980 Single dose penicillin prophylaxis against neonatal group B streptococcal infections. New England Journal of Medicine 303: 769–775

Silverman W A, Blanc W A (1957) The effect of humidity on the survival of newly born premature infants. Pediatrics 20: 477–487

Simmons M A, Adcock E Q, Bard H, Battaglia F C 1974 Hypernatremia and intracranial haemorrhage in neonates. New England Journal of Medicine 291: 6–10

Sinclair A J, Crawford M A 1972 The accumulation of arachidonate and docasa-hexaenoate in the developing rat brain. Journal of Neurochemistry 19: 1753–1758

Slack M P E, Mayon-White R T 1978 Group B streptococci in pharyngeal aspirates at birth and the early detection of neonatal sepsis. Archives of Disease in Childhood 53: 540–544

Smallpiece V, Davies P A 1964 Immediate feeding of premature infants with undiluted breast milk. Lancet 1964 ii: 1349–1352

Smith C A 1976 Physiology of digestive tract. In: Smith C A, Nelson N M (eds) The physiology of the newborn infant. Thomas. Springfield, Illinois

Smith M F, Borriello S P, Clayden G S, Casewell M W 1980 Clinical and bacteriological findings in necrotizing enterocolitis: a controlled study. Journal of Infection 2: 23–32

Smith M L, Spencer S A, Hull D 1980 Mode of delivery and survival in babies weighing less than 2000 G at birth. British Medical Journal 281: 1118–1119

Smith P C, Schach E, Dally W J R 1972 Mechanical ventilation of newborn infants. II Effects of independent variation of rate and pressure on arterial oxygenation of infants with respiratory distress syndrome. Anesthesiology 37: 498–502

Southgate D A T, Widdowson E M, Smits B J, Cooke W J, Walker C H M, Mathers N P 1969 Absorption and excretion of calcium and fat by young infants. Lancet i: 487–489

Speer M E, Taber L H, Yow M D, Rudolph A J, Urteaga J, Waller S 1976 Fulminant neonatal sepsis and necrotizing entercolitis associated with a 'nonenteropathogenic' strain of Escherichia Coli. Journal of Pediatrics 89: 91–95

Speidel B P 1978 Adverse effects of routine procedures on preterm infants. Lancet i: 864–866

Stanley F H, Hobbs M S T 1980 Neonatal mortality and cerebral palsy: the impact of neonatal intensive care. Australian Paediatric Journal 16: 35–39

Stahlman M T, Cheatham W, Gray M E 1979 The role of air dissection in bronchopulmonary dysplasia. Journal of Pediatrics 95: 878–882

Stark A R, Bascom R, Frantz I D 1979 Muscle relaxation in mechanically ventilated infants. Journal of Pediatrics 94: 439–443

Starkey R H, Orth D N 1977 Radioimmunoassay of human epidermal growth factor (Urogastrone). Journal of Clinical Endocrinology and Metabolism 45: 1144–1153

Steiner E S, Saunders E M, Phillips E C K, Maddock C R 1980 Very low birthweight children at school age: comparison of neonatal management methods. British Medical Journal ii: 1237–1240

Stevens D C, Schreiner R L, Bull M J, Bryson C Q, Lemons J A, Gresham E L, Grosfield J L, Weber T R

1980 An analysis of tolazoline therapy in the critically ill neonate. Journal of Pediatric Surgery 15: 964–970

Steigman A J, Bottone M J, Hanna B A 1978 Intramuscular penicillin administration at birth. Prevention of early onset group B streptococcal disease. Pediatrics 62: 842–843

Stewart A 1977 Follow up of preterm infants. In: Anderson A, Beard R M, Brudenell J M, Dunn P M (eds) Preterm labour. Royal College of Obstetricians and Gynaecologists, London, p 372–384

Stewart A L, Reynolds E O R 1979 Intensive care and the very low birthweight infant. Lancet ii: 846–847

Stewart A, Reynolds E O R, Lipscombe A P 1981 Outcome for infants of very low birthweight: Survey of world literature. Lancet i: 1038–1040

Stewart A, Turcan D, Rawlings G, Hart S, Gregory S 1978 Outcome for infants at high risk of major handicap. In: Major mental handicap: methods and costs of prevention. Ciba Foundation Symposium No 59. Elsevier: Excerpta Medica, North Holland, Amsterdam, Holland, New York, p 151–163

Stocks J 1980 The effect of nasogastric tubes on nasal resistance during infancy. Archives of Disease in Childhood 55: 17–21

Stoddard R W, Widdowson E M 1976 Changes in the organs of pigs in response to feeding in the first 24 hours after birth. III Fluorescence histochemistry of carbohydrates of the intestine. Biology of the Neonate 29: 18–27

Stoll B S, Kanto W P, Glass R J, Nahmias A J, Brann A W 1980 Epidemiology of necrotizing enterocolitis. A case control study. Journal of Pediatrics 96: 447–451

Sturman J A, Gaull G E 1975. Taurine in the brain and liver of the developing human and monkey. Journal of Neurochemistry 25: 831–836

Sturman J A, Gaull G, Räihä N C R 1970 Absence of cystathionase in human fetal liver: Is cystine essential? Science 169: 74–76

Taeusch H W, Frigoletto F, Kitzmiller J, Avery M E, Hehre A, Fromm B, Lawson E, Neff R K 1979 Risk of respiratory distress after prenatal dexamethasone treatment. Pediatrics 63: 64–72

Taeusch H W, Kamait H, Hehre A, Tulchinsky D 1978 Dexamethsone and its effect on adrenal function in prematures. Pediatric Research 11: 422 (Abstract)

Tautibhedhyangkul P, Hashim S A 1975 Medium chain triglyceride feeding in premature infants. Effects on the fat and nitrogen absorption. Pediatrics 55: 359–370

Tautibhedhyangkul P, Hashim S A 1978 Medium chain triglyceride feeding in premature infants: Effects of calcium and magnesium absorption. Pediatrics 61: 537–545

Thornfeldt R E, Franklin R W, Pickering N A, Thornfeldt C R 1978 The effect of glucocorticoids on the maturation of premature lung membranes. American Journal of Obstetrics and Gynecology 131: 143–147

Tooley W H 1979 Epidemiology of bronchopulmonary dysplasia. Journal of Pediatrics 95: 851–855

Torday J S 1980 Glucocorticoid dependence of fetal lung maturation in vitro. Endocrinology 107: 839–844

Torma M J, DeLemos R A, Rogers J R, Diserens H W 1973 Necrotizing enterocolitis in infants. American Journal of Surgery 126: 758–761

Touloukian R J, Kadar A, Spencer R P 1973 The gastrointestinal complications of neonatal umbilical venous exchange transfusion: A clinical and experimental study. Pediatrics 51: 36–43

Tsang R C 1980 Vitamin D and bone mineralisation in neonates. In: Sunshine P (ed) Feeding the neonate weighing less than 1500 G — Nutrition and beyond. Proceedings of the 79th Ross Conference on Pediatric Research. Ross Laboratories, Columbus Ohio, p 32

Uauy R, Loo S, Gross I 1975 Nasojejunal feeding in the small premature infant: A controlled trial. Pediatric Research 9: 309 (Abstract)

Usher R 1963 Reduction of mortality from respiratory distress syndrome with early administration of intravenous glucose and sodium bicarbonate. Pediatrics 32: 966–975

Usher R H, Allen A C, McLean F H 1971 Risk of respiratory distress syndrome related to gestational age, route of delivery and maternal diabetes. American Journal of Obstetrics and Gynecology 111: 826–832

Visser H R A (ed) 1979 Nutrition and metabolism of the fetus and infant. Nijhoff, The Hague

Vogel L C, Boyer K M, Gadzala C A, Gotoff S P 1980 Prevalence of type specific group B streptococcal and antibody in pregnant women. Journal of Pediatrics 96: 1047–1051

Wald E R, Snyder M J, Gutberlet R L 1977 Group B haemolytic streptococcal colonization. American Journal of Diseases of Children 131: 178–180

Wells D H, Zachman R D 1975 Nasojejunal feedings in low birthweight infants. Journal of Pediatrics 87: 276–279

Wennberg R P, Schwartz R, Sweet A Y 1966 Early versus delayed feeding of low birthweight infants: Effects on physiological jaundice. Journal of Pediatrics 68: 860–866

Wharton B A, Bower B D 1965 Immediate or later feeding for premature babies. Lancet ii: 969–972

Whitby C, De Cates C R, Robertson N R C 1982 Infants weighing 1.80–2.50 kg: Should they be cared for in neonatal units or postnatal wards? Lancet i: 322–325

Whittle M J, Wilson A I, Whitfield C R, Paton R D, Logan R W 1981 Amniotic fluid phospholipid profile determined by two dimensional thin layer chromatography as an index of fetal lung maturation. British Medical Journal 282: 428–430

Widdowson E M, Colombo V E, Artaramis C A 1976 Changes in the organs of pigs in response to feeding for the first 24 hours after birth. II the digestive tract. Biology of the Neonate 28: 272–281

Wigglesworth J S, Keith I H, Girling D J, Slade S A 1976 Hyline membrane disease, alkali and intraventricular haemorrhage. Archives of Disease in Childhood 51: 755–762

Wilkinson A 1979 Personal communication

Wilkinson A, Yu V Y H 1974 Immediate effects of feeding on blood gases and some cardiorespiratory functions in ill newborn infants. Lancet i: 1083–1085

Williamson S, Finucane E, Ellis H, Gamsu H R 1978 Effect of heat treatment of human milk on absorption of nitrogen, fat, sodium, calcium and phosphorus by preterm infants. Archives of Disease in Childhood 53: 555–563

Winick M 1976 Nutrition and brain development. Oxford University Press, London

Woods J R 1979 Effects of low birthweight breech delivery on neonatal mortality. Obstetrics and Gynecology 53: 735–740

Wung J T, Koons A H, Driscoll J M, James L S 1979 Changing incidence of bronchopulmonary dysplasia. Journal of Pediatrics 85: 845–847

Yao A C, Wallgren C G, Sinha S N, Lind J 1971 Peripheral circulatory response to feeding in the newborn. Pediatrics 47: 378–383

Yashiro K, Adams F H, Emmanouilides G C, Mickey M R 1973 Preliminary studies on the thermal environment of low birthweight infants Journal of Pediatrics 82: 991–994

Yeung C Y, Tam A S Y 1972 Gastric aspirate findings in neonatal pneumonia. Archives of Disease in Childhood 47: 735–740

Yeh T F, Amma P, Lilien L D, Baccaro M M, Matwynshyn J, Pyati S, Pildes R S 1979 Reduction of insensible water loss in premature infants under the radiant heater. Journal of Pediatrics 94: 651–653

Young B K, Klein S A, Katz M, Wilson S J, Douglas G W 1980 Intravenous dexamethasone for prevention of neonatal respiratory distress. A prospective controlled study. American Journal of Obstetrics and Gynecology 138: 203–209

Yow M D, Leeds L J, Thompson P K, Mason E O, Clark D J, Beachler C W 1980 The natural history of group B streptococcal colonisation in the pregnant woman and her offspring. American Journal of Obstetrics and Gynecology 137: 34–38

Yow M D, Mason E O, Leeds L J, Thompson P K, Clark D J, Gardner S E 1979 Ampicillin prevents intrapartum transmission of group B streptococcus. Journal of the American Medical Association 241: 1245–1247

Yu V Y H, Hollingsworth E 1979 Improving prognosis for infants weighing 1000 g or less at birth. Archives of Disease in Childhood 55: 422–426

Yu V Y H, James B, Hendry P, MacMahon R A 1979 Total parenteral nutrition in very low birthweight infants: A controlled trial. Archives of Disease in Childhood 54: 653–661

Yu V Y H, Liew S W, Roberton N R C 1975 Pneumothorax in the newborn. Archives of Disease in Childhood 6: 449–453

Zanini B, Paul R H, Huey J R 1980 Intrapartum fetal heart rate: correlation with scalp pH in the preterm fetus. American Journal of Obstetrics and Gynecology 136: 43–47

7. Mother-infant interaction: the bonding of affection

Alfred White Franklin

The behaviour of a mother towards her baby and of a baby towards its mother should no longer be thought of as preordained, instinctive or inevitable. From careful observations and analyses of what really happens when the mother first perceives her baby's existence outside the womb, of what they both do and how they react to each other during the ensuing days and weeks, a complex picture has been constructed. Apart from the immediate effects of these interactions on the well-being of both, evidence has been gathered which strongly suggests that the pattern of those interactions influences the development of the baby and the relationships which it forms for many years if not for the rest of life. This pattern can be influenced by methods of perinatal management for better or for worse.

We think of the process of the development of the baby's first relationships as dependent upon a mother's love compounded of unselfishness, a readiness to sacrifice comfort, the wish to understand what the baby's needs are and the will to satisfy them, and pride in the fulfilment of a biological role on behalf of herself and her family. Unfortunately this kind of love from the mother is not always available.

Two strands of enquiry into both human and animal behaviour have given us insight; one is how the relationship grows and can be observed to grow under both natural and contrived experimental conditions, and the other is why, what is the purpose of the relationship. The strands are often interwoven. Three main groups of observers of behaviour can be identified (Ainsworth, 1969): those concerned with social learning theory, those interested in psychological development and psychoanalytic theories of object attachment, and ethologists. These aspects of behaviour do not exclude each other; nevertheless the work of ethologists especially in relation to attachment, which is the outward manifestation of the bond between mother and baby, seems the most relevant to the area of our concern for a joint approach to the management of the events of the ante-, peri- and postnatal periods by obstetricians, paediatricians and midwives.

To help achieve a balanced view, a selection is presented of the many studies of the newborn baby's sensory system and of interactions between itself and the mother from which so much has been learned. The altered outlook and attitudes attendant on the change from largely domiciliary to almost total hospital delivery are discussed together with some of the practical conclusions that follow.

THE INTERPRETATION OF BEHAVIOUR

Ethology

When Scott Williamson founded the Peckham Health Centre (Pearse, 1979) and began his studies of human ethology almost 50 years ago, his aim was to observe human family behaviour free from the distortion of outside intervention and without any imposed authority. He hoped to discover the core of evolved, biologically based behaviour. Unlike the learning theorists and the psychologists he had no theory except the theory of evolution into which his observations had to be fitted. He tried to be an objective observer.

Human ethology concerns itself with four interrelated aspects of a behaviour, its survival function, its evolution in the species, its development in the individual and by what internal and what external factors it is elicited (Weisfeld, 1979). The attachment of mother or some other adult caregiver and baby for feeding and protection is essential for the baby's survival and also for the survival of the species. In Bowlby's words (1969) attachment to a mother figure is an essential part of the ground-plan for the human species. If there is too little interaction with one principal caregiver the ground plan is unfulfilled. If the baby acquires an inner representation of the mother (caregiver) as generally accessible and responsive, it feels secure. When responses to the baby's needs are belated and inappropriate, it has no confidence in the mother and reacts to stress with anxiety. Ainsworth (1979) using a 'strange situation' technique which enabled her to watch the behaviour of year-old children when removed from mother and then reunited found that differences in behaviour were related to the baby's previous experience of the mother's responses. For example, children in the one group who disliked physical contact had mothers with the same aversion. Ainsworth concluded that 'differences in attachment are attributable to maternal behaviour'. Reviewing the literature she found evidence that these differences persist at least up to the age of six years. A secure baby is able to explore the environment; exploration widens experience and stimulates learning. If it be true that the baby's relationship with the mother provides the working model for the construction of all future human relationships, its importance for emotional development as well as for learning is apparent. That the organisation of attachment is finally fixed in the first year is difficult to believe. The baby must remain sensitive to change in maternal behaviour and to life's experiences, nevertheless the feeling of security and of being loved and valued acquired from birth provides the basis for the development of personality.

The bonding of affection

An important place in the development of attachment between mother and baby, and what seems to initiate it, has been claimed for a process named the bonding of affection. Many words of art, such as bonding, attachment, attachment behaviour, dependence, are intended to clarify concepts and to aid the understanding of observed phenomena. Unfortunately such words are quickly seized by various protagonists to be used with their own special meanings in accordance with a given hypothesis. Semantic problems ensue.

The bonding of affection can be variously interpreted. What it describes is an emotional interaction between a mother and her newborn baby when each accepts the other as an object of love, the dependence of the baby for warmth, feeding and protection being met by the mother's solicitude, milk and care. When bonding fails to take place, the baby's progress certainly can be handicapped with harmful and possibly lifelong effects. Some regard bonding as a critical happening reserved for the first few hours of life. The opportunity denied, the occasion does not recur. Others believe that while an immediate bonding often occurs, delay is possible and, as can be observed in clinical practice, even an immediate rejection on the grounds of baby's appearance, sex or deformity can change to acceptance with all the feeling believed to originate in bonding. No-one has suggested that failure of bonding and problems in the development of attachment between mother and baby are always followed by emotional handicaps but even those who are sceptical about the test methods used accept that 'early, mutually satisfying reciprocal social interactions between infant and care-giver are central to the optimal development of the infant and to the adult's satisfaction with caregiving' (Hock et al, 1979).

Circumstances arise which can certainly prevent the bonding process and impetus has been given to the subject by the realisation that a failure of bonding may play some part in the aetiology of child abuse and neglect. Among the possible preventive measures there is some hope that the removal of obstacles to bonding might make a valuable contribution. As so often happens in medicine, knowledge gathered in the study of severe abnormality produces unexpected insights into normal processes.

Accepting that bonding of affection is important to normal family life, all those circumstances which might place obstacles in the way of its development must be identified and examined. Taken one step further, sufficient knowledge should enable those responsible for maternity care positively to encourage bonding. In applying to practice the knowledge that exists, the paediatrician may well take the lead, but obstetricians, midwives and social workers all have their parts to play.

HISTORICAL PERSPECTIVE

The paediatrician now occupies a recognised place in maternity departments and needs to make no apology for his presence. The modern obstetrician must find it difficult to understand that it could ever have been otherwise. Yet the irruption of paediatricians into the departments in the United Kingdom only followed the establishment of the National Health Service in 1949, although there were exceptions. Observation combined with the increasing availability of investigative and laboratory methods suitable for the newborn baby and the fetus has increased knowledge both of physiology and pathology, paving the way for preventive as well as curative successes. Not all effects have been good. In some departments the obstetrician has washed his hands entirely of the product of his efforts, relinquishing the baby to the care of the paediatrician. Following tradition, many of the details of the care of mother and baby remain in the hands and at the discretion of the midwife. What should surely be a co-operative enterprise is too often conducted by three virtually independent professions, obstetric, paediatric and midwifery, largely in ignorance of each other's practice and point of view. Relevant knowledge of family circumstance is not always communicated to obstetric staff from the general practitioner, the health visitor or the social worker.

Recently other professionals have begun to concern themselves with what happens in maternity departments. Sociologists, anthropologists and ethologists are turning some of their attention from studies of animals and primitive tribes to westernised human families, and pushing back their frontiers at least as far as the labour ward if not to the antenatal department. Psycho-analysts, too, have begun to reach back in their adult patients' histories to neonatal experiences and psychiatrists to interest themselves in other perinatal problems than puerperal psychosis. And above all the mothers themselves are seriously reviewing the influence which they believe that they should exercise.

The obstetrician's responsibility

Through all these changes the obstetrician remains in primary charge of the obstetric department with the responsibility for securing, so far as it is possible, the birth of a healthy, normal baby to a mother unharmed by her obstetric experience. In recent history the first contributions to greater safety were made following Eardley Holland's improved understanding of the mechanics of labour (Holland & Lane-Claypon, 1926), enabling midwives as well as obstetricians to be better trained. The second contribution came from avoidance of preventable complications through antenatal supervision and care. Baird (1960) realised early the importance to the outcome of pregnancy of socio-economic status and the physical environment, including diet, housing and working career. Smoking and the consumption of drugs were added later. Preparation for breast feeding led in some departments to the appointment of special nurses, although many details of technique remain in dispute. In a fourth phase the paediatricians arrived to take over the care of the baby from the time of birth instead of at the time of discharge from hospital.

Antenatal paediatrics was pioneered through Parsons (1946), who made this the subject of his Blair Bell Lecture. At that time the vigour and growth of the baby and its immunity against disease, and the pregnant woman's diet held pride of place, while the danger to the fetus of rubella, recognised in 1941, raised hopes that some forms of congenital malformation acquired in utero might be preventable. The thalidomide tragedy, like the epidemic of retrolental fibroplasia, taught the sad lesson that iatrogenic damage was certainly possible.

Avoiding emotional damage

In all of this the emphasis was on the physical state of the baby. Health was equated with the absence of obstetric injury, of infection, of malformation or of such perinatal complications as disorders of respiration, haemolytic disease and immaturity. The last decade has seen the understanding grow of the importance of emotional reactions and of the need to recognise a sixth phase, in which the object is to avoid emotional damage and attitudes and management techniques that might prevent the establishment of happy relationships within the family when the new member returns home.

Just as the dangers of pregnancy and childbirth in terms of mortality and morbidity for mother as well as baby had to be recognised and studied before maternal deaths could be prevented and the fetus and the neonate protected from physical injury, so now the dangers of emotional damage need recognition and study. New observations and inferences compel us to re-examine in detail the whole management and care provided in maternity departments. 'Obstetric responsibility is now seen to begin at conception, to continue through the ante-, peri, and immediate postnatal periods and then to pay some regard to what will happen to mother, baby and the family when united at home . . .' (Franklin, 1980). This requires a team, but it is surely incumbent on the obstetrician to see that the total service is available within his department.

Handling and separation

Bonding of affection between mother and baby should not be regarded as an isolated phenomenon but rather as occupying a place, albeit a very important one, in the emotional interactions first between mother and baby and then between all the family members. That the newborn baby responds to its handling and management has long been known to those who have had the time to sit and study its behaviour. Bakwin (1949) noted that 'sight, hearing and equilibrium, taste, smell, the skin senses, the internal sensations are all functionally active at or soon after birth'. In those days fear of infection still dominated practice because penicillin was not always available and this fear ordained minimal handling of the baby. Deprived of sensory stimuli, especially of skin sensations and kinaesthetic sense, many babies failed to thrive. When routine methods in the baby ward at the Bellevue Hospital, New York, were changed so that babies were handled, the case fatality fell from between 30 and 35 per cent to under 10, and the fear of infection from this cause was shown to be without foundation. In most maternity departments the handling of newborn babies after forceps or Caesarian delivery was routinely forbidden, and it still is in some, with 24 or even 48 hours of so-called cot-nursing however normal the baby's condition. It is not clear what danger is avoided by depriving the baby of body contact, kinaesthetic experience and sensory stimuli which are the main sources of emotional reactions and 'set in motion processes that appear to be essential for the child's well-being' (Bakwin, 1949).

Bowlby (1956) drew attention, in his classical observations on the effects of mother-child separation, to the damage done to emotional development and to the child's subsequent behaviour. At that time he was concerned with the first three or five years of life when, it was accepted, 'the child is making his first social relationships — those with his parents.' Bowlby's work caused a revolution in ideas and more practically in the management of children in hospitals and other institutions but many years passed before doctors and nurses recognised that increasing hospital delivery meant that more and more newborn babies, as soon as they were born, were in one sense being admitted to hospital and then being separated from their mothers. Truly being born at home also means arrival in a new and strange environment, even if that is the mother's bed. Nevertheless the handling of the baby and contact with the mother present considerable differences both in quality and quantity in the two environments. The question arises of whether these differences can be sufficiently appreciated by the newborn baby to affect his development. The answer appears to be yes.

What constitutes good and bad maternal care is difficult to assess by any objective measurement. What is important is whether mother and baby satisfy each other. Doctors and nurses feel competent to recognise who is good at mothering and who is not in the absence of a quantitative unit of measurement for love. Measurable information has been sought through noting and counting the actual operations performed by the mother. Rheingold (1960) used 30 maternal and 12 infant items and recorded every fifteenth second for the first ten minutes of every consecutive quarter hour for eight hours (1280 observations). Comparing five babies at home with five in institutions she found statistically significant differences with four and a half times the amount of attention given to the former compared with the latter.

Talking, patting, adjusting baby's position, changing napkins occupied more of the mother's time at home. Bathing, dressing and showing affection did not differ significantly. Care by the mother as opposed to a number of caregivers produced consistency and life was considerably richer in the more complex family environment.

THE NEONATAL SENSORY SYSTEM

Since Bowlby's original report, more attention has been paid to the baby's first human relationships at the time of birth. A new look at the baby's behaviour suggested strongly that it should not be regarded as a kind of natural reflex reaction but that it had a pattern which grew out of his experiences. More than this, his behaviour could and did influence the reactions of his mother with a continuing flow of behavioural reactions and emotional responses between them. This raises questions of the baby's appreciation of sensory stimuli and of his adaptability.

Attentive behaviour
The gathering of evidence about the newborn baby's sensory system either for clinical or research purposes requires an understanding of the baby's attention span. The newborn baby is capable of attentive behaviour at birth, but this is fitful and the baby seems to go away into a world of its own, of inattention, between sleeps. Wolff (1959) made continuous observations on four normal newborns and later (1965) regular though intermittent observations on ten normal bottle-fed infants for the first month after birth. He distinguished four states: regular sleep, irregular sleep, alert inactivity and alert activity, and found that the baby was in its most responsive state during alert inactivity. The baby is fully awake, quiet, breathing regularly 50 to 60 a minute, eyes wide open with muscles relaxed. In this state appropriate stimuli were best able to produce auditory responses and conjugate eye movements. The time of alert attentiveness is short, the maximum for a specific task limited to five minutes in the first week and 30 minutes at one month. At first attentive behaviour is incompatible with muscular activity. After two weeks, muscular activity can accompany the performance of a familiar but not a new or complicated task. As well as responses to external stimuli the baby has inner needs like hunger, calls for food or for the relief of pain, which produce tension. If sleep be the natural state, wakefulness is initiated not only by external stimuli but also by an inner need.

Interpreting need states
These need states require interpretation by the mother or caregiver. A smile or the expression that precedes crying shows low tension of need, crying and kicking high tension. Hunger produces 'rhythmic braying' and kicking, and wind pain sporadic screeching (Wolff, 1959). Crying antedates speech as a means of communication. Cries from hunger, frustration and pain are audibly as well as spectrographically different. Many mothers soon learn to interpret the meaning as well as to recognise the cries of their own baby, sleeping through the crying of others but wakened by their own.

How far does the mother or caregiver understand this language, accept the cues and give the positive answer? To a greater or lesser extent the mother and the caregivers can either impose their own programme on the baby or else they must depend on looking for instructions provided by the baby's crying or movements. Crying initiates interaction and is interpreted as a request for mother or caregiver to come close, to stay close and to attend to needs (Lozoff et al, 1977). Proximity and body contact form important elements in the interaction. The future behaviour of the baby reflects the mother's success or failure in understanding and making the right response to the crying. Crying can be relieved when the baby is lifted upright on to the mother's shoulder and in this position the baby is quiet and visually alert, scanning the environment. Unravelling the skein of possible reasons is difficult. Motor activity is prevented by holding, there is the comfort of body contact and proprioceptive stimuli come into play.

Vision

What the baby sees appears to be very important. Many mothers describe their first eye to eye contact, when the baby 'looks deeply into their eyes' as a moment of first feeling love, of recognition of the baby as a real person, the mother's own baby. Brazelton (1961), using a moving red ring, demonstrated that the baby's ability to follow a moving object and to fixate, when in an alert attentive state, lasts for some hours after delivery. The baby can focus at 30 to 40 cm. Indeed following and fixation are among the first acts of the infant that are intentional and subject to his own control (Robson, 1967). He can withdraw visual attention. These visual responses are not automatic and many observations prove a baby's ability to discriminate. Goren et al (1975) in a study of 40 normal newborn babies at a mean age of nine minutes (3 to 27) after birth found that they were more likely to turn the head and follow with the eyes a drawing of a face than the drawings of the same features arranged in two different ways, for example, with mouth uppermost, both equally complex and bright. All three patterns received higher scores than a blank. By the age of two weeks the infant is more responsive to the mother's than to a stranger's face.

Newborn babies react differently towards an object and a person. Brazelton and his colleagues (1975) watched the interactions of twelve mothers and their infants. When face-to-face, something seemingly of great value to the baby, the baby's reaction is rhythmical, a phase of attention and approach alternating with non-attention and withdrawal. When the mother's face is unresponsive, the baby's movements change becoming jerky, he turns his face away and then tries to gain the mother's interest once more. If several attempts fail he curls up, movements cease and the face is averted. When mother once more looks interested, baby returns to the original reactive phase. If the breast feeding mother wears a mask some babies become distressed, feed and sleep poorly and avoid looking at her.

Confirmation of the importance of facial expression comes from observations on a family suffering from myotonic dystrophy which affected a mother and her baby (Lynch et al, 1979). Their inability to use facial expression effectively as a means of communication led to bonding failure. Fortunately the mother could be taught ways of overcoming the difficulty.

Visual skills are available for learning through gaining acquaintance with the environment and play a stimulating part in cognitive development. For the psycho-analyst they provide the clearest example observable in the neonate of 'primary autonomous ego function' (Korner & Grobstein, 1966).

Hearing

The newborn baby can respond non-verbally to the speaking voice, more to the female than to the male voice, and shows a preference for its own mother's voice.

Smell

Macfarlane (1975) investigated the newborn baby's sense of smell to discover whether smell can be used to locate the food source. He found that at two days 17 out of the 32 babies turned preferentially to the mother's breast pad and at six days the number had risen to 22. The baby can discriminate between olfactory stimuli as well as between visual stimuli.

Individuality and adaptability

The fundamental question, whether there are temperamental differences between newborn babies which can be observed before the mothers handle them and which might evoke different responses in the mother and affect her mothering, was studied by Korner et al (1968).

They analysed movements, recorded on film, of 32 normal, bottle-fed female infants 45 to 88-hours-old. Finger sucking and hand-mouth and hand-face contact were interrelated and correlated to high motility, endurance of crying and high levels of arousal. Mouthing showed only a correlation with hunger. These workers concluded that although babies exhibited innate individual characteristics which influenced the caregiver's reaction, they did adapt to the impact of experience and the influence of the environment in ways that were independent of individuality.

The legitimate conclusions from these studies seem to be that the newborn baby has not only its own individuality but also a complex system of responses to sensory as well as motor stimuli, that it does discriminate and that it can adapt to experience. In the light of these conclusions the details of care and management of the neonate must be perceived as influencing development and as being either advantageous or detrimental.

THE NEED FOR THE BONDING OF AFFECTION

The satisfaction of need

The idea is now generally accepted that the development of a newborn baby requires stimulation and the satisfaction of its emotional as well as its physical needs. The baby must be in a satisfactory state of mind to make use of stimulation. The traditional measure of a baby's progress has been by assessing physical growth and motor activity. Sensory input and opportunity for sensory exploration have not always been given due importance. The programme of physical development is laid down from head control, through sitting and standing to walking. Delays causing this development to get out of programme can produce handicaps. Undoubtedly emotional development can be distorted in a similar way.

Winnicott (1958) taught that creativity and confidence grow in the child when the mother is enough in tune with her baby to satisfy and to comfort as the need arises and before the need becomes too urgent. The baby cries and is comforted. The baby feels pleasantly hungry and food arrives giving rise to the illusions that satisfactions follow activity and that the baby has control over what happens. Later in infancy when the mother begins to separate from the baby, he can tolerate his loss and her gradual withdrawal while retaining his confidence and trust. Good mothering takes account of the principle that the baby's environment must be good enough yet not perfect, since the ultimate aim is the rearing of an independent person able in his turn to cope with life while benefitting from the support which a loving relationship can be relied upon to provide. This first loving relationship is now regarded as the model for all future human relationships. Mishandling of this first relationship can damage the personality in ways that continue for a whole life.

The failure to bond may be responsible for the affectionless psychopath, unable to make relationships with others and dangerous to society. The breaking of a bond is stressful but it does not always lead to breakdown. As in so much in life, parents need to keep in mind the Greek warning 'nothing too much'. Johnson and colleagues (1979) have drawn attention to the dangers of too intense attachment. Working with nine Vervet monkey pairs he observed that the offspring of the mothers who were least responsive and who had the most time off in the first three months were socially more competent at six months. Babies as well as mothers can be rejecting. This could simplify the baby's eventual autonomy and detachment; processes almost as important in development as the formation of the bond in the beginning. Mothering styles vary between frustrating, satisfying and promoting infant exploratory behaviour. Too intense attachment to the mother interferes with adequate growth of later and other social bonds. Nevertheless good bonding and attachment remain the ideal.

The effects of separation

Short-term

Evidence now exists that shows how easily the establishment of this relationship in the perinatal period can be disturbed to the detriment of mother and baby. When baby immediately after birth is separated for even so short a time as three weeks the mother feels less competent and her attachment behaviour decreases. Leiderman & Seashore (1975) found that the altered attitude and behaviour may take a month to recover. A follow up at 11, 12 and 15 months after discharge from hospital showed that despite the return to the 'normal' attitude the mothers who had been separated touched their infants less, suggesting incomplete recovery.

Long-term

The long-term effects of failure of mother and newborn baby to adapt to each other are not so clear cut as those immediately apparent in the early weeks and months of life. Yet they are serious when they do occur and must always be considered in relation to obstetric and nursing techniques in the perinatal period. Reference is made below to the relationship between outright child abuse and emotionally stressful events like neonatal separation.

Non-organic failure to thrive

A general failure of development is another sequel to neglect. Growth in height and weight provide important indices of emotional adaptation. Growth retardation has been the subject of several studies. Powell and his colleagues (1967a,b) investigated 13 children believed to be suffering from idiopathic hypopituitarism whose growth accelerated in a remarkable way when admitted to a convalescent home. They were not given hormone treatment although some were deficient in ACTH and growth hormone. Their histories revealed considerable occasion for emotional stress. The children showed evidence of psychiatric disturbance and tended to be isolates, to bite themselves, to have bizarre eating and drinking habits and foul-smelling, bulky stools. When removed from the emotionally disturbed environment, the level of growth hormone returned spontaneously to normal. However, Whitten & colleagues (1969) proved to their own satisfaction that growth delay is the result of insufficient intake of food. The growth of seven deprived children accelerated at home when their diets were corrected, the only other change being the interest of the dietician and 11 out of 13 others similarly accelerated when given adequate diets during a trial period away from home but in a seriously deprived and unstimulating environment. These children, of course, had been removed from home and the emotional stress of rejecting parents. The similar acceleration of growth and relief of coeliac-like gastrointestinal symptoms that follow hospital or foster home admission for the abused child supports the idea that it is in fact the relief from a battering, abusing and rejecting home that is responsible.

Bullard & colleagues (1967) reviewed children who were failing to thrive. For 101 some physical explanation such as congenital heart disease or a neurological defect could have been the explanation. Fifty had no primary organic illness. Not only were the children very far below expected height and weight, but mental development was slow, with frequent feeding difficulties and gastro-intestinal disturbances. In social behaviour the children were apprehensive, frightened, apathetic and withdrawn. Healed or healing fractures were revealed by X-ray in 10 per cent and these would currently be classed as suffering from child abuse. When parenting fails in infancy, rejection and emotional deprivation delay growth in the same way.

THE VULNERABLE MOTHER

Prediction of vulnerability

Rejection, emotional deprivation and abuse are often predictable and possibly preventable. Since the majority of women find their way into maternity departments, attendance there provides an excellent opportunity for seeking predictive information. Many of the mothers in the studies had been brought up in foster homes or institutions. Other prominent features in the history were instability of character, erratic living habits, fitful employment, marital strife and deficient finances. Personal and socio-economic problems combined to damage the mothering process and destroy the normal mother-child relationship.

The obstetric details that might complicate the birth of a baby are matters of such importance that the experience of family life that preceded the birth tends to be overlooked. The prime purpose of antenatal supervision is to reveal any condition of the pregnant woman that might lead to an obstetric problem. The list can be made and the items ticked one by one. Routine enquiry seldom contains data on which can be based the assessment of a mother's likely ability to discharge her mothering responsibilities to the baby that she is expecting. Making such an assessment should be part of the routine study of the expectant mother during the antenatal period.

Child abuse and neglect

Information about predisposing factors comes mainly from failure and most clearly from studies of families in which the emotional relationships within the family are so disordered as to produce incontrovertible evidence of child abuse and neglect. A comparison made by Lynch & Roberts, working with Ounsted at the Park Hospital, Oxford (Lynch, 1975; Lynch & Roberts, 1977), between 25 abused children and their 35 unbattered siblings revealed six factors as highly significantly over represented in the abused group. Three concerned obstetric management: abnormal pregnancy, abnormal labour/delivery and separation of the newborn for 48 hours or more. They also showed the value of flow charts of the parents' life histories in predicting vulnerable families who will find special difficulty in coping with their babies. When 50 abusing mothers were compared with 50 control mothers, more abusing mothers were less than 20 years old when their first children were born, more had been emotionally disturbed in the past, more had been referred to a social worker and more of their babies had been admitted to the special care baby nursery. Predictive factors include illegitimacy, early sexual experience, a variety of consorts but, much earlier in life, rejection by their own parents, cruelty and battering, life in institutions, school truancy and delinquent behaviour. The inclusion of data of this kind in histories might be at least as important for the baby as the history of the mother's physical illnesses and the records of her blood pressure. It is necessary to emphasise that the prediction resulting from this collection of details is not of which families will abuse or neglect their child but which are likely to need help in coping with the stresses of family life and the rearing of children. The prediction is of vulnerability.

Questions in the labour ward

Kempe (1977) has drawn attention to the usefulness of posing three simple questions, in the labour ward. When the mother is given her baby immediately after birth, how does the mother look? What does the mother say? What does the mother do? Avoiding looking, making an unkind comment clearly not in jest, and holding at arm's length are of ill omen. Allowance must be made for the mother's state in relation to general anaesthesia or drugs. Nursing staff are inclined to believe that no mother rejects her baby once she has seen it and may claim never to have noticed an unwelcome reception. After attention has been drawn to the significance of the three questions, they become aware that occasionally they do observe it. Naturally the evidence should be correlated with the mother's life history, but everyone concerned with the mother should be alerted to her need for special help and support.

Maternal intelligence

With attention focused on the personality of the mother and its possible distortion through rejection by her own parents and unbearable emotional stresses during her life, her level of intelligence has been somewhat overlooked. Sheridan (1956) studied a hundred mothers who had been charged with wilful neglect of their babies finding that they lacked the 'nice combination of insight and foresight which is ordinary common sense . . . (they) fail to appreciate either the socially unacceptable nature of their actions and omissions or the possible results'. They acted on the spur of the moment, and they were not able to learn from experience, or to accept any rule of life but their own immediate wishes. When given intelligence tests fourteen scored 105 to

125, but the majority 65 to 95. Fifty-seven were rated feeble-minded and six imbecile according to the classification at that time. It is now realised that mild mental handicap is found mainly in the lower social classes as a result of poor language stimulation, emotional deprivation and disadvantaged ante- and perinatal care. The fault lies with the circumstances of the grandparents' generation. This fits in with Baird's (1980) correlation between stature and reproductive competence (p. 174).

Maternal depression

Puerperal depression and, because so frequently missed, post-puerperal depression have profoundly disturbing effects on the mother-infant relationship. Those charged with responsibility for supervising mother's care of her infant should bear these possibilities in mind. Depression can contribute to child abuse and neglect and once recognised is treatable (Tylden, 1978).

Drugs and anaesthetics

Effects on interaction

How far can the important early interactions between mothers and their newborn babies be harmed by damping down the reaction of either or both by drugs given to the mother at the latter end of pregnancy, especially in the perinatal period or given to the baby after birth? Ploman & Persson (1957) showed in fetuses legally aborted by hysterotomy that maternal and fetal blood levels of barbiturates came approximately into equilibrium 30 minutes after injection into the mother. The drug accumulated in the placenta and in fetal liver and brain.

Brazelton (1961) observed decreased responsivity to breast feeding in his studies of the effect of maternal medication with barbiturates on the behaviour of the human newborn. This has also been found in mammalian studies of the kind that have contributed so much to the present understanding of the early attachment of infant and mother. Whittlestone (1978) at the Ruakura Animal Station, Hamilton, New Zealand, considered that in his animals a critical period was present immediately after parturition. The level of prolactin and oxytocin in the bloodstream may activate the mother's drive to attachment. The maternal solicitude response is at its highest immediately postpartum and is under hormonal control, reinforced by eye to eye contact and augmented by the suckling process. The hungry infant should be rewarded pleasurably by the mother's ejection of milk. Suckling reassures and alleviates fear and with the comfort of contact reduces stress responses. If the mother and the baby are under sedative drugs at birth the baby's suckling reflex is affected and its suckling capability reduced for four days. Eye contact is also less likely.

Effects on the baby

The question that follows is whether the effect of drugs in humans is transient or whether the immediate effect of the drug, apart from inducing the failure of suckling, causes an alteration in the interaction between mother and baby which upsets the future development of their relationship with long-lasting effects. The baby's adaptive mechanisms during the first week which are affected by the nature and duration of the delivery, and by immaturity, are also adversely affected by drugs and anaesthetics given to the mother before and during delivery. Brazelton (1961) found a relative state of disorganisation of the baby's behaviour from 24 to 48 hours of age when the mother had been given drugs. This state lasted for three or four days, the period when lactation is likely to become established. From observations on 41 multiparae breast feeding for the second or third time, he noted that satisfactory breast feeding began earlier, as did the start of weight gain, when the mother had no drugs. Some explanation for the difference was provided by Kron et al (1966). They showed that newborn babies sucked at significantly lower rates and pressures and took less nutrient for the first four days when the mothers had been given even a single dose of sedative during labour compared with mothers who had none.

Babies of low birth weight
The immature baby of very low birth weight requires an intensive care nursery. Apart from natural difficulties in sucking, the baby's special life support technology makes handling, body contact or changes in position virtually impossible. A group of workers at University College Hospital, London (Blake et al, 1975) where great success with low birth weight babies has been obtained, reported on 160 babies with birth weight below 1.5 kg. The maternal emotional crisis compounded of anxiety, feeling of failure and guilt varied in amount and in kind, but did not resolve until the baby had returned home; a lesson here for the general management of all immature babies for whom departments insist that a weight of 2.5 kg is obligatory before a return home is allowed.

Over thirty years ago, Miller in Newcastle showed that premature babies fared no worse at home than in hospital and the mother was spared from receiving after four to six weeks 'an unknown infant, feared and strange' (Miller, 1948). Blake and colleagues (1975) observed that a rigid or distorted maternal personality, or psychiatric disorder, contributed to failure, but support and sympathy from the father to eventual success. Some of the children were noted at follow-up to be mildly over-dependent, shy and anxious. Even before these technological triumphs mothers lost confidence and remained anxious for much of the childhood of their premature babies, who had been hospitalised for weeks. This was especially the case when the mother was given little or no opportunity in the hospital to play any part in the baby's care or feeding. That the baby is losing important experience through separation and the absence of handling, movement and body contact must always be kept in mind when plans are being made for special care for the baby.

IMPLICATIONS FOR PRACTICE

The encouragement of bonding and attachment
That early separation of newborn baby from mother is stressful to both and can jeopardise the interaction between them, especially the loving relationship on which so much of the future success and happiness of family life depends, is now generally agreed. Linguistic as well as attachment behaviour are likely to be impaired. Since separation has potentiality for damaging effect, is there some positive method of encouraging what is now generally called the bonding of affection?

Klaus & Kennell (Ringler et al, 1975) have studied the effects of increasing the contact between a mother and her newborn baby. Their usual routine plan was for a mother to glimpse her baby shortly after birth, have a brief contact between six and 12 hours, and four-hourly visits for feeding for 20 to 30 minutes. For the test group the extra contact comprised nude contact for one hour within the first three hours with five extra hours of contact each afternoon for three days. They were satisfied that the test group's reciprocal reactions were better on review at one month and one year of age. At two years they observed that the test group mothers asked twice as many questions and adopted a teaching attitude as compared with the controls who gave basic information and more commands to the infants. They concluded that extra contact with the mother 'may change the linguistic environment she provides her child in the first few years of life, and this in turn may affect the child's language and learning far into the future'.

Extra contact

De Chateau & Wilberg (1977) following up the ideas of Klaus & Kennell found that extra skin contact when added to even good perinatal care did have a positive effect. An extra 15 minutes of skin contact was allowed the test babies in the first hour of life. They had already noted that the babies of multiparae behaved differently from those of primiparae when observed breast feeding at 36 hours. Test and control babies were selected, who had been delivered spontaneously at term under optimal obstetric conditions. There were 22 primiparae in the test with 20 primiparous and 20 multiparous controls. Follow-up assessment at three months of age based on mother-infant free play and personal interview showed that the test babies cried less, smiled more, spent more time en face and kissing. More were still breast feeding. Boys showed a greater difference than girls.

In another study infants who had face-to-face interaction and early interaction through physical contact during the first three months of life, who were secure and whose mothers were sensitive to infant signals, showed a better quality of attachment at one year of age (Waters et al, 1980). The mothers cooperated rather than interfered with ongoing infant behaviour, were more readily available and responsive at one year. The infants were better able to use an adult as a secure base from which to explore.

Socio-economic influences

Baird (1980) has recently suggested that neonatal death rates are related to the period at which the mother herself was born and reared and therefore to the type of care provided by grandparents. While improved obstetric care will probably further reduce the perinatal mortality rate, the key to the problem lies in improvements in socio-economic conditions and involves the two generations. A woman's reproductive efficiency as measured by the incidence of stillbirth and perinatal death is significantly related to her stature. Social class differences in stature (Illsley, 1955) suggest environmental and socio-economic deleterious effects which must be prevented before optimal results can be achieved. Attachment failure likewise interferes with growth. These facts tally with the present belief that primary prevention of child abuse and neglect depends to a large extent on the grandparents' care of the parents from the time of their birth. Both the physical and the emotional health of the baby seem to require a similar response from society and the caring professions.

The total family

The total family situation needs to be considered in other ways. The mother's reaction to the baby involves the father whose supportive role is now recognised by his presence in the labour ward. For multiparae visiting by siblings is now encouraged. The arrival of the new baby, especially the first, and the mother's interaction with it alter the balance of relationships within the whole family. This shift in relationships affects the father and the grandparents and other socially important family members whose support may be vitally necessary. Psychiatrists have observed that child-birth-related psychosis can result (Ketal & Brandwin, 1979). Stress capable of inducing psychosis must be capable of producing a need for adaptation.

BREAST FEEDING AND IMMUNOLOGY

The arguments in favour of breast feeding used to rely on somewhat dubious evidence. The balance struck between encouraging it as natural and leading to a happy relationship and not discouraging the minority of mothers, who found the task beyond their powers, shifted periodically and at one time no advice was offered to the expectant mother; she could suit herself. The higher infant death rates, mainly from gastro-enteritis, lost their significance as the production of artificial feeds improved along with hygiene and environmental conditions. Unfortunately in the developing world the serious dangers of bottle feeding are again evident. Meanwhile immunological research has provided more scientific and therefore probably more influential reasons against the giving of cows' instead of human milk in the early months of life. Johnstone & Soothhill (1981) summarise the development of knowledge since Glaser & Johnstone (1953) showed that feeding influenced the occurrence of allergic diseases in genetically vulnerable infants. Exclusive breast feeding has been shown to produce a low incidence of atopic dermatitis and possibly of later respiratory allergy. Various explanations include the provision of potential protective mechanisms in human milk. The susceptibility may be due to late development of effective immune exclusion of antigen by the mucosal surface. Starting weaning at four months appears then to be relatively safe. The physiological immunologic immaturity of the early months of life makes it important to *exclude if possible even single supplementary cows' milk feeds in this period*. Inasmuch as a mother's willingness and ability to breast feed her baby is influenced by her attitude towards her baby, this newer knowledge provides yet another argument in favour of thoughtful, sensitive and sympathetic ante- and perinatal care.

REVIEWING GENERAL POLICY

What practical conclusions can be drawn from the results of these observations and studies?

The original policy of selecting certain categories of pregnant women for hospital delivery has been replaced by selecting the few who are deemed safe for home delivery and encouraging hospital admission for the rest. One result is that many perfectly normal women in the reasonable expectation that delivery will be normal come under hospital jurisdiction with consequent loss of independence, of choice and of responsibility. Yet they are expected to return home on their discharge with the total responsibility for the care of a young baby and for the choices and the decisions which are inevitable and often urgent.

There is good agreement between the view of Baird (1980), who is concerned with physical aspects, and of those whose major interest is the prevention of child abuse and neglect. We need a whole generation of mothers who were themselves well cared for physically and emotionally, from the time of their own conception, before optimal obstetric results will become possible, however much perinatal care improves.

The methods of antenatal supervision, like those of peri- and postnatal management, do not result from controlled trials. Tradition, the habits of particular departments, the outlook of influential members of staff have all contributed. There should therefore be no serious objection to reviewing practices, exploring their rationale and their scientific basis, and making the test for their survival or discarding how far they contribute to the health, the well-being and the comfort of mother and baby. The touchstone should be the success of that sixth phase referred to earlier, the settling down of the family at home.

Routine practices in hospital have a greater protective value for the staff than for the patient. Their adoption relieves individuals of responsibility and of the need to think. They are easy to introduce but tend to outlive their original purpose. Lack of courage, fear of responsibility and dislike of change make them difficult to stop. *All routines should be subjected to regular periodic review and we should work towards stopping all practices which separate mother and baby and which have not been shown to hold any benefit for either.*

The authoritarian and hierarchical structure which forms the basis for the institutional hospital system was developed for the care and safety of the sick and dying. Such a structure needs to be reviewed in all its details and adapted for the very different functions of a maternity centre. It is here that the foundations are to be laid for the optimal development of the new baby in body and in mind, which bonding of affection makes possible.

Unhelpful arrangements

New information about the value of breast feeding has been described above. Successful breast feeding is not an essential for bonding of affection and satisfactory mother/infant attachment, but is both desirable and helpful. Hospital practices that militate against the establishment of successful breast feeding and at the same time, not surprisingly, interfere with bonding include the following:

Intrapartum drugs
Delayed suckling
Giving supplementary bottles
Enforcing four-hourly feeds
Weighing before and after feeds
Excluding father, and above all
Separating mother and baby, and
Failing to support and encourage breast-feeding mothers.

Helpful arrangements

In order to avoid these discouraging practices, some helpful arrangements are

Giving the baby to the mother at birth
Ensuring skin contact in the labour ward
Suckling early within the first hour
Eliminating supplementary feeds
Encouraging eye-to-eye contact and
The face-to-face position
Involving the father

The kind of women who are in danger of failing to cope with the responsibilities of motherhood can often be singled out by suitable enquiries in the antenatal department, both about their own childhood experiences and their attitude to the pregnancy. Such women need careful handling since they are likely to be isolates with low self-esteem and a fear or a hatred of authority. The principle is that the staff of the department should do everything possible to receive them graciously and to ease the stress of hospital attendance and examination. Similarly in the labour ward and after the birth, the mother should be given as much responsibility and as big a part in choices of what is done as is possible. Many of the details have been discussed by Franklin (1980) after a survey of practice in a number of maternity departments.

Proposals
The following proposals are based on those in the review of the mother-newborn relationship by Kennell & Klaus and their colleagues (Lozoff et al, 1977) who have stimulated so much new thinking on the subject. Decisions about perinatal care not based on sound scientific evidence should be left as far as possible to parental choice. Our new awareness that the newborn baby is a highly complex bundle of capabilities should be shared with families (as well as midwives and obstetricians). We should recognise the great significance of the interaction between mother and baby and how much each depends on the other for the development of a good relationship. Klaus & Kennell in 1970 posed three questions: Is there a critical or sensitive period for the formation of a bond between human mother and her baby as there is in animals? What are the needs of most normal mothers with normal full-term babies in the first hours after delivery and during the first week? Has the hospital culture produced disorders of mothering which can last a lifetime?

CONCLUSION

The weight of evidence supports the idea that the interaction between the mother and her new baby at birth with the opportunity for the bonding of affection is important and that this is a sensitive period. So far it cannot be asserted that it is critical in the sense that, if the moment for bonding at birth is missed, lifelong damage results. Close contact and access to the baby, confidence, responsibility for making decisions and for much of the care of the baby, together with support from staff and other family members are important needs. Elements in hospital management, which place obstacles to the bonding of affection, can damage a mother's competence in ways that can last a lifetime. Mother/infant attachment, in the development of which the bonding of affection plays its part, is too important to place in jeopardy.

The prediction that a mother will find difficulty in coping with the job of motherhood can be based on knowledge of the mother's life story, of her attitude to her pregnancy and of her behaviour towards the baby at the time of birth. Such vulnerable women and their families need especially sensitive handling and support. In this way child abuse and neglect may be avoided. These families are a small minority. The lessons learned from them and the enlargement of our knowledge gained in recent years need to be applied to the majority. The maternity department has an important part to play in helping to establish for the new baby emotional security as well as physical health.

REFERENCES

Ainsworth M D S 1969 Object relations, dependency, and attachment: a theoretical review. Child Development 40: 969–1025

Ainsworth M D S 1979 Infant-mother attachment. American Psychologist 34: 932–937

Baird Sir D 1960 The evolution of modern obstetrics. Lancet 2: 557–567

Baird Sir D 1980 Environment and reproduction. British Journal of Obstetrics and Gynaecology 87: 1057–1067

Bakwin H 1949 Emotional deprivation of infants. Journal of Pediatrics 35: 512–521

Blake A, Stewart A, Turcan D 1975 Parents of babies of very low birth weight: long-term follow-up. In: Porter R, O'Connor M (eds) Parent-infant Interaction, Ciba Foundation Symposia No 33 Associated Scientific Publishers, Amsterdam p. 271–281

Bowlby J, Ainsworth M, Boston M, Rosenbluth D 1956 The effects of mother-child separation: a follow-up study. Britsh Journal of Medical Psychology 29: 211–247

Bowlby J 1969 Attachment and Loss. Vol I The Hogarth Press and the Institute of Psycho-analysis, London

Brazelton T B 1961 Effect of maternal medication on the neonate and his behaviour. Journal of Pediatrics 58: 513–518

Brazelton T B, Tronick E, Adamson L, Als H, Wise S 1975 Early mother-infant reciprocity. In: Porter R, O'Connor M (eds) Parent-infant Interaction, Ciba Foundation Symposia No 33 (n.s.) Associated Scientific Publishers, Amsterdam p. 137–149

Bullard D M, Glaser H H, Heagarty M C, Pivchik E C 1967 Failure to thrive in the 'neglected' child. American Journal of Orthopsychiatry 37: 680–690

de Chateau P, Wiberg B 1977 Long-term effect on mother-infant behaviour of extra contact during the first hour post-partum. Acta Paediatrica Scandinavica 66: 137–143

Franklin A W 1980 A fresh look at childbirth. Journal of Maternal and Child Health 5: 26–32, 58–63

Glaser J, Johnstone D E J 1953 Prophylaxis of allergic disease in the newborn. Journal of the American Medical Association 153: 620–622

Gordon A H, Jameson J C 1979 Infant-mother attachment in patients with non-organic failure to thrive syndrome. Journal of the American Academy of Child Psychiatry 18: 251–259

Goren C C, Sarty M, Pyk W 1975 Visual following and pattern discrimination of face-like stimuli by newborn infants. Pediatrics 56: 544–549

Hock E, Christman K, Stewart L, Weinhaus E 1979 Mother-neonate bonding: further theory development and research. Journal of Pediatrics 94: 166–167

Holland E, Lane-Claypon J 1926 A clinical and pathological study of 1673 cases of dead-births and neonatal deaths. MRC Medical Report Series No. 109 HMSO, London

Illsley R 1955 Social class selection and class differences in relation to stillbirths and infant deaths. British Medical Journal 2: 1520–1524

Johnson C K, Gilbert M D, Herdt G H 1979 Implications for adult roles from differential styles of mother-infant bonding. Journal of Nervous and Mental Disease 167: 29–37

Johnstone D E J, Soothill J F 1981 Immunological aspects of infant feeding. In Paediatric Immunology eds. Hayward A R, Soothill J F, Wood C B S Blackwell Scientific Publications, Oxford

Kempe C H 1977 Mother's introduction to her newborn baby. In Child Abuse: Prediction, Prevention and Follow-up ed. Franklin A W Churchill Livingstone, Edinburgh, London & New Yrok ch 9 p 79

Kennell J H, Trause M A, Klaus M 1975 Evidence for a sensitive period in the human mother. In Porter R, O'Connor M (eds) Parent-infant Interaction, Ciba Foundation Symposia No 33 (n.s.) Associated Scientific Publishers, Amsterdam p 87–101

Ketal R M, Brandwin M A 1979 Childbirth psychosis and familial symbiotic conflict. American Journal of Psychiatry 136: 190–192

Klaus M H, Kennell J H 1970 Mothers separated from their newborn infants. Pediatric Clinics of North America 17: 1016–1037

Korner A F, Chuck B, Dontchos S 1968 Organismic determinants of spontaneous oral behaviour in neonates. Child Development 39: 1145–1157

Korner A F, Grobstein R 1966 Visual alertness as related to soothing in neonates: implications for maternal stimulation and early deprivation. Child Development 37: 867–876

Kron R E, Stein M, Goddard K E 1966 Newborn sucking behaviour affected by obstetric sedation. Pediatrics 37: 1012–1015

Leiderman P H, Seashore M J 1975 Mother-infant neonatal separation: some delayed consequences. In: Porter R, O'Connor M (eds) Parent-infant Interaction, Ciba Foundation Symposia No 33 (n.s.) Associated Scientific Publishers, Amsterdam p 213–231

Lozoff B, Brittenham G M, Trause M A, Kennell J H, Klaus M H 1977 The mother-newborn relationship: limits of adaptability. Journal of Pediatrics 91: 1–12

Lynch M A 1975 Ill-health and child abuse. Lancet 2: 317–319

Lynch M A, Roberts J 1977 Prediction of child abuse: signs of bonding failure in the maternity hospital. British Medical Journal 1: 624–626

Lynch M A, Roberts J, Ounsted C 1979 Myotonic dystrophy and bonding failure. Archives of Disease in Childhood 54: 807–808

Macfarlane A 1975 Olfaction in the development of social preferences in the human neonate. In: Porter R, O'Connor M (eds) Parent-infant Interaction, Ciba Foundation Symposia No 33 (n.s.) Associated Scientific Publishers, Amsterdam p 103–113

Miller F W J 1948 Home nursing and premature babies in Newcastle-on-Tyne. Lancet 2: 703–705

Parsons L G 1946 Ante-natal paediatrics. Journal of Obstetrics and Gynaecology of the British Empire 53: 1–16

Pearse I H 1979 The Quality of Life: the Peckham Approach to Human Ethology. Scottish Academic Press, Edinburgh

Ploman L, Persson B H 1957 On the transfer of barbiturates to the human fetus and their accumulation in some of its vital organs. Journal of Obstetrics and Gynaecology of the British Empire 64: 706–711

Powell G F, Brasel J A, Blizzard R M 1967a Emotional deprivation and growth retardation simulating idiopathic hypopituitarism Part I New England Journal of Medicine 276: 1271–1278

Powell G F, Brasel J A, Raiti S, Blizzard R M 1967b Part II New England Journal of Medicine 276: 1279–1283

Rheingold H L 1960 The measurement of maternal care. Child Development 31: 565–575

Ringler N M, Kennell J H, Jarvella R, Navojosky B J, Klaus M H 1975 Mother-to-child speech at 2 years — effects of early postnatal contact. Journal of Pediatrics 86: 141–148

Robson K S 1967 The role of eye-to eye contact in maternal-infant attachment. Journal of Child Psychology & Psychiatry 8: 13–25

Sheridan M 1956 The intelligence of 100 neglectful mothers. British Medical Journal 1: 91–93

Thomas H P 1980 Role of the pediatrician in fostering good parenting. Pediatrics 65: 371–372

Tylden E 1978 Personal communication

Waters E, Vaughn B E, Egeland B R 1980 Individual differences in infant-mother attachment relationships at age one: antecedents in an urban economically disadvantaged sample. Child Development 51: 208–216

Weisfeld E 1979 An ethological view of human adolescence. Journal of Nervous & Mental Disease 167: 38–55

Whitten C F, Pettit M G, Fischoff J 1969 Evidence that growth failure from maternal deprivation is secondary to undereating. Journal of the American Medical Association 209: 1675–1682

Whittlestone W G 1978 The physiology of early attachment in mammals: implications for human obstetric care. Medical Journal of Australia 1: 50–53

Winnicott D W 1958 Collected Papers: Through Paediatrics to Psychoanalysis. Tavistock Publications, London

Wolff P H 1959 Observations on newborn infants. Psychosomatic Medicine 21: 110–118

Wolff P H 1965 The development of attention in young infants. Annals of the New York Academy of Sciences 118: 815–830

SUGGESTIONS FOR FURTHER READING

Seminars in Perinatology January 1979 Vol 3 (1) Parent-infant relationships (ed) P M Taylor

Clinics in Developmental Medicine 1978 No. 68 & Separation and special care baby units. Brimblecombe F S W, Richards M P M, Roberton N R C (eds) Heinemann, London

8. Fertility after childbirth

Peter W. Howie   Alan S. McNeilly

INTRODUCTION

In recent years, Western society has largely discounted the natural contraceptive effect of breast feeding on the grounds that it is an ineffective and largely irrelevant method of birth control. There has however, been a renewed research interest in lactational infertility for a number of reasons. Firstly, it is now recognised that the birth-spacing effect of lactation is of major demographic importance in developing countries; (Short, 1976). Secondly, an understanding of the mechanisms responsible for this naturally evolved method of fertility control might lead to new initiatives in contraceptive research (NcNeilly, 1979), thirdly, the resurgence of enthusiasm for breast feeding in Western Society (Coles et al, 1978) has created the need in breast feeding mothers for effective contraceptive methods which do not have adverse effects on lactation and, fourthly, there are mothers who wish to know how they can maximise the natural contraceptive effect of breast feeding and reduce their dependence on other methods of family planning. In this Chapter, we discuss the demographic importance of breast feeding, the clinical factors which control the return of ovulation after childbirth and the endocrine mechanisms of lactational infertility.

BIRTH SPACING EFFECT OF LACTATION

A number of studies have indicated that fertility after childbirth returns more quickly in non-nursing than in lactating mothers (for references see Buchanan, 1975). In one such study, Berman et al (1972) investigated fertility rates after childbirth in Alaskan Eskimos because they were a population who used no contraception and did not practise any sexual taboo during lactation. The non-lactating mothers conceived rapidly after delivery and 50 per cent were pregnant at four months postpartum (Fig. 8.1). In the breast-feeding mothers, fertility was substantially delayed and 19 months elapsed before 50 per cent had conceived again. If these patterns of fertility were repeated in successive pregnancies, non-lactating mothers would have more than twice as many pregnancies as lactating mothers.

The impact of reducing the birth-spacing effect of lactation was illustrated dramatically by Cox (1978) who reported on an Aboriginal family living near a mission station in West Queensland. The young Aboriginal mother progressively decreased the duration of full breast feeding from six months after her first pregnancy to two months after her fifth by using the formula milk supplied by the mission station. Conception invariably occurred after weaning and she had six children (including twins) before she was 21 years old. In each case, the introduction of supplementary

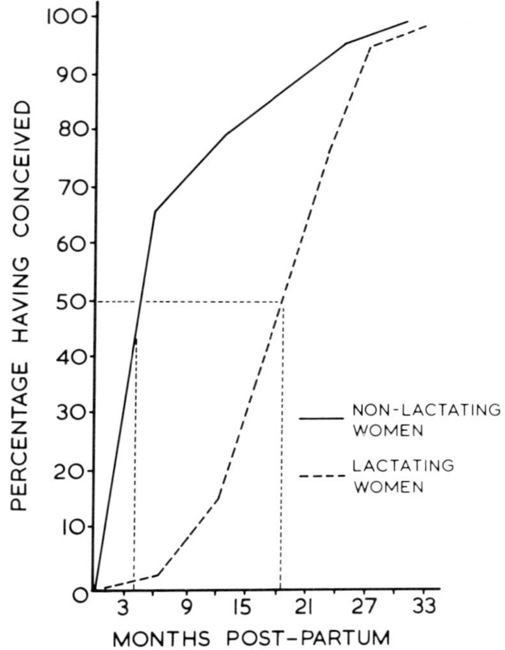

Fig. 8.1   Cumulative percentages of lactating and non-lactating mothers become pregnant postpartum; data from Alaskan Eskimos, Berman et al, 1972.

food was associated with gastro-enteritis and a flattening of the infants' growth curves which failed to return to normal even after the diarrhoea was treated.

Rosa (1975) attempted to quantify the impact of lactational infertility in the non-communist developing world and a summary of his calculations are shown in Table 8.1.

Table 8.1   Couple-years protection from breast-feeding and contraception in developing countries, 1973 (from Rosa, 1975)

Area	Total population ($\times 10^6$)	Mothers breast-feeding (%)	Fertility protection (months)	Couple-years protection
Rural	1378	85	8	31 300 000
Urban	459	75	4	3 400 000
		Total protection by lactation		34 700 000
		Estimated protection by contraception		24 000 000

From published data, which showed that in rural communities of the developing world 85 per cent of mothers breast fed, Rosa estimated that this resulted in eight extra months of fertility protection compared with non-lactating mothers; in urban populations, where 75 per cent of mothers breast fed the increased fertility protection was 4 months. From these figures, breast feeding would be responsible for 33.7 million couple years of infertility compared with an estimated 24.0 million couple years of protection over the same time period from all other methods of artificial contraception put together. Rosa's calculations emphasise clearly the major impact which lactational infertility has on population growth in the developing world.

Assessment of lactational infertility

The two indicators which have been used most extensively to estimate the effect of breast feeding on fertility have been the inter-birth interval and the duration of lactational amenorrhoea. While there is no doubt that breast feeding is associated with an increase in the inter-birth interval, it cannot be assumed that inhibition of ovulation is the only factor to influence the date of conception (Thomson et al, 1975). In many communities, especially in Africa, sexual taboos are imposed during breast feeding and reduced frequency of intercourse would impair fertility. Furthermore, it is essential to have exact information on contraceptive practices which vary widely between communities.

As an alternative to the interbirth interval, the duration of lactational amenorrhoea has been used as a convenient marker to indicate the probable return of fecundity (potential for fertility). In support of the use of lactational amenorrhoea as a marker, the duration of postpartum amenorrhoea is related to the length of lactation and is longer in rural than in urban communities (van Ginneken, 1977). Since the interbirth interval also tends to be longer in rural communities despite lower use of contraception, it seems reasonable to use lactational amenorrhoea as a guide to fecundity on a population basis. The relationship between lactational amenorrhoea and the interbirth interval is, however, less reliable for individuals than for total populations because between 2 and 10 per cent of mothers conceive during the period of lactational amenorrhoea (for references, see Badraoui & Hefnawi, 1979). Another source of error is that menstruation during lactation may be associated with anovular cycles so that the return of menses does not necessarily indicate the return of normal fecundity. After lactating women resume menstruation, they often have irregular cycles and are less likely to conceive than non-lactating women who are menstruating (Sharman, 1951). It is clear that a precise marker of first ovulation during lactation would greatly facilitate the understanding of how breast feeding acts to achieve its natural contraceptive affect.

Ovulation during lactation

Most studies which have investigated the resumption of ovulation during lactation have used basal body temperature, cervical mucus changes and endometrial biopsies as indicators of ovulation (Sharman, 1951). The most detailed investigation was that of Perez et al (1972) who studied the return of ovulation in 200 Chilean mothers after childbirth. They reported that ovulation returned between 36 and 77 days postpartum in bottle feeders compared with a mean of 112 days postpartum in the breast feeders: they also found that 78 per cent of mothers ovulated before first menses. Not all reports, however, have agreed with the findings of Perez et al (1972). For example, Udesky (1950), while agreeing that ovulation returned promptly after delivery in bottle feeders, found that ovulation before first menses occurred in only 14 per cent of lactating mothers. El-Minawi and Foda (1971) studied a group of Egyptian mothers who experienced prolonged lactational amenorrhoea and found that 96 per cent of their endometrial biopsies during lactation showed an anovular pattern. The reasons for these discrepant results are not clear but one factor may be the difficulty of interpreting endometrial biopsies taken from lactating mothers (El-Minawi and Foda, 1971). Another, and possibly more important, factor may be the widely different infant feeding patterns in the populations which have been studied because the stronger the suckling stimulus, the more likely are menstruation and ovulation to be suppressed for prolonged periods.

Urinary steroid excretion during lactation

An alternative method of studying ovarian activity during lactation is the sequential measurement of urinary steroid excretion, interpreting a rise of total urinary estrogens as evidence of ovarian follicular development and a rise of urinary pregnanediol as evidence of ovulation (McNeilly et al, 1980). In a longitudinal study of 10 bottle feeding and 27 breast feeding mothers, we have defined first ovulation and related it to first menstruation, infant feeding patterns and basal prolactin levels (Howie et al, 1981a).

The relationships between these factors are illustrated by a typical bottle feeding (Fig. 8.2) and breast feeding mother (Fig. 8.3). In the bottle feeding mother, basal

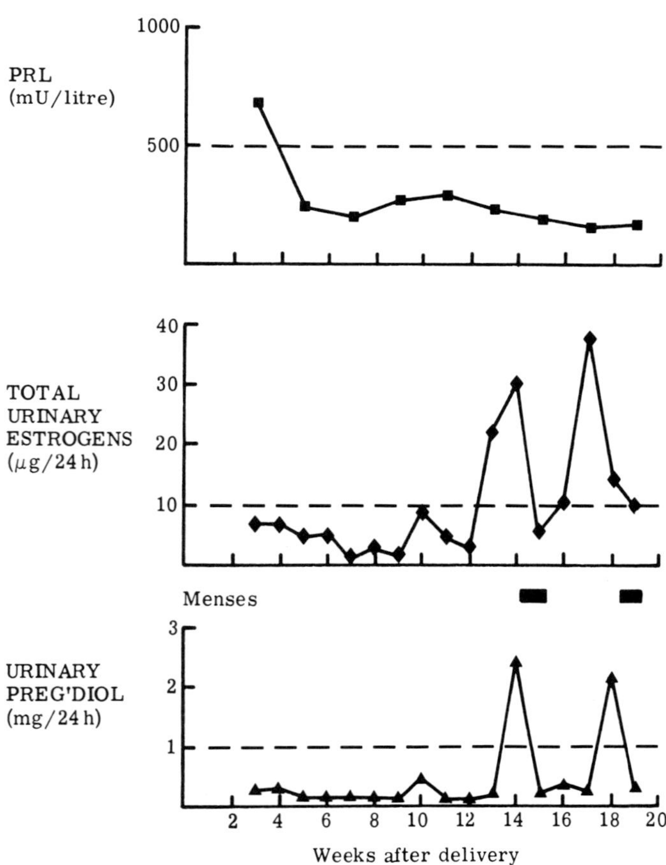

Fig. 8.2 Changes in serum prolactin (PRL), total urinary oestrogens and urinary pregnanediol in a bottle feeding mother, indicating their relationships to the return of menstruation.

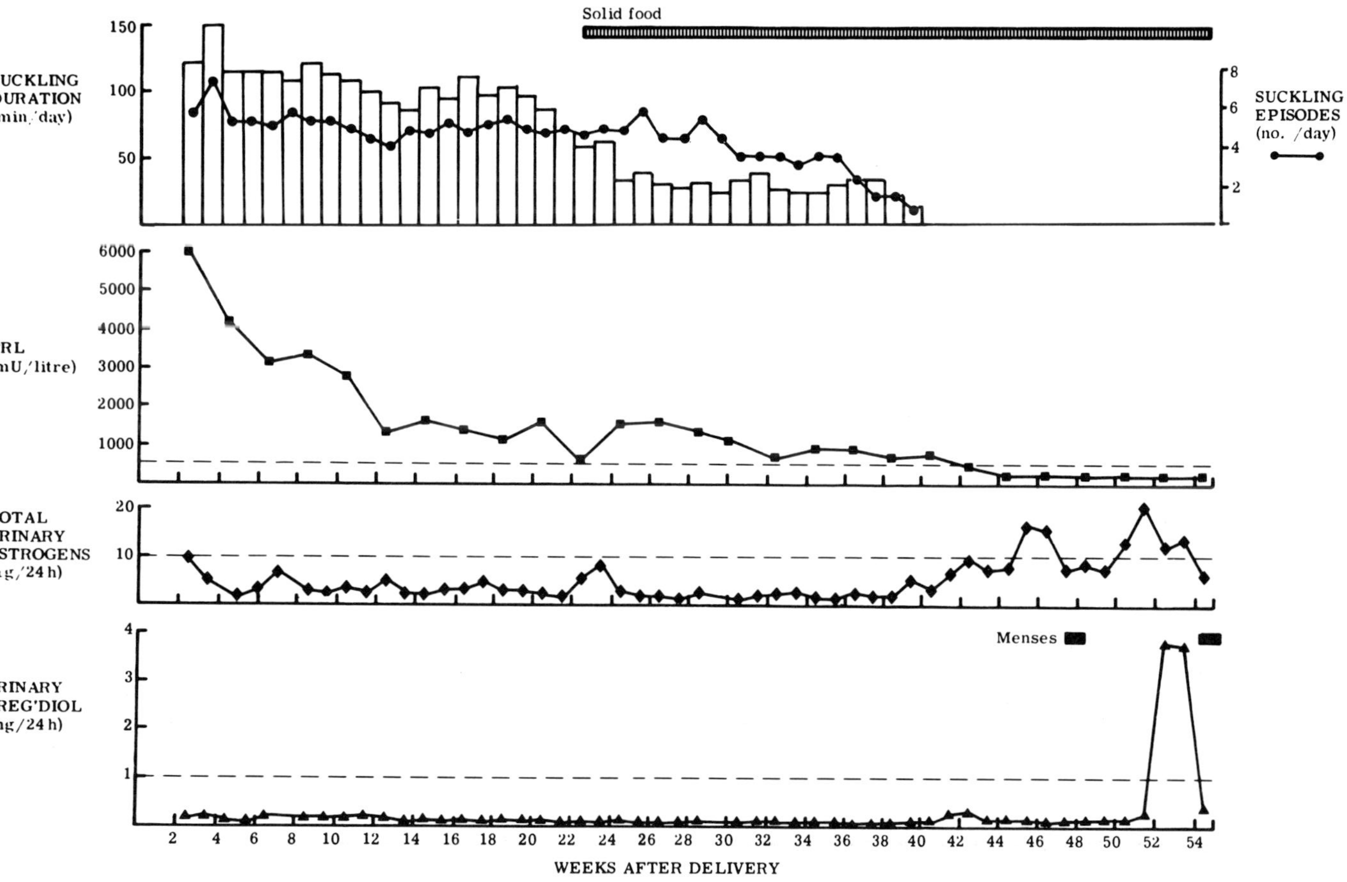

Fig. 8.3   Changes in suckling frequency, suckling duration, serum prolactin, total urinary oestrogens and urinary pregnanediol in a breast feeding mother, indicating their relationships to the use of solid food and the return of menstruation.

prolactin levels had returned to the non-pregnant range four weeks postpartum. Thereafter, there was cyclical ovarian follicular development (total urinary oestrogens > 10μg/24 hrs) followed by menstruation on each occasion. Ovulation (pregnanediol > 1 mg/24 hrs) did not occur in the first cycle but did so in the second and third cycles. By contrast, the sequential pattern in a breast feeding mother is presented in Figure 3. This mother breast fed for 40 weeks, during which time there were progressive falls in suckling frequency and duration which were reflected in the basal prolactin levels. Basal prolactin, however, remained above the non-pregnant range until complete weaning and both menstruation and ovarian activity were suppressed during lactation. After breast feeding stopped, ovarian follicular activity returned and after one anovular cycle ovulation resumed in the second menstrual cycle.

Relationship of first menstruation to first ovulation

This study confirmed that breast feeding delays the resumption of menstruation and ovulation and showed that, even among well-nourished mothers from Western Society ovulation could be delayed for up to one year or more (Fig. 8.4). Although the

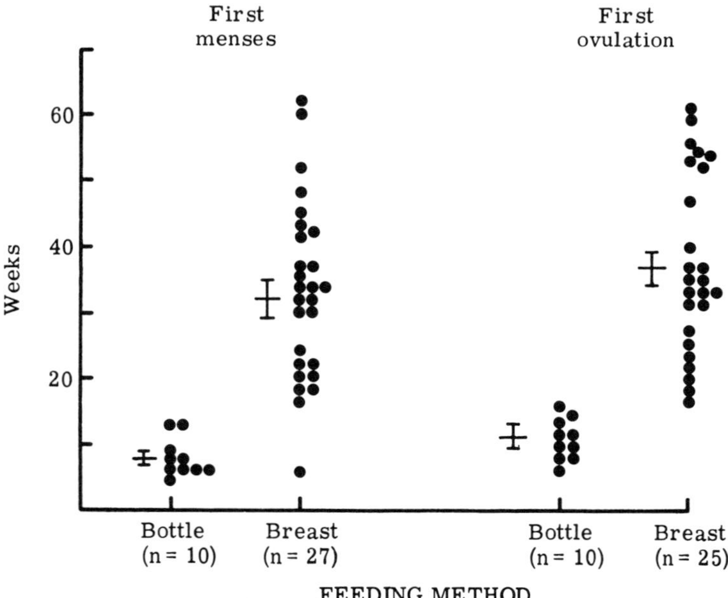

Fig. 8.4   Differences between bottle-feeding and breast feeding mothers in respect of the time to first menstruation and to first ovulation after childbirth.

time to first ovulation correlated positively with the duration of lactational amenorrhoea on a population basis, the relationship was not an exact one in individual cases. Among the 10 bottle feeding mothers eight failed to ovulate before first menses but all resumed ovulation within a few weeks thereafter (Fig. 8.5). Among the breast feeders, 12/27 ovulated before first menses but the remainder had intervals varying from four to 35 weeks between first menses and first ovulation (Fig. 8.5).

It is clear, therefore, that menses during lactation is not a reliable marker of ovulation and that first menses cannot be relied on to indicate when breast feeding mothers should resume contraception. Rolland et al (1975a) conducted a similar study to our own and reported comparable findings during the early puerperium but did not continue observations beyond 120 days. Perez et al (1972) showed that ovulation before first menses was most likely to occur when lactational amenorrhoea was prolonged, a finding which was confirmed in our own study. The most probable explanation of this finding is that there is a progressive reduction of suckling over time and that this reduction allows ovulation to occur before first menses.

RELATIONSHIP BETWEEN FIRST MENSES AND
FIRST OVULATION

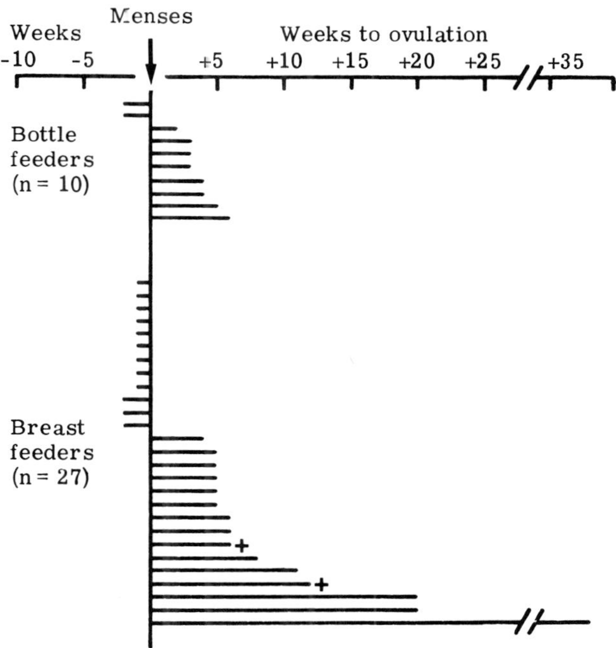

Fig. 8.5 The relationship of first ovulation to first menstruation after childbirth in 10 bottle feeding and 27 breast feeding mothers. (+) indicates two mothers who had not ovulated before observations were discontinued.

RELATIONSHIP OF FIRST OVULATION TO INFANT FEEDING

The most striking finding to emerge from our longitudinal study of breast feeding mothers was the relationship between infant feeding and ovarian activity. In Figure 8.6, the mean levels of basal prolactin, suckling frequency, suckling duration and supplementary feeds are shown over 40 weeks for the total cohort of 27 breast feeding mothers. During this time, basal prolactin levels rose to peak values at week 6 post-partum and then fell progressively towards the non-pregnant range. The mean basal PRL levels correlated positively with the mean suckling frequency ($r = 0.946$) and mean suckling duration ($r = 0.949$) and inversely with the mean number of

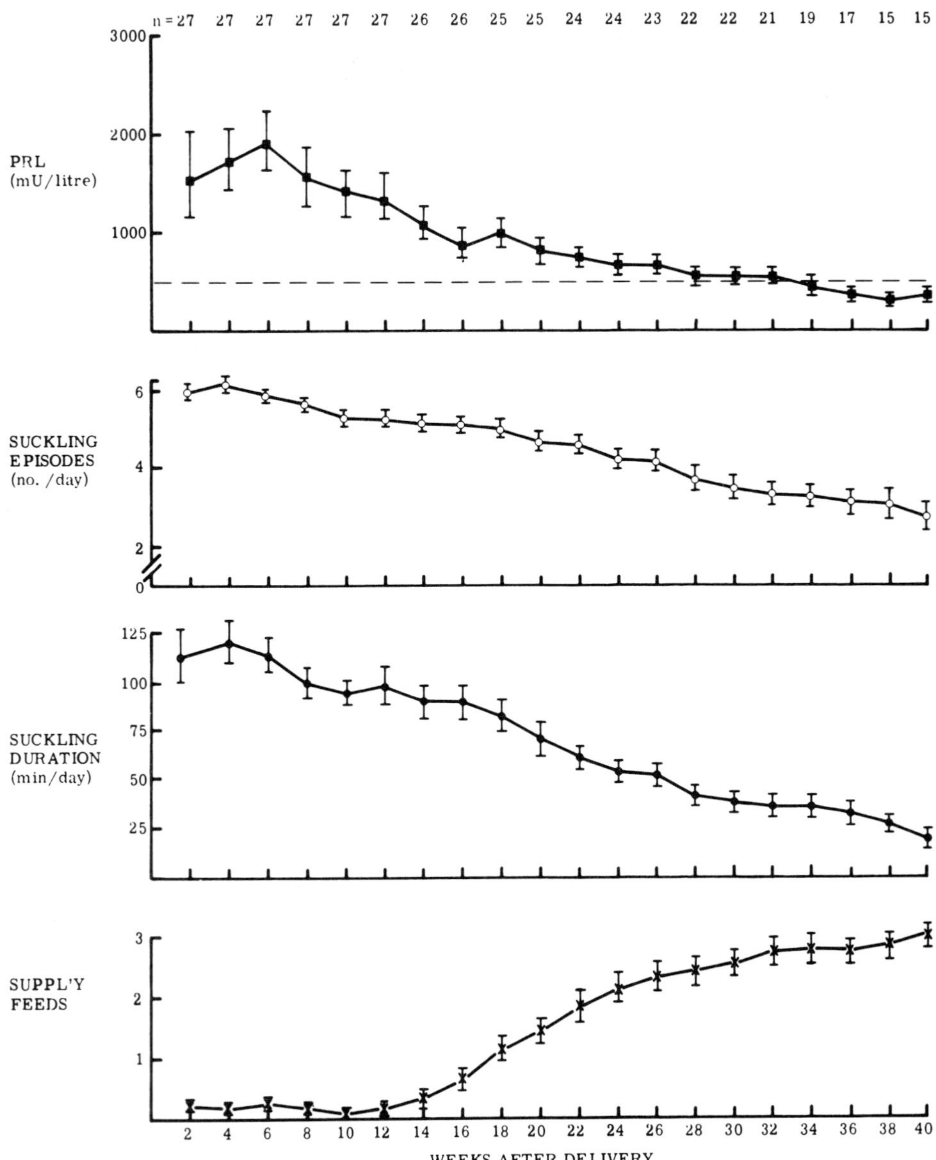

Fig. 8.6   Changes (Mean ± S.E.M.) in suckling episodes, suckling frequency, basal PRL (log normal) and supplementary feeds in 27 breast feeding mothers after delivery (from Howie et al, 1981a, reproduced by kind permission of the Editor, British Medical Journal).

supplementary feeds (r = −0.923). This suggested that basal prolactin levels reflected the strength of the suckling stimulus which in turn was inversely influenced by the frequency of supplementary feeds.

The importance of supplementary feeding is even more clearly illustrated by examining suckling patterns and ovarian activity before and after the introduction of supplements. As can be seen in Figure 8.7, suckling duration and suckling frequency were relatively constant until the introduction of supplementary food, after which they both showed an immediate and progressive decline. Before the introduction of supplements, only two mothers had shown evidence of ovarian follicular development and none had ovulated. After supplements were introduced, there was a progressive increase in the number of mothers who had evidence of follicular development and ovulation. Sixteen weeks after the introduction of supplements, 52 per cent of the mothers had ovulated and these were the mothers who had introduced supplements most abruptly and reduced suckling most quickly.

Ovulation and supplementary food

In contrast to the above findings, Perez et al (1972) reproted that 24/170 (14 per cent) of the breast feeding mothers in their study ovulated while fully nursing. This indicates that even full nursing is not a guarantee against pregnancy but Perez et al (1972) did not define the suckling characteristics in those mothers who ovulated before the introduction of supplements. There is now a growing body of evidence that the strength of the suckling stimulus is the most important variable in determining the duration of lactational infertility. Several reports have shown that menstruation returns more quickly in mothers who are partially nursing compared with those who are fully nursing (Sharman, 1951; McKeown & Gibson, 1954; Perez et al, 1971; Chen et al, 1974). In a detailed study of the infant feeding practices among the !Kung hunter-gatherers of the Kalahari desert, Konner & Worthman (1980) have shown that these nomadic mothers suckle their babies very frequently for short periods during the day and sleep with their babies at night. This pattern of frequent feeding continues for several years and the !Kung mothers experience prolonged inter-birth intervals of up to four years without use of artificial contraception.

In a large cross-sectional study of mothers in Rwanda, Delvoye et al (1978a) found that basal prolactin levels were related to the number of suckling episodes per day and that the association persisted beyond the first postpartum year. The duration of lactational amenorrhoea was also related to basal prolactin and, by extrapolation, to suckling frequency, suggesting that the infant feeding patterns were of central importance in controlling the return of fertility. Further support for the critical role of suckling comes from population studies among the rural and urban women of Rwanda. In that country, rural mothers breast fed on demand and 50 per cent conceived again within 23 months after delivery; among the urban mothers, however, a more rigid schedule of feeding was practised with fewer suckling episodes, and 50 per cent of women conceived again within nine months postpartum (Bonte et al, 1974). These epidemiological studies were supported by our own data when we compared the mothers with early and late postpartum ovulation. The late-ovulating mothers had higher levels of suckling duration and frequency, had maintained night feeds for longer and had introduced supplementary food later and more slowly. (Howie et al, 1981b). These data are consistent with the view that the suckling stimulus plays a major part in controlling ovarian activity and fertility after childbirth.

Supplementary food and contraception

If suckling patterns and the efficiency of lactational infertility are dependent upon the use of supplementary food, it must be a matter for concern that more and more

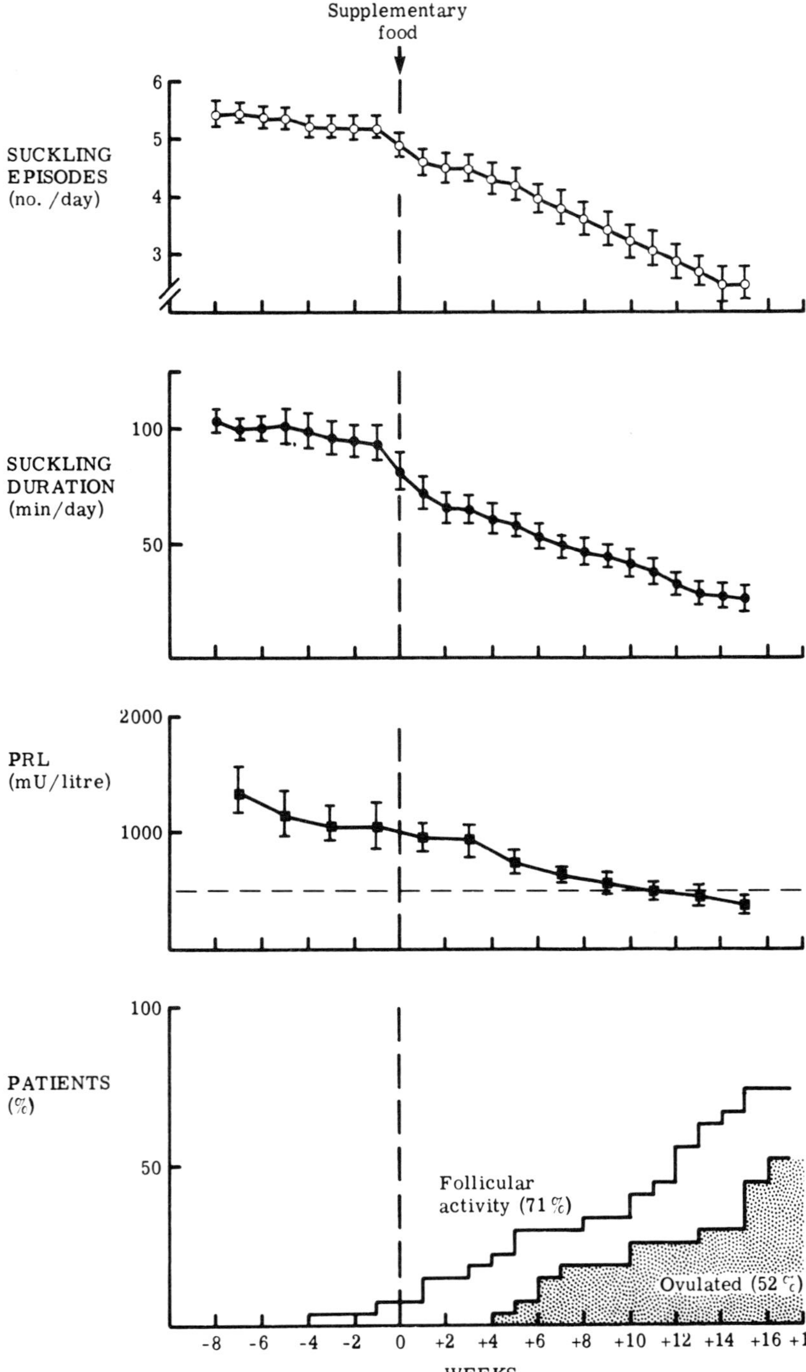

Fig. 8.7   Changes (mean ± S.E.M.) in suckling episodes, suckling duration, basal PRL and ovarian activity in 27 breast feeding mothers before and after the introduction of supplementary food (from Howie et al, 1981a, reproduced by kind permission of the Editor, British Medical Journal).

mothers in developing countries are resorting to the early introduction of supplementary food. This trend was clearly illustrated by the WHO collaborative study on breast feeding (1979) which reported on infant feeding among 25 different sub-groups drawn from nine different countries. A high proportion of mothers were using supplements at two to three months and the great majority were giving supplements at six months postpartum (Table 8.2). The notable exceptions were

Table 8.2   Percentage of breast-feeding mothers giving supplements (occasional or regular) in EA/economically advantaged) UP (urban poor) and R (rural) groups of nine different countries (from WHO Collaborative Study on Breast feeding 1979)

Country	Group	2–3 months	6–7 months
Hungary	All	46.8	96
Sweden	All	30.7	100
Ethiopia	EA	67.8	—
	UP	49.2	38.6
	R	49.3	85.3
Nigeria	EA	86.1	100
	UP	63.5	91.7
	R	35.0	86.3
Zaire	EA	38.3	84.4
	UP	36.0	95.8
	R	49.0	76.0
Chile	EA	60.0	90.9
	UP	59.0	100.0
	R	59.0	95.5
Guatemala	EA	91.3	—
	UP	51.9	87.1
	R	13.8	65.4
Philippines	EA	84.7	—
	UP	36.1	90.9
	R	41.9	95.0
India	EA	52.3	82.3
	UP	5.5	22.3
	R	1.8	12.4

among the poorer mothers of Ethiopia and India and it is of interest that these mothers have prolonged inter-birth intervals despite low contraception usage. If mothers in developing countries undermine the contraceptive effect of breast feeding by the early use of supplements, it will be of great importance to balance this effect by efficient use of contraception. The use of supplementary food among infants is a complex issue with implications for nutrition (Waterlow & Thomson, 1979) and infection (Jelliffe & Jelliffe, 1978) as well as for birth-spacing. The subject urgently requires more intensive investigation.

Ovulation and malnutrition
It has been suggested that chronic malnutrition contributes to the duration of amenorrhoea associated with prolonged breast feeding and consequently to reduction of fertility (Delgado et al, 1978). Poorly nourished women tend to have a late

menarche and an early menopause, both of which would reduce fertility, but it is less clear whether chronic malnutrition per se has any additional effect on lactational amenorrhea. Assessment of the effect of chronic malnutrition is made difficult by the tendency of poorly nourished mothers to breast feed for longer and suckle more frequently as compared with well nourished mothers (Prema et al, 1979). Bongaarts (1980) has recently reviewed the evidence and concluded that chronic malnutrition has only a minor effect on fecundity and fertility. For example, he quoted a study from Bangladesh which found the median duration of amenorrhoea in low, medium and high nutrition status groups to be 21.2, 20.4 and 20.2 mothers respectively and also found that weight for height ratios were similar in amenorrhoeic and menstruating nursing mothers (Huffman et al, 1978). From his detailed analysis, Bongaarts concluded that the age at menarche and the duration of lactational amenorrhoea were the major determinants of fertility in non-contracepting populations. In contrast to the relatively minor effect of chronic malnutrition, extreme food deprivation during famine was invariably associated with large but temporary reductions in fertility (Bongaarts, 1980).

Lunn et al (1980) reported on a study among Gambian mothers which compared a group of nursing mothers receiving a calorie supplement with a group of controls who received no such supplement. The mothers who received no supplement had higher prolactin levels than those mothers receiving the supplement and Lunn et al speculated that the higher prolactin levels might be related to their calorie deficiency. This study did not quantify suckling frequency or duration but demonstrated that further controlled studies were required before the relationships between maternal nutrition and postpartum amenorrhoea could be fully defined. The relationship of chronic maternal malnutrition to fertility is of practical importance in determining whether food supplements in areas of food shortage should be given primarily to the nursing mother or directly to the baby.

From a consideration of these studies, it is evident that the strength of the suckling stimulus plays a major part in determining the resumption of ovulation after childbirth. It is logical that this should be so because the infant who has been displaced from the breast by a new sibling is placed at a serious disadvantage (Morley, 1977). Nature has designed an exquisitely balanced mechanism that has placed within the infant's mouth the means by which it preserves for itself the natural advantages of breast feeding. It is appropriate that the mechanisms by which this is achieved should now be discussed.

LACTATION AND RESUMPTION OF OVULATION

Sensitivity of the breast

During pregnancy, there is a relative loss of skin sensitivity in the breasts and areola which persists until delivery has occurred (Robinson & Short, 1977). After delivery, tactile sensitivity returns to normal and this ensures that suckling provides a steady stream of afferent impulses to the hypothalamus. These afferent impulses stimulate prolactin release which, apart from being required for lactogenesis (Tyson et al, 1972) may contribute to the suppression of ovarian activity during lactation. It is not yet clear whether lactational infertility is mediated through the hypothalamic pituitary axis, or through a direct effect on the ovary but it is possible that both mechanisms are involved.

Gonadotrophins during lactation

Follicle stimulating Hormone (FSH)

During pregnancy, FSH levels are suppressed by the high levels of circulating oestrogens and progesterone which are secreted by the placenta. After delivery the placental steroids fall abruptly and, after an interval of 15 to 20 days, FSH returns to the normal range of the follicular phase in both bottle and breast feeding mothers (Reyes et al, 1972; Bonnar et al, 1975; Rolland et al, 1975a). It would appear that the mechanism of lactational infertility is not mediated through changes in circulating levels of FSH.

Luteinising hormone (LH)

Because of cross-reaction with HCG, it is not possible to measure LH accurately during pregnancy or the early puerperium. It is probable that LH is low during pregnancy, because the pituitary content is less than 1 per cent of normally cycling women (de la Lastra and Llados, 1977). In non-lactating mothers, plasma LH concentrations return to normal cyclic levels about the third week postpartum when prolactin concentrations fall to the non-pregnant range (Bonnar et al, 1975). In lactating mothers, LH concentrations rise more slowly and by 15 to 20 days are in the low normal range where they remain until after weaning has taken place (Reyes et al, 1972; Bonnar et al, 1975). The action of LH, however, may depend upon its release in a normal pulsatile pattern from the anterior pituitary and it has been suggested that this may be absent or reduced in lactating women (Bohnet and Schneider, 1977). The pulsatile release of gonadotrophins at different stages during lactation has been studied by Glasier et al (1981) in 20 breast feeding mothers and a typical series from one mother is illustrated in Figure 8.8. Blood samples were collected at 15 minute intervals over a six-hour period (1) during full breast feeding at nine weeks postpartum (2) during partial breast feeding at 49 weeks and (3) after complete weaning at 58 weeks postpartum.

During these three phases there was no significant change in FSH levels but there was a progressive rise in basal LH concentrations and an increase in the amplitude and frequency of LH pulses. These change in LH were associated with a fall in basal prolactin levels and a rise in the levels of ovarian activity as indicated by ovarian steroid excretion. These results are consistent with the hypothesis that failure of pulsatile LH release may play a part in the suppression of ovarian activity during lactation.

Hypothalamic sensitivity during lactation

The reason for the reduced pulsatile LH secretion during full lactation is probably due to an increased sensitivity of the hypothalamus to the negative feedback effect of ovarian steroids. Baird et al (1980) administered oestrogen to lactating and non-lactating mothers at seven, 30 and 100 days postpartum. The oestrogen suppressed LH and FSH concentrations to a greater extent in the lactating than in the non-lactating women and failed to induce positive feedback in the lactating women. This evidence suggests that a failure of a normal hypothalamic feedback response to oestrogen may be the central feature in maintaining lactational amenorrhoea although it is not known whether this mechanism is mediated by prolactin itself or by some other means.

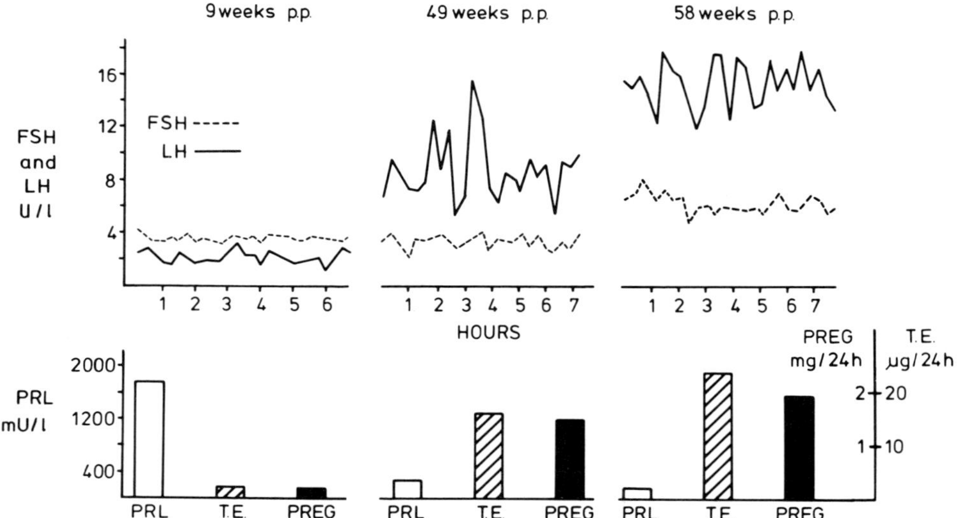

Fig. 8.8   Patterns of plasma FSH and LH over six hour periods and their relationships to basal prolactin (PRL), total urinary estrogen (T.E.) and urinary pregnanediol (P) in a breast feeding mother, (1) nine weeks postpartum during full breast feeding, (2) 49 weeks postpartum during partial breast feeding and (3) 58 weeks postpartum after complete weaning. Urinary steroid levels indicate peak volumes reached during the cycle.

Gonadotrophin response to LHRH

During the first seven days postpartum in both lactating and non-lactating mothers, the FSH and LH responses to luteinising hormone releasing hormone (LHRH) are diminished or absent. After this initial phase, non-lactating women exhibit exaggerated LH and FSH responses to LHRH which are equivalent to those seen in the normal follicular phase of the cycle. In fully-breast feeding mothers at six to eight weeks postpartum, LHRH induces a normal FSH response but a diminished LH response, (Jeppsson et al, 1974; Le Maire et al, 1974; Andreassen & Tyson, 1976) while, in long-term lactation, the FSH response remains exaggerated and the LH response is similar to that seen in the normal luteal phase (Delvoye et al, 1978b). These data support the concept that it is a failure of LH secretion rather than of FSH, which contributes to the maintainance of lactational amenorrhoea.

Ovarian sensitivity during lactation

During the first 15 days postpartum, the ovaries are refractory to gonadotrophins whether given exogenously or secreted endogenously by LHRH (Zarate et al, 1972; del Pozo et al, 1975). After this refractory phase, gonadotrophins are capable of inducing ovarian follicular development and oestrogen secretion (Andreassen & Tyson, 1976). Although the ovaries can respond in this way to pharmacological stimulation by gonadotrophins, it is still possible that there is a diminished ovarian responsiveness in vivo to the physiological stimulation of normal gonadotrophin release. In eight of the 20 mothers studied by Glasier et al (1981) there was absent ovarian activity despite apparently normal FSH and LH release during lactational amenorrhoea. In vitro studies have shown that raised prolactin levels inhibit progesterone production by granulosa cells (McNatty et al, 1974) so the hyperprolactinaemia during lactation might induce a state of partial or complete ovarian insensitivity to physiological concentrations of gonadotrophin.

Further evidence of diminished ovarian response comes from a study of the incidence of anovular cycles and the adequacy of the luteal phases in ovulatory cycles

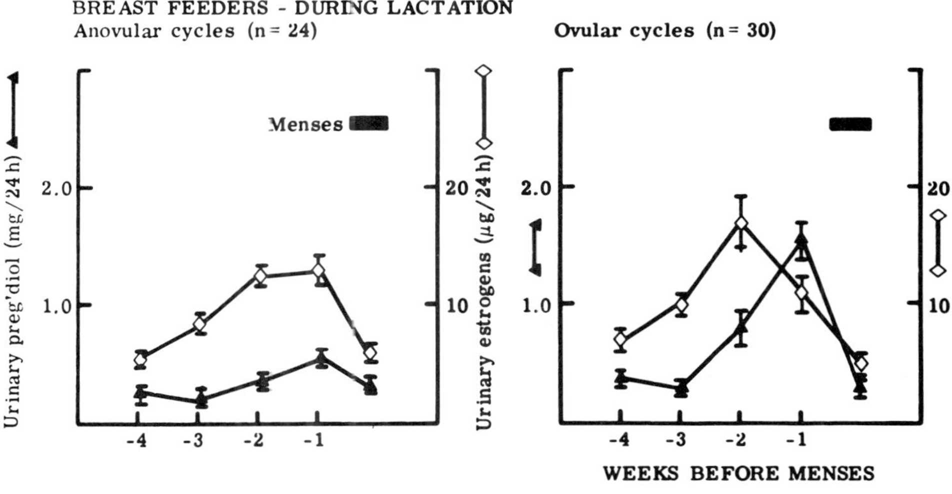

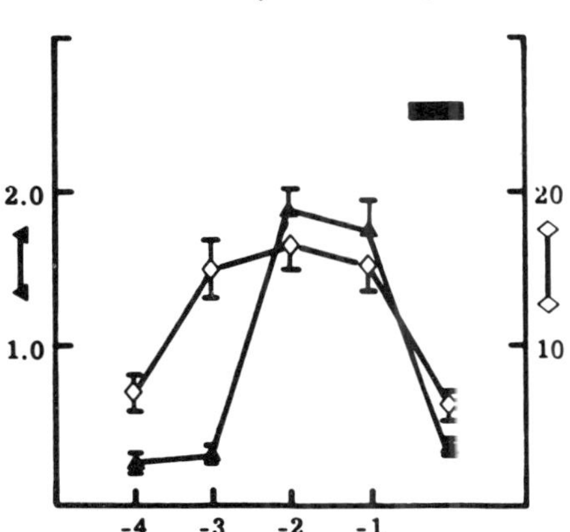

Fig. 8.9   Mean levels of urinary pregnanediol and total urinary oestrogens in anovular and ovular cycles during lactation compared to cycles after lactation.

during lactation (McNeilly et al, 1981). Fifty-four cycles were observed during lactation in 27 breast feeding mothers and 24 (44 per cent) of these were anovular (urinary pregnanediol < 1 mg/24 hrs). The urinary pregnanediol and total urinary oestrogen levels during lactation were compared with those in 27 cycles after lactation (Fig. 8.9). The levels of pregnanediol in the ovulatory cycles during lactation were lower when compared with those in the cycles after lactation, suggesting that even when the gonadotrophins were sufficient to induce ovulation, the ovarian response was deficient during lactation. It is likely that the adequacy of the corpus luteum reflected the adequacy of follicular development because total urinary estrogen levels corresponded with the pregnanediol levels, being lowest in the anovular cycles during lactation (see McNeilly, 1980).

From the information presented above, a hypothesis of the mechanism of lactational infertility can be presented. During suckling, afferent neural impulses are sent to the hypothalamus which becomes more sensitive to the negative feedback effect of ovarian steroids and less sensitive to positive feedback. The change in hypothalamic sensitivity leads to a failure of normal LH pulsatile release from the pituitary although FSH levels are unaffected. The failure of normal LH release causes impairment of ovarian follicular development, amenorrhoea and infertility. After recovery of LH production from the pituitary, there may be a phase of relative ovarian insensitivity, during which time there may be a progression from complete gonadal inactivity to anovular cycles or ovular cycles with defective luteal phases before normal ovarian activity is finally restored.

Prolactin and lactational amenorrhoea

Several studies, using cross sectional data, have shown that the amenorrhoea associated with prolonged lactation is associated with hyperprolactinaemia and suppression of ovarian activity (Delvoye et al, 1978b; Duchen & McNeilly, 1980). It is well known that pathological hyperprolactinaemia in non-pregnant women is associated with infertility and menstrual disturbances which return to normal after treatment of the hyperprolactinaemia (Thorner et al, 1974). Furthermore, the use of bromocriptine in non-nursing mothers leads to more rapid normalisation of prolactin levels and an earlier resumption of ovulation (Rolland et al, 1975b). From these considerations, it is tempting to assume that prolactin must play a part in the mechanisms of lactational infertility, but it is not yet certain whether prolactin per se mediates the contraceptive effect of lactation or merely acts as a convenient marker of the suckling stimulus. Further studies are required to elucidate the exact role of prolactin but an attempt has been made to reinforce the contraceptive effect of breast feeding by the use of sulpiride which raises circulating prolactin levels (Badraoui and Hefnawi, 1979). This study showed that menstruation and ovulation were slower to return in lactating mothers taking sulpiride compared with controls but, although the pregnancy rate was lower in sulpiride-users nine months postpartum, this difference had disappeared at one year. Further trials are required to evaluate this potentially valuable approach to contraception.

Contraception during lactation

There is some evidence that combined oestrogen-progestogen oral contraceptives may reduce milk production in lactating women (for review see Buchanan, 1975), although the degree to which this occurs depends on type and dose of the pill and the time at which it is started. Progestogen only contraceptive pills do not appear to have an adverse effect on milk production and are usually preferred to the combined preparations (Gupta et al, 1977). Alternatively intrauterine devices or barrier methods of contraception can be used during lactation.

For many women, however, none of these methods of contraception ideally suit their individual needs and it would be of great value if they could be given guidelines about their chances of conception in relation to differing patterns of suckling duration and frequency. Potter et al (1979) has evaluated alternative strategies for starting contraception in Bangladesh and recommended beginning contraception at six months postpartum when fewer than one in 200 women would have become pregnant before beginning contraception. If similar information was available for developed countries, a proportion of mothers might wish to use the natural contraceptive effect of lactation as a birth-spacing method, accepting the small possibility of an unexpectedly early conception associated with a practice of frequent nursing. Carefully collected information among non-contracepting breast feeding mothers in both developed and developing countries should be made a research objective of high priority.

SUMMARY AND CONCLUSIONS

1. There is strong epidemiological evidence to indicate that breast feeding acts as a natural contraceptive and that this effect is of major demographic importance in developing countries.

2. The most important determining factor in the success of lactational infertility is the strength of the suckling stimulus, which is, in turn inversely dependent upon the introduction of supplementary food to the infant.

3. The mechanism of lactational infertility is complex involving changes in hypothalamic sensitivity, a loss of normal pulsatile LH release from the pituitary and a probable change in ovarian sensitivity to gonadotrophins.

4. Menstruation is an unreliable guide to ovulation during lactation and more information is required to develop practical guidelines for mothers who wish to maximise the natural contraceptive effect of breast feeding.

REFERENCES

Andreassen B, Tyson J E 1976 Role of the hypothalamic-ovarian axis in puerperal infertility. Journal of Clinical Endocrinology and Metabolism 42: 1114–1122

Badraoui M H H, Hefnawi F 1979 Ovarian function during lactation. In: Hafez E S E (ed) Human Ovulation. Elsevier North Holland Biomedical Press Ch 13, p 233

Baird D T, McNeilly A S, Sawers R S, Sharpe R M 1980 Failure of estrogen-induced discharge of luteinising hormone in lactating women. Journal of Clinical Endocrinology and Metabolism 49: 500–504

Berman M L, Hanson K, Hellman I L 1972 Effect of breast feeding on postpartum menstruation, ovulation and pregnancy in Alaskan Eskimos, American Journal of Obstetrics and Gynaecology 114: 524–534

Bohnet H G, Schneider H P G 1977 Prolactin as a cause of anovulation. In: Crosignani P G, Robyn C (eds) Prolactin and human reproduction. Academic Press, London, New York, p 153

Bongaarts J 1980 Does malnutrition affect fecundity? A summary of evidence. Science 208: 564–569.

Bonnar J, Franklin M, Nott P N, McNeilly A S 1975 Effect of breast feeding on pituitary-ovarian function after childbirth. British Medical Journal 4: 82–84

Bonte M, Akingeneye E, Gashakamba M, Nbarutso E, Nolens M 1974 Influence of the socio-economic level on the conception rate during lactation. International Journal of Fertility 19: 97–102

Buchanan R 1975 Breast feeding — aid to infant health and fertility control. Population Reports Series J No. 4: 49–67

Chen L C, Ahmed S, Gesche M, Mosley W 1974 A prospective study of birth interval dynamics in rural Bangladesh. Population Studies 28: 277–297

Coles E C, Cotter S, Valman H B 1978 Increasing prevalence of breast feeding. British Medical Journal 2: 1122–1123

Cox J 1978 Effect of supplementary feeding on infant growth in an aboriginal family. Journal of Biosocial Science 10: 429–436

Delgado H, Lechtig A, Martorell R, Brineman E, Klein R E 1978 Nutrition, Lactation and postpartum amenorrhea. American Journal of Clinical Nutrition 31: 322–327

del Pozo E, Varga L, Schulz K D, Künzig H J, Marbach P, Lopez del Campo G, Eppenberger U 1975 Pituitary and ovarian response patterns to stimulation in the postpartum and in galactorrhea-amenorrhea: the role of prolactin. Obstetrics and Gynaecology 46: 539–543

Delvoye P, Badawi M, Demaeged M, Robyn C 1978a Serum prolactin, gonadotrophins and estradiol in menstruating and amenorrheic mothers during two years of lactation. American Journal of Obstetrics and Gynaecology 130: 635–639

Delvoye P, Badawi P, Demaeged M, Robyn C 1978b Long lasting lactation in association with hyperprolactinaemia and amenorrhoea. In: Robyn C, Harter M (eds) Progress in Prolactin Physiology and Pathology. Elsevier/North Holland Biomedical Press, p 213

Duchen M, McNeilly A S 1980 Hyperprolactinaemia and long-term lactational amenorrhoea. Clinical Endocrinology 12: 621–627

El-Minawi M F, Foda M S 1971 Postpartum lactation amenorrhoea. American Journal of Obstetrics and Gynaecology 111: 17–21

Glasier A, McNeilly A S, Howie P W 1981 Unpublished data

Gupta A N, Mathur V S, Gorg S K 1977 Effect of oral contraceptives on the production and composition of human milk. Journal of Biosocial Science Supplement 4: 123–133

Howie P W, McNeilly A S, Houston M J, Cook A, Boyle H 1981a Effect of supplementary food on suckling patterns and ovarian activity during lactation. British Medical Journal 283: 757–759

Howie P W, McNeilly A S, Houston M J, Cook A, Boyle H 1981b The relationship of infant feeding patterns to the timing of ovulation during lactation. Submitted for publication

Huffman S L, Chowdhury A M K, Chakborty J, Mosley W H 1978 Postpartum amenorrhoea: How is it affected by maternal nutritional status? Science 200: 1155–1157

Jelliffe D B, Jelliffe E F P 1978 Human milk in the modern world. Oxford University Press, Oxford. ch 5, p 84

Jeppsson S, Rannevik G, Kullander S 1974 Studies on the decreased gonadotropin response after administration of LH/FSH-releasing hormone during pregnancy and the puerperium. American Journal of Obstetrics and Gynaecology 120: 1029–1034

Keye W R, Jaffe R B 1976 Changing patterns of FSH and LH response to gonadotrophin releasing hormone in the puerperium. Journal of Clinical Endocrinology and Metabolism 42:1133–1138

Konner M, Worthman C 1980 Nursing frequency, gonadal function and birth spacing among !Kung hunter gatherers. Science 207: 788–791

Lastra M de la, Llados C 1977 Luteinizing hormone content of the pituitary gland in pregnant and non-pregnant women. Journal of Clinical Endocrinology and Metabolism 44: 921–923

LeMaire W J, Shapiro A G, Riggall F, Yang N S T 1974 Temporary pituitary insensitivity to stimulation by synthetic LRF during the postpartum period. Journal of Clinical Endocrinology and Metabolism 38: 916–918

Lunn P G, Prentice A M, Austin S, Whitehead R G 1980 Influence of maternal diet on plasma prolactin levels during lactation. Lancet i: 623–625

McKeown T, Gibson J A 1954 A note on menstruation and conception during lactation. Journal of Obstetrics and Gynaecology of the British Empire 61: 824–826

McNatty K P, Sawers R S, McNeilly A S 1974 A possible role for prolactin in control of steroid secretion by the human graafian follicle. Nature 250: 653–655

McNeilly A S 1979 Effect of lactation on fertility. British Medical Bulletin 35: 151–154

McNeilly A S 1980 Paradoxical prolactin. Nature 284: 212

McNeilly A S, Howie P W, Houston M J 1980 Relationship of feeding patterns, prolactin and resumption of ovulation postpartum. In: Zatuchni G I, Labbok M H Sciarra J J (eds) Research Frontiers in Fertility Regulation. Harper And Row, New York Ch 12: p 102

McNeilly A S, Howie P W, Houston M J, Cook A, Boyle H S Adequacy of the luteal phase in menstrual cycles during lactation 1981. Submitted for publication

Morley D 1977 Biosocial advantages of an adequate birth interval. Journal of Biosocial Science Supplement 4: 69–81

Perez A, Vela P, Potter R G, Masnick G S 1971 Timing and sequence of resuming ovulation and menstruation after childbirth. Population Studies 25: 491–503

Perez A, Vela P, Masnick G S, Potter R G 1972 First ovulation after childbirth: The effect of breast feeding. American Journal of Obstetrics and Gynecology 114: 1041–1047

Potter R G, Kobrin F E, Longstern R L 1979 Evaluatory acceptance strategies for timing of postpartum contraception. Studies in Family Planning 10: 151–160

Prema K, Naidu A N, Kumari S N 1979 Lactation and Fertility. American Journal of Clinical Nutrition 32: 1298–1303

Reyes F I, Winter J S D, Fairman D 1972 Pituitary-ovarian interrelationships during the puerperium. American Journal of Obstetrics and Gynaecology 114: 589–594

Robinson J, Short R V 1977 Changes in human breast sensitivity at puberty, during the menstrual cycle and at parturition. British Medical Journal 1: 1188–1191

Rolland R, Lequin R M, Schellekens L A, De Jong F H 1975a The role of prolactin in the restoration of ovarian function during the early postpartum period in the human female I. Study during physiological lactation. Clinical Endocrinology 4: 15–25

Rolland R, de Jong F H, Schellekens L A, Lequin R M 1975b The role of prolactin in the restoration of ovarian function during the early postpartum period in the human female II. A study during inhibition of lactation by bromergocryptine. Clinical Endocrinology 4: 27–38

Rosa F W 1975 The role of breast feeding in family planning. Protein Advisory Group Bulletin 5: 5–10

Sharman A 1951 Menstruation after childbirth. Journal of Obstetrics and Gynaecology of the British Empire 58: 440–445

Short R V 1976 Lactation — the central control of reproduction. In: Ciba Foundation Symposium 45, Breast Feeding and the mother. Elsevier, North Holland p 73–86

Thomson A M, Hytten F E, Black A E 1975 Lactation and reproduction. Bulletin of the World Health Organisation 52: 337–349

Thorner M O, McNeilly A S, Hagen C, Besser G M 1974 Long-term treatment of galactorrhoea and hypogonadism with bromocriptine. British Medical Journal 2: 419–422

Tyson J E, Hwang P, Guyda H, Friesen H 1972 Studies of prolactin secretion in human pregnancy. American Journal of Obstetrics and Gynaecology 113: 14–20

Udesky I C 1950 Ovulation in lactating women. American Journal of Obstetrics and Gynaecology 59: 843–848

van Ginneken J K 1977 The chance of conception during lactation. Journal of Biosocial Science Supplement 4: 41–54

Waterlow J C, Thomson A M 1979 Observations of the adequacy of breast feeding. Lancet ii: 238–241

World Health Organisation Collaborative Study on Breast Feeding 1979: Preliminary Report.

Zarate A, Canales E S, Soria J, Ruiz F, MacGregor C 1972 Ovarian refractoriness during lactation in women: Effect of gonadotropin stimulation. American Journal of Obstetrics and Gynecology 112: 1130–1133.

9. Trends in perinatal mortality in the developing world

R. L. TambyRaja

INTRODUCTION

Perinatal mortality and morbidity have been likened to an iceberg where handicap remains the submerged and unknown moiety. Several decades ago in Asia and Africa most of the neonates with serious problems died. As improvements in maternity care reach the third world we may be faced with a fall in the number of deaths but an increasing number of infants of low birthweight with serious physical and mental handicaps. In a few fortunate countries of South-East Asia like Singapore and Japan, perinatal care has reached the stage where morbidity as well as mortality has decreased. The major contributions towards this have come from socio-economic changes, improvement in health care, decrease in family size and a move towards the delivery of infants in maternity hospitals under optimal circumstances.

The major health problems of mothers and children in the third world arise from the synergistic effects of malnutrition, infection and high fertility, combined with lack of adequate obstetric care and bad communications. Poor living conditions and ineffective public health services afford little protection during pregnancy and delivery against an uninhibited stream of parasitic, viral and bacterial infections.

A complete study of perinatal mortality and morbidity in South-East Asia is not possible for two main reasons. First, the definition of perinatal mortality in these countries has not been uniform. It is assumed to imply the number of late fetal deaths (stillbirths) and deaths in the first week of life (early neonatal deaths) per 1000 live and stillbirths. Second, collection of basic data in many of these countries is incomplete and incorrect statistics have often been reported, e.g. the perinatal mortality rate of Thailand 1973–1974 was reported in the World Health Organisation Statistics as four to six per 1000. More than 80 per cent of the population in South-East Asia lives in rural areas, where registration of births and deaths is inaccurate. This chapter will confine itself to experiences reported by reputable workers and will demonstrate that South-East Asian countries, given the time and opportunity, should be able to reduce their perinatal mortality to levels reached by the developed countries.

Table 9.1 illustrates the magnitude of the problem. Whereas two thirds of the world population is distributed in the less developed regions, one third is sited in the WHO South-East Asia region, and the 1980 population of the countries illustrated in Table 1 will have increased considerably by 1985. The annual growth rates of these developing countries have contributed considerably to their high perinatal mortality with governments trying to meet the important and urgent need of food while forgetting the roles of public health and family planning.

Countries with vast populations like Bangladesh, India, Thailand, Indonesia and the Philippines have widespread poverty in rural areas and in urban slums, with lack of sanitation, pure water, food, education and health services. Nearly 80 per cent of

Table 9.1 Total population and rates of growth by world total and countries in WHO South-East Asia region

Region and country	Population (millions)		Annual rates of growth (%)	
	1980	1985	1975–80	1980–85
1. World Total	4373.2	4815.6	1.95	1.93
2. More developed regions	1181.1	1230.8	0.85	0.83
3. Less developed regions	3192.1	3584.8	2.37	2.32
4. WHO South-East Asia region	1068.1	1209.3	2.54	2.51
(a) Bangladesh	84.8	98.0	2.79	2.89
(b) Burma	35.2	39.7	2.38	2.40
(c) India	682.2	782.9	2.48	2.40
(d) Sri Lanka	15.5	18.0	2.01	1.88
(e) Thailand	49.5	57.8	3.23	3.11

women in these countries go through pregnancy and delivery without receiving any form of antenatal care. Further, only about half the children reach the age of five years due to the vicious cycle of malnutrition, infection, and high fertility. To talk about perinatal care and to expend limited public funds on expensive technology would be putting the cart before the horse. In these countries priority must be given to reducing the high infant mortality by the provision of food, sanitation, immunisation and health education. Apart from governmental dedication, the people have to be open to the acceptance of new ideas some of which may be contrary to their cultural traditions and religious beliefs. Projects in perinatal care have failed in these developing countries because systems functioning well in the industrialised world were copied and transferred without considering the indigenous social, cultural and religious environment.

PERINATAL MORTALITY IN THE DEVELOPING WORLD

Figure 9.1 shows the perinatal mortality as a league table and may give an erroneous impression. This is true of any international comparison of perinatal mortality. It is meaningless to compare a small island city like Singapore with a country composed of hundreds of islands like Indonesia or the Philippines. Many factors are responsible for the perinatal mortality rates of any country.

Hospital and field-based studies and birth registrations from third world countries reviewed by the WHO in the 1960s revealed perinatal mortality rates ranging between 80 and 100/1000 live births, with low birthweight as the underlying cause in at least one third. If low socioeconomic groups form 90 per cent of the population this is hardly surprising. Perinatal mortality reported for the Indian subcontinent by the Registrar General was reviewed by Menon (1971) and showed a reduction from 182/1000 in 1930 to 78/1000 in 1960. Sepsis was a major cause. The infections arose principally from prolonged infected labour and from tetanus neonatorum which remains a serious problem with almost 100 per cent mortality. By the mid-1970s perinatal mortality was considerably reduced and as shown in Figure 9.1 mortality rates varied from 14–15 in Japan and Singapore to 55 in India. This decrease could be directly coupled with socioeconomic progress in the first two which are industrialised nations. The details of late fetal, neonatal and post-neonatal mortality rates in the Asian region given in Table 9.2 bring to light the following:

1. Countries like Singapore and Japan which have reduced their infant mortality

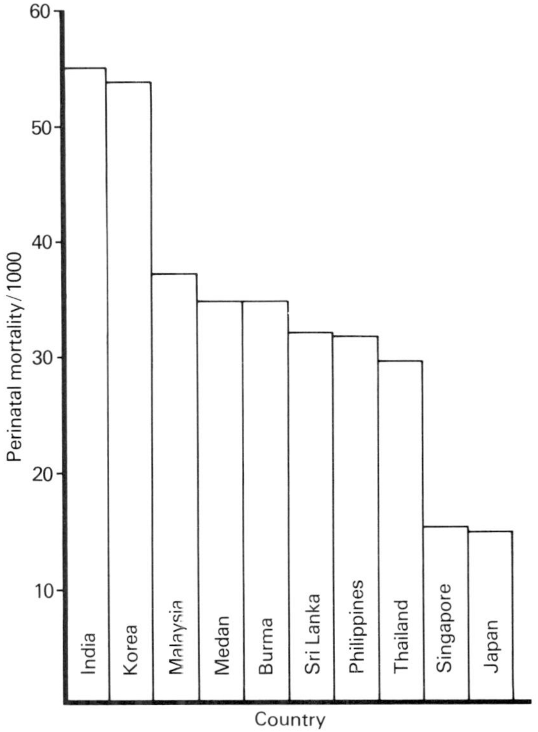

Fig. 9.1 Perinatal mortality in Asian countries.

are now in a position to improve further their perinatal mortality and morbidity by the selective use of new technology.

2. Countries like the Philippines, Malaysia and Thailand should embark on programmes of infant care and immunisation, combating sepsis and gastro-enteritis by public health measures. They should inprove their perinatal services and concentrate their efforts on delivering high risk pregnancies in hospitals rather than at home.

Table 9.2 Late fetal, infant, neonatal, post-neonatal and perinatal mortality per 1000 births in Asian region, 1976

	Late fetal	Perinatal	Neonatal	Post-neonatal	Infant
Japan	9.7	14.8	6.4	3.0	9.3
Malaysia	19.3	34.6	22.0	13.4	35.4
Philippines	10.7	32.07	16.7	28.9	53.3
Thailand	1.7	5.4	7.7	18.0	25.7
Singapore (1978)	7.0	15.2	9.7	3.0	12.6

PERINATAL MORTALITY IN INDIVIDUAL COUNTRIES OF ASIA

India

With a population of nearly 700 million people, India had a perinatal death rate of 182 per 1000 in 1930. By 1960 the figure was around 78 per 1000, with a range 60–109/1000 (Menon, 1976). Trauma and stress of labour were responsible for nearly a third of fetal deaths while another third was due to pre-eclampsia and antepartum haemorrhage. Maternal illnesses like anaemia, acute infections, hepatitis and dysentery contributed to the toll.

Recently Ajit Mehta and Jayant (1979) collected 3500 cases of perinatal death from 42 centres and compared their results with 4546 controls delivered during the same period. There was an average perinatal mortality of 55 per 1000. Seventy-four per cent of perinatal deaths weighed less than 2500 g compared to only 33 per cent of the survivors. An important factor responsible for perinatal mortality was inadequate antenatal care. Significant antenatal problems included antepartum haemorrhage, polyhydramnios and premature rupture of membranes.

Korea

The perinatal mortality in a Korean hospital declined from 92.2 in 1967 to 53.8 in 1977 (Nicholson et al, 1979). The most significant change was in the neonatal death rate which decreased from 50.8 to 24. The major reasons were decreases in birth asphyxia and syphilis. Improvements in antenatal care in keeping with socioeconomic changes contributed to the improvement.

Indonesia

National figures are not available. Rangkute et al 1979 reported that perinatal mortality was 128.9/1000 in Pirngadi Hospital. The perinatal mortality rate was related to antenatal care. It was 203.4 per 1000 when mothers had no antenatal care and 34.0 per 1000 when the mothers received care. The main causes of perinatal death were asphyxia, low birthweight and septicaemia.

Sri Lanka

In the 1960s perinatal mortality ranged between 70 and 80 per 1000. In 1970, Rajanayagam reported a two year analysis and a perinatal mortality in the region of 62 per 1000. Sixty per cent of neonatal deaths were due to the respiratory distress syndrome. Birth trauma and congenital malformation made up the remainder. Five years later Raja Kaariyar (1975) reported that preterm births accounted for approximately 64.5 per cent of all perinatal deaths. This was followed by neonatal infection (gastroenteritis and septicaemia). Small for dates babies accounted for 25 per cent of perinatal mortality. Full term babies accounted for 10.5 per cent of perinatal mortality. Asphyxia, particularly intrapartum, seems to be the leading cause of death and should be a cause for concern in this country. Every year nearly 1000 mothers die in Ceylon leaving nearly 5000 infants motherless. If progress is to be made, government supported health and family planning programmes in the rural areas are essential.

Thailand

Accurate perinatal mortality figures at a national level are urgently required (viz. four to six per 1000 in WHO statistics). The most accurate report by Snidvongs 1979 was a retrospective study of 606 stillbirths from nearly 70 000 births in a teaching hospital. The stillbirth rate was 8.71/1000 births. Maternal medical diseases including syphilis and hypertension accounted for 10 per cent of all stillbirths and 15.8 per cent of cases had obstetric complications, the chief of which was antepartum haemorrhage.

Philippines
In this country composed of hundreds of islands over a million babies are born each year; 70 per cent of these births occur in the rural areas, the majority being delivered by traditional birth attendants. The infant mortality of above 100 (per 1000 live births) in 1950 has steadily declined to 53 in 1975 when the perinatal mortality was 32. Physicians from this region report at perinatal conferences that local ingenuity and the motivation of groups such as the Maternal and Child Health Association and the Obstetric and Paediatric Associations, have gone further than government policies in reaching the rural populations. The setting up of base hospitals and early referral of problems will see further success in lowering the neonatal mortality rate of 24.4.

Malaysia
A neighbour of Singapore has a land area of 312 633 sq km and 14 million inhabitants. Overall there has been a significant reduction in perinatal mortality from 58.7 (1969) to 34.6 (1976), but little change in neonatal mortality — 23.4 and 22 respectively. Teaching units in the capital, Kuala Lumpur, have reported lower figures. Infant mortality rates in Peninsular Malaysia, Sabah and Sarawak are still above 36 per thousand live births. Training courses for midwives in the rural areas are of limited value in the face of ill-equipped, poorly staffed base hospitals. A WHO field study in Perak is at present underway. The setting up of a national conference on perspectives in perinatal medicine would see a new era of perinatal care.

Japan
The perinatal mortality rate was 46.6 per 1000 live births in 1950 and decreased to 13 per 1000 in 1978. The committee on perinatal statistics under the chairmanship of Sakamoto (1979) has reported annual statistics since 1974. Published data for 1974, 1975 and 1976 show a decrease in the stillbirth rate from 9.72 to 8.96 and 8.67 and low neonatal death rates 4.38, 6.18 and 5.51. The number of deaths due to placenta praevia and respiratory distress syndrome shows a clear decrease. The figures from this industrial giant compare favourably with most other developed nations.

MORTALITY FROM LOW BIRTHWEIGHT (LBW) IN THE DEVELOPING WORLD

About 22 million LBW babies are born each year, one-sixth of the global number of live births. Only 5 per cent of these, mostly preterm, are in developed countries. Of the 21 million in developing countries 16 million are believed to be small-for-dates (Petroz-Barvazian and Behar, 1978). Reports from Indonesia, Malaysia and Singapore lead to an estimate of 3 million LBW infants born in South-East Asia during 1980. From Table 9.3 it is seen that in countries such as India a third of the infants weigh less than 2500 g (Menon 1976) while the proportion is only 7.6 per cent in Singapore and 16.8 per cent in Malaysia and most other South-East Asian countries. An explanation of low birthweight purely as a consequence of maternal nutrition is too naive (Bonham, 1979). The 2500 g cut-off point has perhaps served its purpose and a fifth percentile definition of low birthweight for each race in each developing country, though more complex, would be of more practical value. Among the multiplicity of

Table 9.3 Low birth-weight in South-East Asia

Area	Percentage weighing 2500 g or less	Median birthweight (g)	Median gestation period (weeks)
India	28.0	2771	40.6
Malaysia	16.8	2986	39.8
Philippines	14.2	2889	39.6
Japan	11.3	3029	40.2
Singapore	7.6	3180	40.0

factors influencing birthweight, ethnic characteristics have been shown to persist despite improved economic circumstances among immigrant Chinese and Dravidian communities who have lived for generations in the mixed societies of Singapore, Malaysia, Indonesia and Fiji. The literature has been replete with attempts to identify standards for LBW which relate to the median birthweights found among differing communities in Singapore, India, Indonesia, the Philippines and elsewhere (Millis, 1953; Erwinn et al, 1966; Madhavan & Tasker, 1969; Cheng et al, 1972). The important issue from the point of view of management is to distinguish the small yet fully mature term baby from the immature preterm baby and from the baby with intrauterine growth retardation. A concerted effort has been made in Singapore to reduce perinatal mortality from preterm birth (TambyRaja & Ratnam, 1980).

Low birthweight and its economic impact on developing countries
The ultimate implications of a high incidence of LBW babies depend on the adverse effect of LBW on mortality, morbidity and postnatal development. Low birthweight babies are less likely to survive the first year of life than normal birthweight babies (Chase, 1969; Mata et al, 1971; Lechtig et al, 1976). It is clear that in addition to its human and emotional implications, higher mortality entails heavy economic waste since the average productive employment period in a population is notably reduced as a consequence of early death. This produces a decreased return on the investments made by the family and society during pregnancy and the early postnatal years.

What is the cost of those LBW babies who survive? These babies carry an increased risk of physical growth retardation and impaired mental development. This is of importance in the developing world because maternal resources are strained and the cumulative addition of handicapped children and adults will further deplete limited resources. The association between low birthweight and suboptimal learning during childhood and adolescence may contribute to lower productivity, lower income and poor quality of life (Baldwin, 1974).

In summary, a high incidence of low birthweight babies may create an economic burden heavy enough to become a major public health problem and a serious obstacle to development in many countries of the developing world. Stickney et al (1976) conducted long-term prospective studies in Guatemala and showed that a nutritional programme for pregnant women reduced the risk of low birthweight by 50 per cent. From this it may be inferred that investment in programmes oriented to decreasing the incidence of LBW babies may yield an economic return important enough to justify policies designed to stimulate social and economic development (TambyRaja & Ratnam, 1981).

COULD SINGAPORE BE A MODEL OF PERINATAL CARE FOR DEVELOPING COUNTRIES?

Singapore is a small island with a multi-racial society of 2.36 million people, comprising 76 per cent Chinese, 15 per cent Malays, 7 per cent Indians and 2 per cent other races.

The perinatal mortality has declined through the years from 25.5 in 1965 to 14 in 1980. From 1965 to 1970, there appears to have been no significant change in perinatal mortality. However along with rapid socio-economic progress, the most important influence appears to have been the establishment of the Singapore Family Planning Board, and liberalised sterilisation and abortion laws. This was accompanied by social disincentives in the form of higher delivery fees, reduction of paid maternity leave, lower priority for choice of school for children and higher income tax with higher parity. The importance of small, spaced families in perinatal outcome in South-East Asia cannot be doubted. From 1971 with further socio-economic progress, a new pattern of perinatal care was instituted by setting up Maternal and Child Health Clinics. The service is based on a chain of clinics strategically placed around the island Republic. Spread over an area of 518 sq kilometers, a total of 30 Maternal and Child Health Clinics has been established (SFPPB Report 1979). The aim is to ensure that the clinic services are brought almost to the doorsteps of those who need them. The clinics are staffed by physicians, nurses and midwives. The more serious and complicated cases are singled out and referred for specialised care at the hospitals.

Domiciliary after-care services

The Kandang Kerbau Hospital in the early 1970s delivered nearly 40 000 babies a year and was featured in the Guinness Book of Records. With such a large turnover and limited beds, a system of early discharge had to be developed for apparently normal patients. The average bed-occupancy at the Kandang Kerbau Hospital is estimated at 3.2 days but about 60 per cent of the patients without any complications are discharged from the hospital within 24 hours. The hospital through the Maternal and Child Health Clinics maintains a domiciliary aftercare service for the discharged patients. Midwives visit the mothers and infants daily in their homes advising the mothers on how to care for themselves and their babies. Mothers and infants developing complications are returned immediately to the hospital for attention.

Causes of perinatal death in Singapore

In analysing perinatal deaths, the cause of death needs to be determined if preventive measures are to be instituted. Many factors have militated against such studies in Singapore and all South-East Asian countries. In the perinatal period an autopsy is often required to determine the actual cause of death. Few perinatal pathologists are available in the developing world. In a five year analysis of perinatal deaths in Singapore (Chan et al, 1978) an avoidable factor was identified in 31 per cent. These included failure in booking, uncooperative patients and poor obstetric or neonatal care. Over 60 per cent of deaths were related to low birthweight and were significantly associated with low socio-economic status, preterm birth and obstetric complications resulting in antepartum and intrapartum asphyxia.

The causes of stillbirth and neonatal deaths in Singapore in 1960 were compared

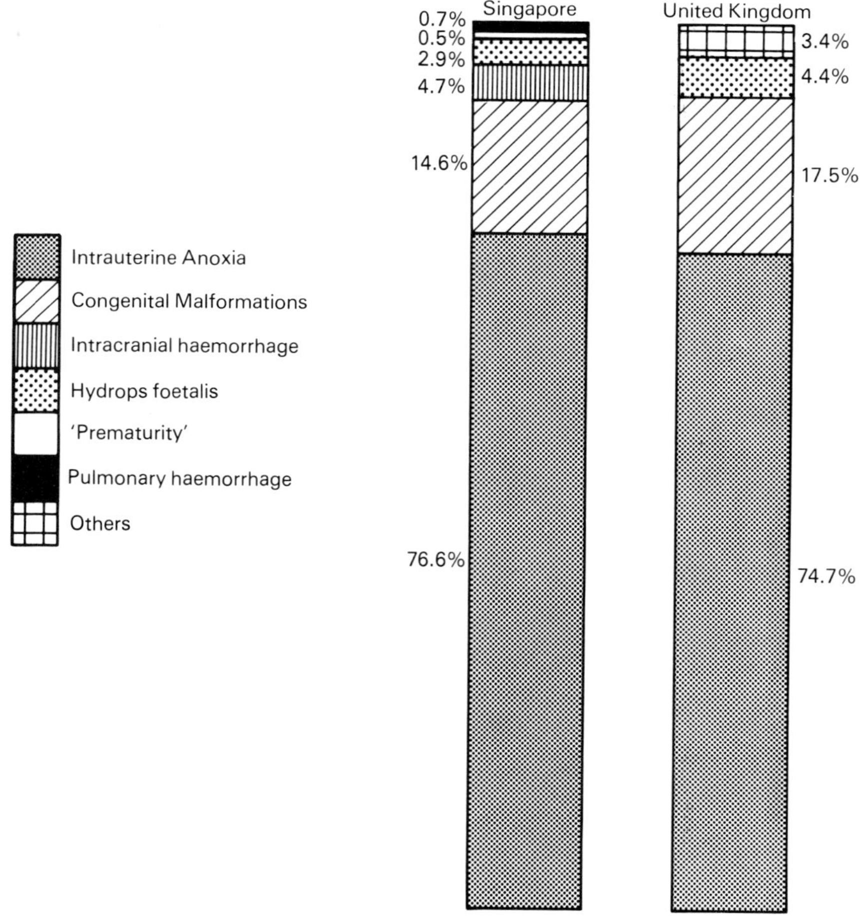

Fig. 9.2 Comparison of stillbirths in Singapore and the United Kingdom.

with those reported in the British Perinatal Mortality Survey and interesting similarities were seen. The perinatal mortality rate in 1965 in Singapore was 25.5 and in the United Kingdom 33.2. Figure 9.2 shows that intrauterine anoxia was responsible for nearly 75 per cent of all stillbirths and congenital malformation for about 15 per cent in both the United Kingdom and Singapore. Hydrops foetalis was responsible for 3 per cent of stillbirths in Singapore and for 4.5 per cent in the United Kingdom. In Singapore, hydrops foetalis was the result of homozygous alpha thalassaemia, while in the United Kingdom, it was due to rhesus incompatibility. There appears to have been a remarkable similarity in causes of stillbirths in the two countries (Wong, 1979). For deaths during the first week (Fig. 9.3), however, RDS was responsible for as many as 28 per cent in Singapore (TambyRaja & Ratnam, 1980) but for only 15 per cent in the United Kingdom, intracranial haemorrhage for 25 per cent in Singapore and 6 per cent in United Kingdom, while congenital malforma-tions accounted for 13.6 per cent in Singapore compared to 21.6 per cent in the United Kingdom. A combination of factors including the rise in per capita income,

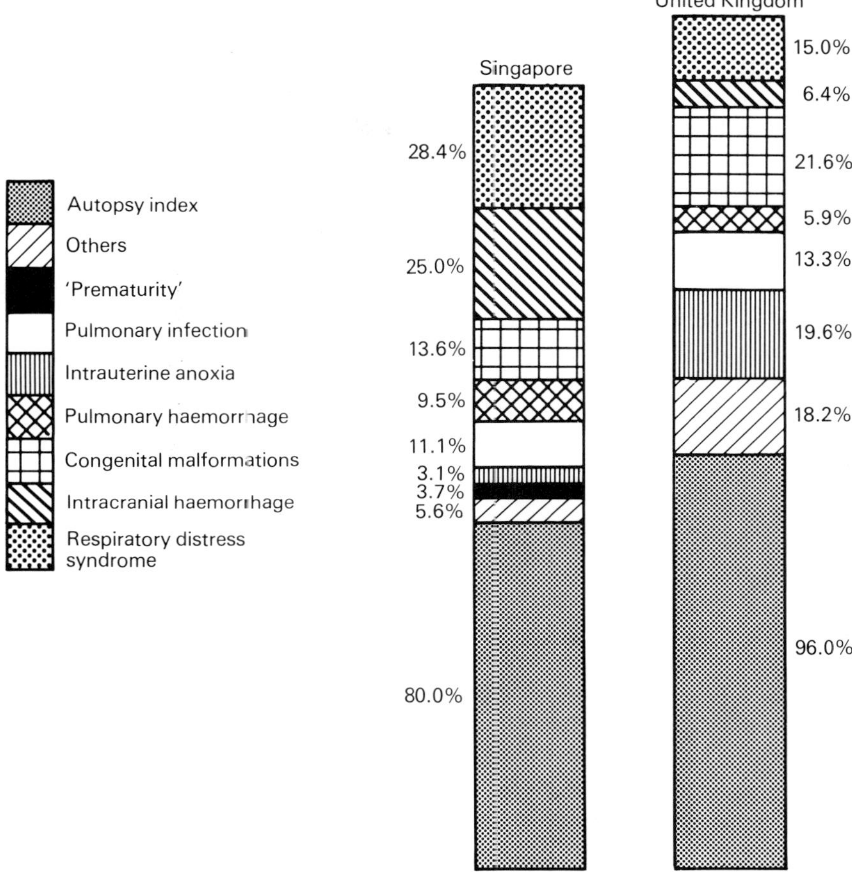

Fig. 9.3 Comparison of first week deaths in Singapore and the United Kingdom.

effectiveness of health education, family planning and better obstetric and paediatric care accounted for the decline in perinatal mortality. In contrast, several other countries in the region have made little progress in improving perinatal care.

CONCLUSION

In developing countries, health services for maternal and child care, with screening and referral of high risk cases to better-equipped institutions, have to be integrated into social development schemes and be designed in such a way that they are appreciated and utilised by the people. Clinical services on the Western model are often mistrusted since there is no bridge to indigenous medicine which in turn is closely associated with cultural and religious patterns. Financial and medical resources are usually too scarce to allow for sufficient density or quality of services. As a result, the services are confined to major cities reaching very few mothers, and seldom those in most need. In many rural parts of the developing world only about 10 per cent of the families have any contact with the maternal and child health services.

Resources will not suffice within the foreseeable future to develop a health service system based on doctors, trained midwives and nurses and on clinics and hospitals that can adequately cater for the total population.

There should be participation of the community members themselves, reaching out into the village homes, and collaborating with indigenous midwifery and health care. Unconventional health service systems have to be developed within existing resources. A key element in such health service systems would be education of the adult population to improve sanitation, hygiene and nutrition and to accept and practise pregnancy planning. International agencies like WHO and UNICEF recognise the need for such low cost schemes of primary health care, adapted to local resources, to priority needs and to socio-cultural conditions of the developing nations.

Further reduction of maternal and perinatal mortality and morbidity in a few of the developed countries with existing low rates would require sophisticated laboratory facilities and expensive technology. Such investments would be ill-advised in the under-privileged areas already characterised by high mortality rates. In these areas elementary preventive measures aimed at reaching the whole population should have priority.

In countries like Singapore and Japan there is a need for sustained and increased emphasis on prevention in order to avoid risk situations. In Singapore nearly 60 per cent of mothers do not attend for antenatal booking until 20 weeks and this group accounts for a high proportion of perinatal deaths (TambyRaja & Ratnam, 1981). The South-East Asian countries given time and adequate resources can reduce their perinatal mortality to levels reached by developed countries. No race or country can be decried for having a predisposition to a high perinatal mortality. Martin (1979) showed that in Australian aborigines, the perinatal mortality of 11.9 per 1000 in hospital booked women was not significantly different from that of Caucasian women. The conclusions of the recent Parliamentary perinatal report from the United Kingdom by Beard et al (1980) are as true for the developing world as for Britain. Firstly, medical intervention has to be aimed at women at high risk, secondly minimum standards of equipment and staffing have to be provided so that deprived areas are no longer underprovided and thirdly, there should be improvements in data collection and analysis.

The contribution of the long-term sequelae of perinatal complications and low birthweight to deficits in childhood in developing countries is complex difficult to identify. Many neonatal problems known to be detrimental to the central nervous system occur in the large population of low birthweight infants born in South-East Asian countries. These infants are more liable to apnoea, respiratory distress syndrome, jaundice and hypoglycaemia, contributing significantly to permanent handicaps. Motivation not only of patients but also of Governments to provide adequate care by the provision of regional neonatal intensive care units is an urgent necessity. Maternal care in the developing world should aim at improving nutrition and basic antenatal needs. This should not only lead to a reduction in incidence of low birthweight babies but also possibly to a decrease in the incidence of neural tube defects (Lawrence, 1980) and congenital abnormalities. If support continues for the present trends in health services the future of some 80 per cent of the world's children will be safe-guarded and their physical and mental growth improved. Perinatal care in the developing countries must be designed to meet the needs of an entire stratum of the population that does not benefit from existing facilities. The governments and the doctors of these countries should realise that resources devoted to Maternal and Child Health are a national investment that will reap a rich harvest in the next generation.

What of the future? In developing countries there should be advances in obstetric research which will be fundamental to understanding prevalent high risk conditions such as pre-eclampsia, abruptio placentae and low birthweight. The prevention of perinatal mortality and morbidity is not when the problem is recognised in pregnancy but at an earlier stage. The studies from Singapore illustrate that provision of continuing care between pregnancies, nutrition and pregnancy spacing are invaluable for an optimal pregnancy outcome. Finally although it is important to evaluate high risk, there is no substitute for expert clinical evaluation of a motivated mother who attends early and regularly for her antenatal care. The obstetrician and paediatrician of the developing world should play a vital role in the primary health care team to ensure a healthy mother and a quality baby'.

Acknowledgements

I am grateful to the editor for allowing me to highlight some of the problems in the developing world. Teachers in Britain and Ireland, Sir John Stallworthy, Sir Norman Jeffcoate, Sir John Dewhurst, Professor John Bonnar, Professor Richard Beard amongst others have devoted much effort to the understanding of the problems in training doctors from these countries. This chapter would not have been possible without the reports of the World Health Organisation and contributions to the Congresses of the Federation of Asia-Oceania Perinatal Societies. I am indebted to Professor S S Ratnam and Professor Wong Hock Boon for the use of statistics compiled in the University departments of Obstetrics and Paediatrics and their encouragement in expanding the concept of perinatal care in the region.

REFERENCES

Ajit Mehta, Kasturi Jayant 1979 Epidemiology of Perinatal Mortality in India. In: Karim S M M (ed) Problems in perinatology. MTP, Lancaster, p 161–167

Beard R W, et al 1980 Perinatal and Neonatal Mortality. Second Report from the Social Services Committee HMS 663–1

Bonham D G 1979 The Epidemiology of Perinatal Mortality and Morbidity. In: Karim S M M (ed) Problems in perinatology. MTP, Lancaster, p 113–128

Baldwin R, Burton A W 1974 Disease and labour productivity. Economic Development and Cultural Change 22: 414–435

Butler N R, Bonham D G 1963 Perinatal mortality. Livingstone, Edinburgh

Chan T, Doshi U, TambyRaja R L, Ratnam S S 1978 A 5-year analysis of Perinatal deaths in Singapore. Unpublished data

Chase H C 1969 Infant Mortality and Weight at birth 1960 United States birth cohort. American Journal of Public Health 59: 1618–1628.

Chase H C 1973 A study of risks, medical care and infant mortality. American Journal of Public Health 63 Suppl 3.

Cheng M C E, Chew P C T, Ratnam S S 1972 Birth-weight distribution of Singapore Chinese, Malay and Indian infants from 34 weeks to 42 weeks gestation. The Journal of Obstetrics and Gynaecology of the British Commonwealth 79: 149–153.

Erwinn S, Dewoonoto O, Sugri S 1966 Birth-weight and birth length of newborns in Bandung. Paediatrics Indonesia 6: 79–88

Lawrence K M 1980 Increased recurrence of pregnancies complicated by fetal Neural Tube defects in mothers receiving poor diets and possible benefits of dietary counselling. British Medical Journal 281: 1592–1595

Lechtig A, Delgado H, Yarbrough C, Habicht J P, Martorell R, Klein R E 1976 A simple assessment of the risk of low birth weight to select women for nutritional intervention. American Journal of Obstetrics and Gynaecology 125: 25–34.

Madhavan S, Tasker A D 1969 Birthweight of Indian babies born in hospital. Indian Journal of Paediatrics 36: 193–204

Martin J D 1979 The Obstetric performance of an urban Australian aboriginal population. In: Karim S M M (ed) Problems in perinatology MTP, Lancaster, p 216–221

Mata L J, Lechtig A, Urrutia J J 1971 Infection and nutrition of children of low socio-economic rural community. American Journal of Clinical Nutrition 24: 249–259.

Menon M K K 1969 Obstetrics in India. In: Kellar R J (ed) Modern trends in obstetrics. Butterworth, London

Menon M K K 1971 Perinatal Mortality in India. Proceedings of 5th Asian Congress of Obstetrics and Gynaecology. Dajkarta, Indonesia 31–38

Menon M K K 1976 Perinatal Mortality in India. In: Perinatal care in developing countries. WHO Workshop GIMO. 81–92

Millis J 1953 Birthweights among different racial groups in Singapore. Medical Journal of Malaysia 7, 169–187

Nicholson E N, Young S K, Donald E M 1979 Changes in the pattern of Perinatal Mortality over 10 years in a Korean Hospital. In: Problems in Perinatology (ed) Karim S M M. MTP, Lancaster 205–211

Petros-Barvazian A, Behar M 1978 Low birthweight — what should be done with this global problem. WHO Chronicle 32: 231–232

Raja Kaariyar S 1975 Report of Department of Neonatal Paediatrics Castle Street Hospital

Rajanayagam S 1972 Perinatal Mortality. Proceedings of Obstetrical and Gynaecological Society of Singapore 2: 60–70

Rangkute S M, Ramayati R, Siregar H 1979 Perinatal Mortality rate and causes of death in low birthweight infants at Dr Pirngadi Hospital Medan in 1978. In: Karim S M M (ed) Problems in perinatology. MTP, Lancaster, p 193–204

Rosa F W 1974 Birthweight in Fiji and Western Samoa — a Pacific prescription for pregnancy? American Journal of Obstetrics and Gyanecology 119: 1121–1124

Sakamoto S, Maeda K 1979 Perinatal Statistics from 200 Hospitals in Japan. In: Karim S M M (ed) Problems in Perinatology. MTP, Lancaster, p 179–182

Snidvongs, Wongkulpat 1979 Stillbirths — five years' experience in Chulalongkorn Hospital, Thailand. In: Karim S M M (ed) Problems in perinatology. MTP, Lancaster, p 183–187

SFPPB (1979) Fourteenth report of Singapore Family Planning and Population Board, p 125

Stickney R E, Beghin I D, Urrutia J J, Mata L J, Arenales P, Habicht J P, Lechtig A, Yarbrough C 1976 Systems analysis in nutrition and health planning: Approximate model relating birth-weight and age to risk of deficient growth. Archivos Latinoamericanos de Nutricion 26: 177–201

TambyRaja R L 1980 Challenges in Perinatal Care. In Proceedings of the Maternal and Child Health Association of the Philippines (MCHAP) Manila, Philippines

TambyRaja R L, Ratnam S S 1980 Factors contributing to the reduction of perinatal mortality from preterm birth in Singapore. In: Ballabriga A, Gallart A (eds) Proceedings of the 7th European Congress of Perinatal Medicine, Barcelona. Industria grafica Sa Provenza, p 152

TambyRaja R L, Ratnam S S 1981 The small fetus, preterm and growth retarded. In: Philpott R M (ed) Clinics in obstetrics and gynaecology 9, 3 (In Press)

Wong H B 1965 Perinatal mortality in Kandang Kerbau Hospital Bulletin of Kandang Kerbau Hospital 4, 41–46

Wong H B 1979 Perinatal morbidity and mortality in South-East Asia. In: Karim S M M (ed) Problems in perinatology, MTP, Lancaster, p 129–146

WHO 1970 The prevention of perinatal mortality and morbidity. Report of WHO Expert Committee. World Health Organization Technical Report Series 457, 60

WHO 1973–79 World Health Organization Statistical Annual

WHO 1976 New Trends and approaches in the delivery of maternal and child care. Sixth Report of the WHO Expert Committee on Maternal and Child Health. World Health Organization Technical Report Series 600, 98

WHO 1978 Risk approach for maternal and child health care. World Health Organization offset publication 39 Geneva.

World Health Statistics 1979. World Health Organization, Geneva, p 17

Gynaecology

10. The detection of ovulation for fertility and infertility

John T. France

Historically, it is only comparatively recently that the time when ovulation occurs in the menstrual cycle has been identified. Even in the early part of this century it was still commonly believed that ovulation took place in association with menstruation. It was not until 1930 that the observation was independently made by Ogino (1930) and Knaus (1933) that irrespective of cycle length ovulation preceded the next menstrual period by a time interval of about 14 days. Their observation was made at a time when associated research by other investigators was leading to discoveries of the pituitary and gonadal hormones. From these studies evolved a correct understanding of the physiological basis of the menstrual cycle. However, though in the subsequent 50 years and particularly in the last 10 years this understanding has grown in great detail and sophistication, direct proof that ovulation has taken place still rests on the establishment of a pregnancy or on the recovery of an ovum from the fallopian tubes.

Indirectly there are a number of signs of ovulation that provide presumptive evidence that ovulation may be about to occur or may have occurred. These signs have an important application in the investigation and management of infertility and for those couples who wish to regulate their fertility by periodic abstinence.

HORMONAL MECHANISMS REGULATING OVULATION

The majority of the signs and symptoms of ovulation are a reflection of the hormonal changes that are involved in the ovulatory process. It is therefore important as a basis to discussion of methods of detecting ovulation that the endocrine events of the menstrual cycle be first reviewed. The endocrine control of ovulation involves an interaction between hypothalamus, pituitary and ovary. The hormonal changes and inter-relationships that occur are, in outline, as follows.

In the last few days of the preceding menstrual cycle, blood concentrations of progesterone and oestradiol decline and in a positive feedback on the hypothalamus-pituitary, secretion of the pituitary gonadotrophin, follicle stimulating hormone (FSH), increases. A new group of follicles in the ovary respond to the stimulus of this hormone and begin to grow and develop. During the early pre-ovulatory days of the new menstrual cycle, one of the developing follicles, for reasons that are unknown, becomes dominant, continues to grow to full maturation and then ovulation, while the remainder become atretic.

Pituitary secretion of LH slowly rises from about the beginning of the new menstrual cycle. The primary action of LH at this time is to stimulate the biosynthesis of androstenedione and testosterone in the theca cells of the active follicle. These androgens diffuse into the follicular fluid and are aromatised to oestrogens by the granulosa cells. Ovarian production of oestradiol therefore slowly increases in response to the LH stimulus. As the blood concentration of oestradiol rises, there is a selective negative feedback effect on the hypothalamic-pituitary system resulting in inhibition of FSH secretion but not that of LH. This preferential suppression of FSH may also arise from the action of ovarian inhibin, a protein produced by the granulosa cell of the follicle which has been shown experimentally to inhibit FSH but not LH secretion (Hafez, 1980). This second mechanism, however, has yet to be conclusively demonstrated in the human. Once follicular growth has begun it appears that continuing maturation requires only low levels of FSH.

From approximately seven days before ovulation there is a marked increase in oestradiol synthesis and secretion as the dominant follicle rapidly acquires full maturation. Oestradiol production and its blood concentration reach a peak maximum at about 40 hours before ovulation and then sharply decline. Blood levels of oestrone also show a preovulatory rise and fall though to a lesser degree than oestradiol. Most of the circulating oestrone is derived from peripheral conversion of androstenedione and from metabolism of oestradiol.

The late preovulatory rise in oestradiol levels has a positive feedback effect on pituitary release of LH, triggering a surge in LH secretion. Oestradiol appears to act in several ways in bringing about the LH surge. Early, the slowly rising blood oestradiol levels promote pituitary synthesis and storage of LH, and also increase pituitary sensitivity to gonadotrophin releasing hormone (GnRH). As oestradiol levels rapidly rise to peak values, the higher concentrations stimulate an increase in hypothalamic secretion of GnRH with resulting release of the stored LH. The high levels of LH, which persist for about 48 hours, bring about the final steps in maturation of the follicle and initiate processes resulting in follicle rupture and expulsion of the ovum. Associated with the LH surge is a smaller but significant surge in FSH. However, a role for FSH at this time in the cycle has yet to be identified. The LH surge also causes a redirection of steroid biosynthesis in the follicle from production of oestrogen to production of progesterone. Circulating progesterone levels begin to rise even before ovulation and show a small increase from preovulatory basal concentrations of about 1.6 nmol/l (0.5 ng/ml) plasma to 3.2 nmol/l (1.0 ng/ml) within 12 hours following onset of the LH surge. The small preovulatory change in the level of progesterone may serve to amplify the gonadotrophin surge mechanism. Ovulation occurs about seven to 24 hours after the peak in the blood concentration of LH.

Following discharge of the ovum at ovulation the cells of the follicle are rapidly luteinised and evolve into a new endocrine structure, the corpus luteum. The primary function of the corpus luteum is to produce progesterone but to a lesser extent it also produces oestrogen. In the absence of pregnancy it remains functional for about 14 days.

In the post-ovulatory phase of the cycle circulating blood levels of progesterone and oestradiol rise to reach maximum values about seven days after ovulation. The higher values are sustained for three or four days with levels then falling during the last few days of the cycle as the corpus luteum regresses. In response to the negative feedback effect on the hypothalamic-pituitary system exerted by the elevated concentrations of progesterone and oestradiol, secretion of LH and FSH is reduced during most of the luteal phase of the cycle with blood levels declining to slightly below those of the preovulatory phase.

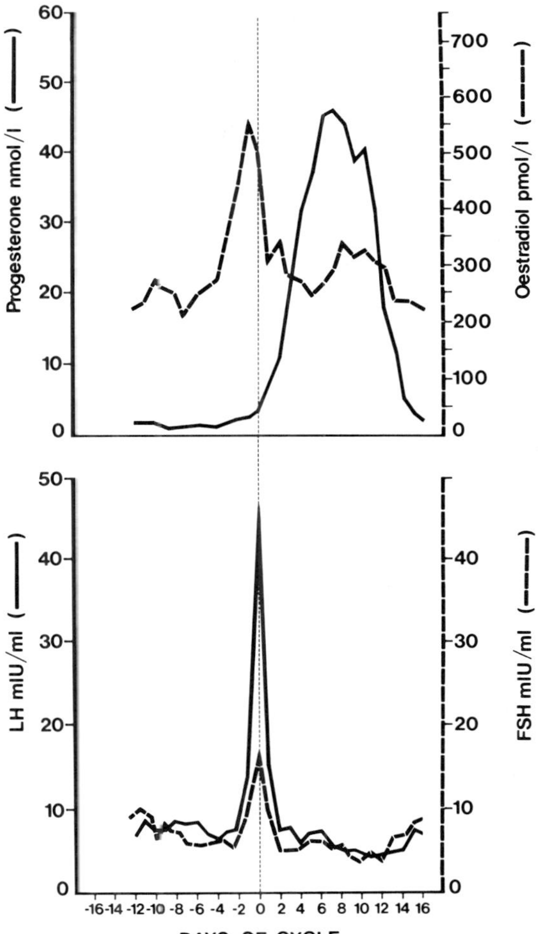

Fig. 10.1   Profiles of daily plasma concentrations of FSH, LH, oestradiol, and progesterone during a normal menstrual cycle. Concentrations are shown relative to the day of the LH peak (day 0).

The day-to-day changes in plasma concentrations of the pituitary gonadotrophins and the ovarian hormones during the menstrual cycle are illustrated in Figure 10.1. For a more detailed account of the endocrine interactions involved in regulating ovulation the reader is directed to the articles of Speroff & Vande Wiele (1971), Fink (1977), Yen (1978), and Pauerstein et al (1978).

Identification of the hormonal changes associated with ovulation by plasma or urine analyses provides a laboratory based approach to ovulation detection. The evaluation of peripheral biological events produced by these hormone changes is an alternative and often simpler approach.

HORMONE ASSAYS AND OVULATION

Plasma progesterone and urinary pregnanediol

Plasma concentrations of progesterone rise rapidly following ovulation, reaching maximum levels, with a mean value of about 48 nmol/l (15 ng/ml), at mid-luteal phase. Thereafter, they decline as the corpus luteum degenerates (Diczfalusy & Landgren, 1977). Though there are differing opinions, plasma progesterone concentration should generally exceed 16 nmol/l (5 ng/ml) to be consistent with normal ovulation and luteal function. However, it is worthy of note that plasma levels of progesterone greater than 16 nmol/l may be observed when there is defective function of the corpus luteum leading to a short luteal phase (Sherman et al, 1974).

The advent of radioimmunoassay has provided a rapid and specific method for determining progesterone in plasma and this assay is now usually available as a laboratory service in most major gynaecological departments. The timing of the blood collection for progesterone analysis is clearly important. Daily sampling is inconvenient to the patient, costly in laboratory charges and the hormone profile that is obtained, while important in research studies, usually offers little of value to clinical management. The common procedure involves the collection of one or two blood samples. Black et al (1972) observed that a single plasma progesterone value of 16 nmol/l or more on a sample taken between 12 and five days before the following menstrual period gave no false positive indication of ovulation but 13 per cent false negative results in the large group of women they investigated. The false negative results they found could be eliminated by increasing the number of samples analysed or by using 32 nmol/l (10 ng/ml) as the delineation level for single samples. Landgren et al (1980), in a recent study of the hormonal profile of the cycle in 68 normal menstruating women, found that 95 per cent of the women exhibited plasma progesterone levels higher than 16 nmol/l for a minimum of five days during the luteal phase, with 90 per cent having levels above 26 nmol/l (8 ng/ml) during the same period.

If the progesterone concentration is to be determined only on a single sample then ideally the collection of the sample should be timed relative to some other index of ovulation, for example, six to nine days after the post-ovulation rise in basal body temperature, to make certain the measurement is made at mid-luteal phase. If a temperature chart is not being kept or other indices of ovulation not observed, two samples collected five days apart between the fourth and tenth day after the expected time of ovulation may reduce the chance of obtaining a misleading result. As a general principle in evaluating progesterone (and pregnanediol) results cognisance should also always be given to when the next menstrual period begins.

A close estimation of the time of ovulation can be made from serial measurements of progesterone made during the periovulatory phase of the cycle. Studies correlating progesterone and other hormone levels with ovulation, timed from visual inspection of the ovary and histological dating of the corpus luteum, have shown that ovulation occurs at a time when plasma progesterone concentrations are between 3.2 nmol/l (1 ng/ml) and 8.6 nmol/l (2.7 ng/ml) (Yussman & Taymor, 1970; Pauerstein et al, 1978). Hilgers et al (1978) have used this observation to provide an estimated time for ovulation in the cycle. They plotted the daily periovulatory progesterone values on semi-log paper to give a linear progression and identified the ovulatory time span as the interval defined by the progesterone values of 3.2 nmol/l (1 ng/ml) and 7.3 nmol/l (2.3 ng/ml). The mid-point of this time span was taken as the estimated time of ovulation.

Pregnanediol-3α glucuronide is the principal urinary metabolite of progesterone and its excretion correlates well with plasma progesterone levels in both 24 hour and overnight collections of urine, with and without correction for creatinine excretion (Stanczyk et al, 1980). Preovulatory excretion levels in women rarely exceed 5 μmol/24 hr. Urinary pregnanediol levels begin to rise significantly at about the time of the LH peak and are markedly elevated by three days after the LH peak; mid-luteal phase maximum levels reach a mean of about 14 μmol/24 hr and may be as high as 25 μmol/24 hr (Barrett & Brown, 1970; Collins et al, 1979; Stanczyk et al, 1980). As a test of ovulation a urinary excretion level greater than 5 μmol/24 hr is generally regarded as indicating ovulation has taken place.

Measurement of urinary pregnanediol has for many years been a routine laboratory test for ovulation. The analytical method described by Klopper, Michie & Brown in 1955, can perhaps be regarded as the first pregnanediol assay that could reliably be used to study relatively large numbers of samples. The method was the basis of a number of investigations that contributed largely to our knowledge of pregnanediol changes during the menstrual cycle. The introduction of gas chromatographic methods in the 1960s, such as those of Cox (1963) and Metcalf (1968), with their potential for processing relatively high sample numbers enabled pregnanediol assays to be offered for the first time as a routine clinical service. Use of overnight or spot samples rather than total 24-hour urine collections further simplified the test procedure (Metcalf, 1973; Stanczyk et al, 1980).

Currently, radioimmunoassay of plasma progesterone has in many centres replaced urinary pregnanediol determinations. Nevertheless, the development of radioimmuno-assay methods for pregnanediol glucuronide (Collins et al, 1979; Stanczyk et al, 1980) and the imminent possibility of an at home 'dip stick' test system based on enzyme immunoassay (WHO, 1980) may see a return in the future to measurment of urinary pregnanediol in assessing ovulation.

Luteinising hormone

The preovulatory surge in release of LH from the pituitary lasts approximately over a 48-hour period and is the most dramatic endocrine event of the menstrual cycle. The peak of the LH surge, as reflected in blood concentrations of LH, has been estimated from histological assessment of corpora lutea to occur from 24 to seven hours before ovulation (Yussman & Taymor, 1969; Pauerstein et al, 1978). The peak in plasma or urinary LH levels serves as a convenient marker for ovulation and is commonly used as a time of reference in endocrine and associated studies of the menstrual cycle.

The urinary excretion level of LH mirrors the plasma concentration. Generally, the peak values are found on the same day though studies involving more frequent blood and urine samples at every four to six hours indicate the peak LH values occur in urine six to 12 hours later than in plasma (Ferin et al, 1973).

When urinary LH changes are studied on a daily basis, analysis of first morning urine samples provides clinical information as useful as a complete 24-hour collection; furthermore, for the patient it is simpler and less likely to be stressful (Collins et al, 1979). Spot urine collections may also be used provided the LH content is expressed as a ratio of the creatinine level (Metcalf & Livesey, 1979).

Most current methods for measuring LH are based on radioimmunoassay and take between one and four days for completion. The time factor associated with these assays restricts their application to a retrospective identification of the time of ovulation. However, more rapid radioimmunoassays and radioreceptor assays for LH have been developed and use of this marker may soon become practical for predicting ovulation. Trouson et al (1980) for example, have recently described a three-hour radioimmunoassay for LH which they have applied for precise detection of ovulation in patients for artificial insemination or embryo transfer.

Several commercial immunoassay systems for urinary LH based on a haemagglutination reaction have been available for several years. While these assays are only semi-quantitative and are relatively costly, they are simple to perform and can provide information on LH levels quite adequate for clinical practice. The Hi-gonavis test system (Mochida Pharmaceutical Co. Ltd., Tokyo) takes approximately $2\frac{1}{4}$ hours and Luteonosticon (Organon, Technica B.V., Oss) approximately six hours to provide a result, so both systems can be employed for predicting ovulation in infertile patients.

Since the LH surge occurs over a very limited time period in the menstrual cycle it could easily be missed unless careful attention is given to deciding when to take samples. Saxena et al (1976) observed that intermittent blood sampling through the cycle including serial samples from day 12 to 16 identified the preovulatory serum LH peak in only 26 per cent of the cycles studied. Daily collection of blood or urine samples throughout the cycle overcomes the difficulty of anticipating correctly when to sample but may not be practical or desirable in clinical practice. When there is a limit to the collection of samples, the time of the LH surge can be predicted mathematically by reference to the previous cycle lengths of the patient (McIntosh et al, 1980). A preferred approach though, as it directly relates to the cycle concerned, is to use the preovulatory changes in cervical mucus as an indicator of when to sample for LH.

Plasma and urinary oestrogens
From approximately six to seven days before ovulation the blood concentration of oestradiol begins to rapidly rise as a consequence of the increased secretion by the maturing follicle. The maximum concentration of plasma oestradiol is generally reached one or two days before the LH peak but occasionally the two peaks coincide (Ferin et al, 1973). Abruptly, oestradiol concentrations then decline, to rise again after ovulation in a broader and less elevated peak around the mid-luteal phase.

The pattern of urinary oestrogen excretion is similar to that observed for blood concentrations. If total urinary oestrogens are measured the maximum excretion level in most cycles will be found to coincide with the peak in LH but it may precede the LH peak or occur one or two days later (Burger et al, 1968; Johansson et al, 1971). When the individual fractions of the total urinary oestrogens are examined separately, slight variations in excretory patterns become evident. Oestrone glucuronide, oestradiol-3-glucuronide, oestriol-3-glucuronide and oestriol-16-glucuronide, all reach maximum levels of excretion following the peak in serum LH, while the maximum urinary level for oestradiol-17-glucuronide, the most abundant of these oestrogens, occurs on the day preceding the LH peak (Stanczyk et al, 1980). The differences presumably are a consequence of variation and clearance of these oestradiol metabolites. The 24 hour excretory level of oestradiol-17-glucuronide, corrected or not corrected for creatinine, correlates well with serum oestradiol concentrations (Stanczyk et al, 1980).

Like the LH surge, the preovulatory rise in oestrogen levels is a convenient marker for timing ovulation. It is important to remember though, that follicular maturation does not always end in ovulation (Adams et al, 1976) and that determination of the oestrogen peak is therefore less reliable in detecting ovulation than determining LH.

When availability of same day rapid assay procedures, the daily monitoring of urinary oestrogen levels or plasma oestradiol concentrations has an important application in the induction of ovulation by administered gonadotrophins. Indeed, rapid oestrogen assays are essential to gonadotrophin therapy in providing feed-back information on the degree of ovarian stimulation and for deciding when ovulation should be triggered with human chorionic gonadotrophin (HCG) (Brown et al, 1969; Brown & Beischer, 1972; Shaaban & Klopper, 1973; McGarrigle et al, 1974; Black et al, 1974). Brown et al (1969) considered a satisfactory response to treatment was indicated by a slow rise in the value of total urinary oestrogens of between 175 nmol/24 hr (50 μg/24 hr) and 350 nmol/24 hr (100 μg/24 hr). Absolute levels of urinary oestrogens might reach as high as 1750 nmol/24 hr (500 μg/24 hr) at the time ovulation was triggered. They suggested a convenient criterion for excessive stimulation to be when oestrogen values exceed 350 nmol/24 hr within five days of commencement of therapy. In such instances administration of HCG should be withheld. Plasma oestradiol concentrations are thought to give a more accurate day to day assessment of ovarian response than urinary oestrogens with values between 735 pmol/l (200 pg/ml and 1470 pmol/l (400 pg/ml) by the fifth day of treatment regarded as indicative of a satisfactory stimulation (Shaaban & Klopper, 1973; Black et al, 1974).

The fertile period of the menstrual cycle is governed to a large extent by oestrogen influences on cervical mucus secretion. Recognition of the preovulatory rise in urinary oestrogen levels has therefore a potential to aid in identifying this period for family planning purposes. Radioimmunoassay methods for direct determination of oestrogen conjugates in urine have been developed (Collins et al, 1979; Stanczyk et al, 1980). This is a first step towards developing an enzyme-immunoassay or immuno-chemical dip stick method for at home testing for oestrogens.

PERIPHERAL PERIOVULATORY HORMONAL EFFECTS AND DETECTION OF OVULATION

The major changes in circulating blood levels of oestrogen and progesterone which occur during the menstrual cycle produce recognisable peripheral effects that can be used as signs of ovulation. These effects include a change in basal body temperature, changes in the cervix and in the mucus it secretes, changes in vaginal cytology, endometrial changes and premenstrual molimina. Some women also experience breast tenderness, a feeling of abdominal distension, vaginal spotting and mood changes near the time of ovulation.

Basal body temperature
Progesterone has a thermogenic action which is probably mediated through the central nervous system (Southam & Gonzaga, 1965). This action becomes evident during the menstrual cycle as a rise in basal body temperature occurring with the appearance of increased blood concentrations of progesterone at the time of ovulation.

The higher temperature is maintained during the postovulatory phase of the cycle until progesterone levels fall to near preovulatory values at menstruation.

In keeping a record of daily temperatures for the purpose of ovulation detection, it is recommended that the temperature be taken in the morning immediately on awakening and before arising. This timing ensures that physiological conditions will be close to basal and that the temperature is taken near the same time each day. When significant variation (>1 hour) in waking times occur, fluctuations due to the diurnal variation in basal temperature will complicate the temperature chart record (Vollman, 1977). A method for correcting temperatures for differing waking times has been proposed recently by Royston et al (1980).

The temperature can be taken orally, vaginally or rectally. Oral temperatures are slightly lower than vaginal or rectal but the biphasic pattern of the ovulatory cycle is similar for all three records. While oral temperature readings are more commonly recorded, they are associated with greater day to day fluctuations and are more likely to be influenced by extraneous factors. Vaginal temperature measurements are recommended for women who consistently present with oral temperature records that are difficult to interpret.

The manner in which the temperature readings are graphically represented is of practical importance in facilitating the study and interpretation of temperature charts. A suitable scale for the coordinates representing the day of the cycle and the temperature must be appropriately selected to allow the higher postovulatory temperatures to be clearly discerned from the lower preovulatory temperature readings. Vollman (1977) recommends that the temperature record chart should have axes with scales in the proportion 0.1°C: 1 day = 1:1 or 0.1°C: 1 day = 2:1.

The shift or rise in basal body temperature that occurs about the time of ovulation is usually of the order of 0.3°C to 0.5°C. The rise may take place rapidly over a period of 24 hours or may be gradual over several days. Marshall (1963), from a detailed study of thermal changes in 1088 menstrual cycles with ovulatory biphasic temperature patterns, concluded that the rise could be one of three types. An acute rise with an elevation of at least 0.4°F (0.2°C) between two consecutive days, a slow gradual rise usually over three to five days but occasionally longer, or a step-like rise. An acute rise is the most usual type of ovulatory temperature shift and was observed in 80 per cent of the cycles in Marshall's study. Temperature charts illustrating the three types of shifts are shown in Figure 10.2.

It is not uncommon to hear reference to an acute temperature dip immediately before the rise in temperature as if it is a feature of all temperature charts. It is also often suggested that the dip is a precise indicator of the time of ovulation. To assume either is incorrect. In the study carried out by Marshall (1963) only 10 per cent of cycles had a dip preceding the temperature rise. In a more recent study with associated hormonal measurements to provide an estimate of the time of ovulation, Hilgers & Bailey (1980) observed the temperature dip in only 10 of 66 hormonally normal cycles and it occurred from two days before to three days after the estimated time of ovulation.

Two methods are commonly used as aids in identifying the ovulatory temperature shift. A WHO Scientific Group (1967) defined the shift as one that occurs in 48 hours or less and in which three consecutive daily temperatures are at least 0.2°C higher than the last six daily temperatures prior to the start of the shift. The sustained shift to a

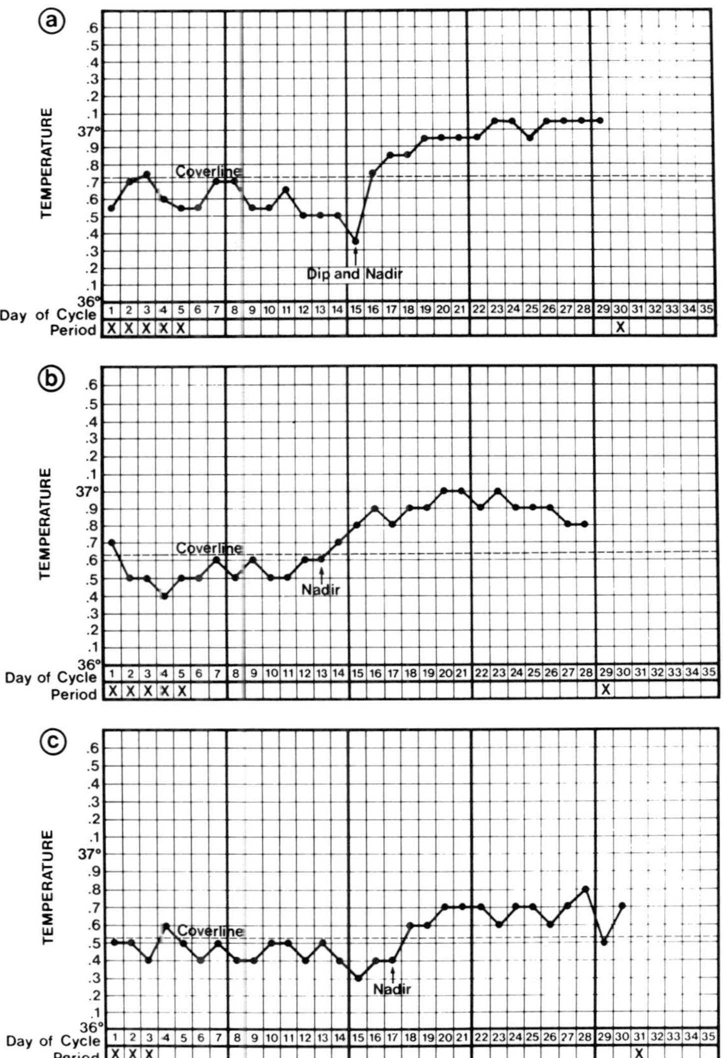

Fig. 10.2   Examples of the three types of ovulatory shifts in basal body temperature: (a) illustrates an abrupt rise; (b) illustrates a slow rise; (c) illustrates a step wise rise. The ovulatory temperature nadir is indicated and the coverline drawn to discern the higher postovulatory temperature readings from the preovulatory readings.

higher temperature level as seen in the three consecutive elevated temperature readings is the criterion for recognising this ovulatory event. The coverline method identifies the day of the temperature shift by drawing a line from left to right across the temperature chart just above the preovulatory readings (excluding temporary elevations due presumably to illness, or other episodic factors). The day before the temperature rises to stay above that line is called the day of the shift with this method (Guerrero, 1974).

The frequency of monophasic temperature charts during the cycles of mature ovulating women would seem to be low. Vollman (1977) estimates a rate as low as

2 per cent. A rate that is supported by the finding of a 4 per cent incidence by Marshall (1963), a 2 per cent incidence by Magyar et al (1978) and more recently a 3 per cent incidence by Hilgers & Bailey (1980). A somewhat higher occurrence rate of 12 per cent was recorded by Johansson et al (1972) and by Morris et al (1976) of 11.4 per cent. Johansson's finding, however, has been questioned by Vollman (1977) who considers that two of the three temperature curves published in Johansson's paper and classified as monophasic were definitely biphasic though with low amplitudes. A relatively high incidence of monophasic temperature patterns was reported by Moghissi (1976) who found that in approximately 20 per cent of ovulatory cycles the basal body temperature failed to demonstrate ovulation. His observation is somewhat anomalous for normal mature woman, and is at variance with the author's own experience of a 7.8 per cent incidence (France & Boyer, 1975).

The temporal relationship between the shift in basal body temperature and ovulation has been investigated by several research workers, all concluding from their observations that the relationship is imprecise. Morris et al (1976) examined the correlation between the temperature nadir and the LH surge in 27 normal menstrual cycles. They defined the nadir as the low point in the temperature curve immediately before the rise to the hyperthermic phase. The LH surge and the temperature nadir occurred on the same day in 44 per cent of the cycles. In 81 per cent of the cycles the LH surge occurred within one day either side of the nadir. In a recent more detailed investigation of various periovulatory basal temperature indices and ovulation, Hilgers & Bailey (1980) looked at the relationship to the estimated time of ovulation (ETO) of the temperature dip, the temperature nadir, the first day of the temperature rise, and the 'coverline' endpoint (the day before the temperature rises above the line). The ETO was deduced from the early rise in plasma progesterone concentrations. Their results are summarised in Table 10.1. In only 10 of the 66 hormonally normal cycles (15.2 per cent) studied was the classic temperature dip observed and in only one cycle (1.5 per cent) did the day of the dip coincide with the ETO. The ETO occurred within a range of ± 2 days of the temperature reference point at a rate 80.3 per cent for the temperature nadir, 77.3 per cent for the coverline endpoint and 65.2 per cent for the first day of the temperature rise. Within the same woman, her cycle to cycle variations for the temperature indices were less than observed for the total population studied but were still extensive. Hilgers and Bailey considered that none of the temperature endpoints tested was precise enough to be a meaningful indicator of the 'day of ovulation' in either research or clinical application. Lenton et al (1977) reached a similar conclusion from a study of temperature charts and hormone profiles in patients attending an infertility clinic.

Despite its imprecision, the daily taking and charting of the basal body temperature is the simplest and most widely used method for detecting ovulation. High motivation, careful instruction and attention to the procedure, and a regular life-style are important in contributing to correct and interpretable readings. A thermometer especially designed for recording basal temperatures with an expanded scale over a limited range and having an easily visualised mercury column is essential. Reading and recording the temperature immediately after it is taken is not necessary provided the procedure followed is consistent from day to day. Attempting to read the thermometer while not yet fully awake may contribute not only to lack of precision but also to arousing antagonism against the method. The advantages of recording the

Table 10.1 Relationship of ETO to 4 BBT endpoints in 66 hormonally normal cycles (from Hilgers and Bailey, 1980)

		None	−6	−5	−4	−3	−2	−1	$\bar{X}$*	+1	+2	+3	+4	Total
BBT dip†	N	56	0	0	0	0	1	1	1	3	2	2	0	66
	%	84.8	0.0	0.0	0.0	0.0	1.5	1.5	1.5	4.5	3.0	3.0	0.0	99.8
BBT nadir‡	N	3	0	1	1	1	7	9	14	13	10	6	1	66
	%	4.5	0.0	1.5	1.5	1.5	10.6	13.6	21.2	19.7	15.2	9.1	1.5	99.9
First day of BBT rise§	N	3	1	2	4	12	17	9	9	4	4	1	0	66
	%	4.5	1.5	3.0	6.1	18.2	25.8	13.6	13.6	6.1	6.1	1.5	0.0	100.0
CoverlineΠ	N	3	0	1	3	3	11	13	16	8	3	4	1	66
	%	4.5	0.0	1.5	4.5	4.5	16.7	19.7	29.2	12.1	4.5	6.1	1.5	99.8

ETO = estimated time of ovulation; BBT = basal body temperature; D = dip; N = nadir; F = first day of BBT rise; C = coverline

* The day of the BBT dip †, BBT nadir ‡, first day of BBT rise §, BBT coverline Π

† X ETO = D + 1.0 days; ETO D − 2 to D + 2 = 12.1%

‡ $\bar{X}$ ETO = N + 0.32 days; ETO N − 2 to N + 2 = 80.3%

§ $\bar{X}$ ETO = F − 1.52 days; ETO F − 2 to F + 2 = 65.2%: ETO F − 3 to F + 1 = 77.3%

Π $\bar{X}$ ETO = C − 0.49 days; ETO C − 2 to C + 2 = 77.3%

temperature at leisure later in the day outweigh any slight error due to very minor contraction of the mercury column. Very rapid electronic thermometers are now available giving an easily viewed reading within 15 seconds. They offer considerable advantages but are currently too expensive for use at home in ovulation detection.

For fertility management, the use of the basal body temperature chart in natural family planning provides a reliable means of recognising the post-ovulatory infertile period of the menstrual cycle when this period is defined as beginning on the evening of the third day of the hyperthermic phase (Marshall, 1968). In the infertility clinic, the temperature chart simply and inexpensively identifies the ovulatory cycle and approximately indicates the time of ovulation. It is useful as an aid to timing progesterone or pregnanediol determinations. Clearly, temperature charts are of no value in indicating to couples desiring pregnancy when is the optimum time for intercourse or when to attend a clinic for artificial insemination.

Changes in cervical mucus

Oestrogen and progesterone exert significant controlling influences on fertility through their hormonal action on the cervix and particularly on the mucosa lining the crypts of the endocervical canal. This latter action brings about cyclic changes in the nature of the mucus fluid secreted by the endocervix that are very important to sperm transport and survival in the female reproductive tract. Detailed accounts are available elsewhere in reviews edited by Elstein et al (1973) and Insler & Bettendorf (1977). In summary, the changes in cervical mucus that take place during the menstrual cycle are as follows.

Early in the cycle, at the time of low oestrogen levels, the mucus secreted by the cervix is highly viscous and small in quantity. The hydrogel glyco-protein constituent of the mucus exists as a complex fibrillar network which forms an effective barrier to sperm penetration. The rising levels of oestrogen accompanying follicular growth and maturation stimulate the profuse secretion of a brilliantly clear, watery mucus of low viscosity and high threadability (spinnbarkeit) which is highly receptive to sperm. The glycoprotein fibrils in the mucus form a micellar structure orientated along the direction of the cervical canal. This structure aids in sperm migration directing them along channels between the micelles towards the uterine cavity and more important into the crypts of the endocervix where reservoirs of sperm are formed. Oestrogenic mucus allowed to dry on a microscope slide produces a classical fernlike pattern. As oestrogen levels fall and progesterone levels rise following ovulation the secretion of mucus rapidly lessens and the character of the mucus reverts back to the highly viscous type seen early in the cycle. This viscous mucus persists through the remainder of the cycle.

Moghissi et al (1972) have studied the properties of cervical mucus and the hormonal profile throughout the menstrual cycle. They found that maximum values for sperm penetration, pH, and ferning and minimum values for viscosity and cell content for the cervical mucus occurred on the same day as the peak in serum LH concentration. The maximum amount of mucus and the maximum value for spinnbarkeit occurred one day before the LH peak and on the same day as the peak excretion of total urinary oestrogens. The authors concluded that while assessment of certain properties were admittedly subjective, the changes in cervical mucus seemed to be an excellent guide to hormonal events during the menstrual cycle and a useful aid in the evaluation of the female reproductive process.

Long before Moghissi's study, cervical mucus changes had of course been recognised as a means of identifying the likely time of ovulation. In contrast to the shift in basal body temperature, the oestrogen induced changes in the mucus and its secretion offer a prediction of the time of ovulation. As well, they give valuable information on potential fertility in regard to sperm transport and survival. However, it should be noted that the appearance of abundant, clear mucus of low viscosity and high spinnbarkeit does not necessarily indicate ovulation. These characteristics merely reflect optimum levels of circulating oestrogens which may occur, for example, in anovulatory cycles or in the lactating woman.

Assessment of spinnbarkeit and of ferning are tests in common use but have been largely confined by gynaecologists to investigation of the patient when attending the clinic or office. A method of scoring the mucus according to its characteristics has been proposed by Insler et al (1970) and found to reliably detect ovulatory cycles (Flynn & Bertrand, 1973). A major advance in fertility management therefore, was the development in the 1970s principally by the Billings and their colleagues in Melbourne, Australia, of methods to teach women themselves to recognise the periovulatory changes in their cervical mucus (Billings et al, 1977; Billings & Westmore, 1980).

The Billings' approach to fertility awareness through self observation of cervical mucus in its practical application in family planning is called the Ovulation Method. The method enables a woman to recognise the infertile and fertile days of her cycle and by timing intercourse accordingly to either avoid pregnancy or enhance the possibility of pregnancy. The mucus symptom is assessed not at the cervix but as the mucus appears at the vulva. The sensation produced by the draining mucus is the most significant component of the symptom and is more important than the quantity or appearance of the mucus. The observations of the mucus are made by the women from wiping the vulva with toilet tissue each time she goes to the toilet. The most fertile symptom of the day is recorded. The major features of cervical mucus symptoms in the menstrual cycle are as follows (Billings et al, 1977; Billings & Westmore, 1980):

1. Menstrual bleeding is followed by a variable number of days on which no vaginal loss of mucus is present. The associated sensation is of dryness. The days are infertile.

2. The onset of fertile mucus symptoms is characterised by the appearance of increasing quantities of 'cloudy' or sticky secretion. The sensation is one of dampness or moistness. The duration of this phase is variable.

3. The immediate preovulatory phase is characterised by the occurrence of clear, slippery, lubricative, stringy mucus having the physical characteristics of raw white of egg. This mucus is most favourable for sperm transport. The last day of the highly fertile, lubricative mucus is called the 'peak symptom'. The 'peak symptom' indicates the day of maximum fertility in the cycle and occurs close to the time of ovulation.

4. After ovulation, the mucus becomes thick, tacky, opaque and of diminished volume. The duration of this mucus symptom is variable and is followed by days when no vaginal loss is observed. Sperm transport in this 'hostile' mucus is poor.

The symptoms are summarised diagrammatically in Figure 10.3. The fertile period of the cycle is considered to commence with the onset of fertile mucus symptoms and end on the evening of the fourth day after the 'peak symptom'.

The teaching of women to recognise the mucus symptoms appears best to be carried out by specially trained instructors who are themselves observing their own symptoms. Teaching is usually on an individual personal basis. Suitably qualified instructors are now providing this service through natural family planning organisations in many countries.

It is claimed by the Billings' that almost all women can be taught to recognise cervical mucus symptoms. Accumulating experience with the Ovulation Method would tend to support this view within the context of a teaching service of good quality. The World Health Organisation recently completed a multicentre, cross-cultural study of the Ovulation Method with a principal objective of determining the percentage of women who are capable of recognising the changes in cervical mucus during the menstrual cycle (WHO, 1981). Centres in El Salvador, India, Ireland, New Zealand and the Philippines participated in the study. The subjects, 869 in total, were regularly ovulating women, of proven fertility, who had not previously used the Method and who represented a spectrum of cultural and socio-economic levels. The teaching was carried out by trained instructors. Subjects were seen by a teacher at monthly intervals. In the first of the three cycles constituting the teaching phase of the study, irrespective of their cultural, social or educational background, 93.1 per cent of the women recorded an interpretable ovulatory mucus pattern and 90.8 per cent were regarded by the teacher as having a good or excellent understanding of the Method. These percentages increased over the subsequent cycles.

The importance of direct teacher-subject contact and personalised instruction to the success of learning mucus symptoms is perhaps demonstrated by Marshall's study of British Women (Marshall, 1975). In his study in which the subjects were instructed by correspondence, only 75 per cent of the women observed interpretable mucus symptoms in every cycle and a further 21 per cent in some cycles.

Absence of sight does not preclude women from making the mucus observations as Sans' study of blind women demonstrates (Sans, 1977).

The scientific basis of the Ovulation Method has been verified by a number of studies showing good correlation between mucus symptoms and the hormonal changes during the menstrual cycle. Billings et al (1972) investigated 22 cycles (22 subjects) and observed that the fertile mucus symptom appeared at a mean of 6.2 days (range three to 10 days) before ovulation, defined as occurring on the day following the mid-cycle peak in plasma LH concentration. The 'peak symptom' occurred at a mean of 0.9 days (range -2 to $+3$ days) before ovulation. Flynn & Lynch (1976) examined the relationship between mucus symptoms and hormonal parameters of ovulation in 29 cycles (nine subjects). They defined the day of ovulation as coinciding with the day of the LH peak and found that mucus symptoms became evident at a mean of 5.2 days (range three to 12 days) earlier. The maximum mucus grade (MMG), defined by Flynn and Lynch as the time of the maximum amount of clear mucus, occurred at a mean of 0.45 days before the serum LH peak and a mean of 0.41 days after the peak in serum oestradiol concentration. The MMG, however, does not always coincide with the 'peak symptom' which is the last day of the fertile mucus. Hilgers et al (1978) in an extensive study of 65 normal cycles found that 64 exhibited a

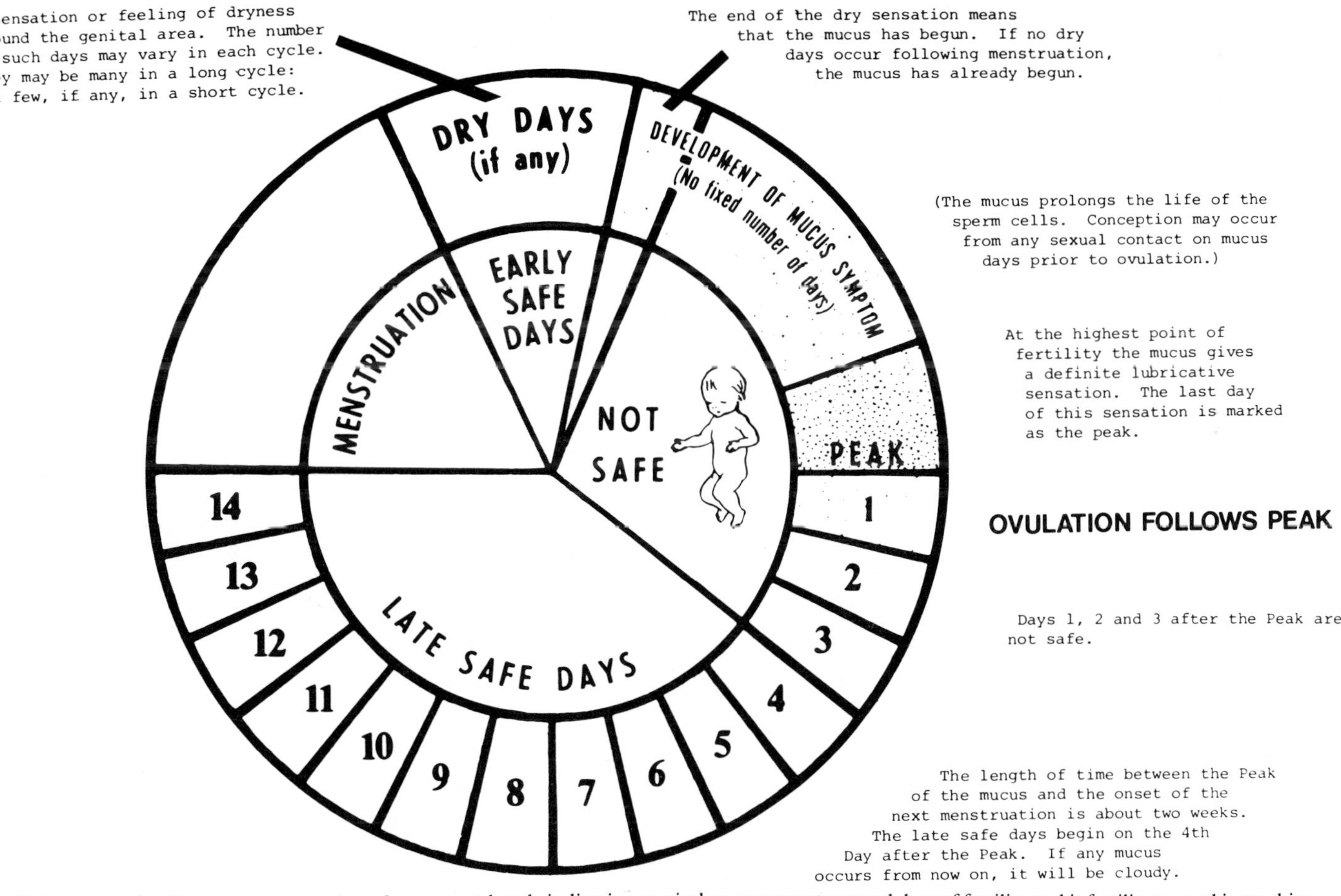

Fig. 10.3 A circular diagram representation of a menstrual cycle indicating cervical mucus symptoms and days of fertility and infertility as used in teaching the Ovulation Method of natural family planning. (Reproduced with the permission of Dr J. J. Billings.)

'peak symptom'. In those cycles the 'peak symptom' occurred on an average of 0.31 days after the time of ovulation as estimated from changing progesterone concentrations, with a range of −3 to +3 days. In 95.4 per cent of the cycles the 'peak symptom' occurred within ±2 days of the time of ovulation; for individual women, the cycle to cycle variation appeared to have a lesser range. The mean number of mucus days preceding the estimated time of ovulation was 5.9 with a range of 0 to 15 days. When allowance is made for the different methods used to define the time of ovulation, the data reported by Hilgers and his co-workers are in very close agreement with those described by Billings et al (1972) and Flynn & Lynch (1976).

The question of whether the woman's vulvar observations are an accurate index of the status of the cervical mucus at the site of secretion, the endocervix, has been investigated by Hilgers & Prebil (1979). As measures of the fertile quality of the mucus taken from the cervical canal, the authors used a fern formation scale and the number of channels appearing in the dried sample. They found that the fertility indices provided by these measurements correlated well with the vulvar observations, both for days of fertility and for days of infertility. The incidence of good positive ferns increased in observations made approaching the 'peak symptom' then decreased as the 'peak' was passed. The highest number of channels was observed on the day of the 'peak symptom'.

In summary, self-recognition of cervical mucus symptoms provides a woman with a simple means of predicting the time of ovulation. Individual cycle variation in the preovulatory duration of the symptoms limits the precision of the prediction, nevertheless, the 'peak symptom' correlates better with the time of ovulation than does the shift in basal body temperature (Hilgers & Bailey, 1980).

Mucus symptoms provide a reliable indication of the fertile period of the menstrual cycle as demonstrated by the method effectiveness values reported for field trials of the Ovulation Method, 0.48 pregnancies per 100 woman years by Weissman et al (1972), 1.2 pregnancies per 100 woman years by Klaus et al (1979) and 3.0 pregnancies per 100 woman years by Ball (1976). While the average duration of preovulatory fertile mucus symptoms is approximately six days, it would seem that the true fertile period would be overestimated when symptoms extend beyond this time interval since sperm survival of longer than five days in the female reproductive tract is rare. The information provided by mucus symptoms obviously is also useful to couples wishing to achieve a pregnancy. The value of teaching mucus symptoms within a service investigating and treating infertile couples has yet to be reported.

Changes in chemical constituents of cervical mucus

Cervical mucus is a complex secretion containing numerous varied constituents (Schumacher, 1973; Moghissi, 1973). Tests for ovulation have been proposed based on daily monitoring of certain constituents that undergo changes or apparent changes in concentration around the time of ovulation. Commercial test-kits have been marketed for determining glucose and chloride. In these test systems the woman obtains a sample of mucus from the cervix by means of a specially designed sampling device or by a swab and observes the interaction of the sample with an appropriate reagent impregnated in absorbent paper.

Glucose content of cervical mucus increases in the immediate preovulatory period of the cycle, reaching mean values above 8.5 mmol/l (150 mg/100 ml) (Birnberg et al,

1958; Weed & Carrera, 1970). It is however, the author's experience and also that of other investigators (Weed & Carrera, 1970) that the majority of women who have attempted to identify ovulation by testing their mucus for glucose have found the test unsatisfactory.

The mucus chloride test for ovulation is based on detecting the associated increased secretion of mucus; as more mucus appears at the cervix, increased quantities are sampled and applied to the test paper. Silver chromate is the reagent impregnated in the test paper and this reacts with chloride ions to form a white spot of silver chloride. From four to five days before ovulation, with the increased amounts of mucus and hence chloride ions available for sampling, a positive test shown by a white spot of high intensity is obtained. A strong positive test may be obtained on the day of maximum mucus secretion. From two to three days after ovulation, negative test responses are again observed.

McSweeney & Sbarra (1964), Hardy et al (1970), and France & Boyer (1975) have investigated the use of the mucus chloride test in a large number of menstrual cycles and found the test responses correlated well with other indices of ovulation and the fertile period. While these studies indicate the test could be useful in indicating the time of ovulation at least in a proportion of women with normal cycles, it would be unreliable if used by itself for defining the fertile period for the purposes of natural family planning.

Activities of the enzymes, alkaline phosphatase (Smith et al, 1970; Moghissi et al, 1976), amylase (Skerlavay et al, 1968), muramidase (Schumacher, 1973) and peroxidase (Shindler et al, 1977) have been investigated in cervical mucus sampled daily during the menstrual cycle. Peroxidase levels showed no consistent pattern during the cycle and appeared uninfluenced by the periovulatory changes in hormone concentrations. Alkaline phosphatase, amylase and muriamidase, however, all showed a decrease in activity just prior to ovulation followed by a marked rise in activity after ovulation. Moghissi et al (1976) thought that the measurement of mucus alkaline phosphatase might have potential as a test for predicting ovulation.

The periovulatory changes in some constituents of cervical mucus could be used to detect ovulation. However, the tests that have already been developed have not found wide acceptance, perhaps partly because of dislike of sampling procedures. Observation of cervical mucus symptoms offers similar information obtained more simply and at negligible cost.

Morphological changes in the cervix

As well as inducing changes in the secretion of cervical mucus, oestrogen also effects changes in the connective tissue and muscle of the body of the cervix. With the preovulatory rise in oestrogens, the tissues of the cervix soften and the cervical os opens. The soft rosy cervix with gaping os from which comes a copious flow of crystal clear mucus is a classic sign to the gynaecologist of an optimum oestrogenic response and of possible impending ovulation. After ovulation, the os closes, the cervical tissues become firm and the cervix returns to a lower position.

Daily self-palpation of the cervix to assess the texture and patency of the os has been advocated by Keefe (1962) as a method of ovulation detection. The technique has been adopted by some users of natural family planning (Kippley & Kippley, 1979) but in general it is not widely practised.

Vaginal cytology

The vaginal epithelium exhibits a sensitive response to oestrogens, progesterone and androgens. The hormonal status of a patient, particularly the oestrogen status can be readily established by cytological examination of exfoliated cells from the vagina. The specimen which should contain freshly exfoliated cells should be taken from the lateral vaginal wall. After staining, the specimen may be evaluated according to several indices, e.g.: Karyopyknotic Index (KPI), Maturation Index, or Eosinophilic Index. The KPI is probably the most commonly used and represents the ratio of mature superficial to mature intermediate cells. The oestrogen stimulated vagina is characterised by a high KPI value (Wied, 1968).

During the menstrual cycle the cytologic pattern undergoes characteristic alterations as hormone concentrations change. Four patterns of cell types can be recognised, (a) the pattern of the menstrual period, (b) the pattern of the proliferative phase, (c) the pattern at the time of ovulation, and (d) the pattern in the secretory or luteal phase. The cell pattern at ovulation is characterised by a maximum sign of proliferation; the KPI reaches its maximum value which is relatively constant from cycle to cycle for the individual but shows significant variation between subjects (Wied, 1968).

Moghissi et al (1972) have investigated the relationship between the variation in vaginal cytology and hormonal parameters of ovulation and showed that the KPI increased gradually to mid-cycle and reached its peak value on the day following the LH surge. Thereafter, the KPI steadily declined to the end of the menstrual cycle, when it reached levels below those observed in the early proliferative phase. The mean peak of the KPI was reached two days after the peak level in total urinary oestrogen excretion. The authors considered there was a lag period required before the vaginal epithelium responded to the increased oestrogenic stimulation. The KPI maximum value coincided with the presumed day of ovulation.

The techniques of vaginal cytology were introduced by Papanicolaou and his co-workers during the 1920s and 1930s. While the test remains of value as a means of assessing the oestrogenic status of a woman, particularly in evaluating the biological response to oestrogen replacement therapy, it is rarely used nowadays for detecting ovulation. More reliable methods are available.

Endometrial histology

Histological examination of the endometrium has been for many years an important investigation in infertility. When the histology is reviewed by an experienced pathologist, the biopsy can be reliably dated in the cycle to within one to two days. The presence of secretory activity in the sample taken during the second half of the cycle usually is indicative of ovulation. Plasma progesterone assays can provide useful additional information when carried out in conjunction with the biopsy (Cooke et al, 1972; Shephard & Senturia, 1977).

Lundy et al (1974) found a good correlation between endometrial dating and corpus luteum dating (r = 0.97), the thermal nadir (r = 0.90), the plasma LH peak (r = 0.97), and the plasma oestradiol peak (r = 0.95). Nevertheless, for the individual specimen, dating the time of ovulation from the histological appearance lacks precision.

SALIVA

Saliva is the most accessible of the body fluids and periovulatory changes in its composition have been recognised. Glucose (Davis & Balin, 1973), alkaline phosphatase (Boyer & France, 1976; Rosado et al, 1977; Cockle & Harkness, 1978), arylsulphatase (Boyer & France, 1976), N-acetyl-β-D-glucosaminidase (Rosado et al, 1977), peroxidase (Cockle & Harkness, 1978), and phosphate ion (Ben-Aryeh et al, 1976) have all been shown to have increased levels in saliva around the time of ovulation. In contrast sialic acid content of whole saliva is at a minimum at mid-cycle (Oster & Yang, 1972). Boyer & France (1976) showed that cells exfoliated from the oral mucosa were a major source of alkaline phosphatase, β-glucuronidase and arylsulphatase in whole unstimulated saliva. The ovulatory peak activities of these enzymes, they thought, were probably due to increase in cell content of the saliva at this time of the cycle.

Recently, oestradiol itself has been serially determined in saliva during the menstrual cycle (Evans et al, 1980). Concentrations were found to be 0.1 to 0.2 per cent of levels found in plasma. The profile of daily saliva oestradiol concentrations resembled that observed for plasma, with a preovulatory surge and a luteal phase peak being clearly discernible. The authors suggested that salivary oestradiol assays could be employed to assess ovulatory function and to determine the hormone profile in individual menstrual cycles.

From a practical point of view, a saliva test could provide a very simple means of detecting ovulation. Foster, Busse and Lorincz at the American Chemical Society Meeting in Washington DC in 1971 presented their findings on the changes in salivary alkaline phosphatase activity during the menstrual cycle and their development of an 'oral diagnostic test tape' as a simple self-administered test system to indicate the fertile period of the menstrual cycle. However, no results of field trials of this test tape have yet been reported.

A wide variation between individual subjects in their levels of activity of alkaline phosphatase (Boyer & France, 1976) and of peroxidase (Cockle & Harkness, 1978) has been observed. A peak value on one woman may be no higher than baseline values in another. Such a variation makes design of a simple, at home, test for ovulation difficult unless it is possible to adjust the sensitivity of the test to the individual woman.

At the present time it seems that a suitable analyte has yet to be identified for a simple saliva based test of ovulation.

MITTELSCHMERZ (INTERMENSTRUAL PAIN)

The occurrence of lower abdominal pain near the time of ovulation, often referred to as mittelschmerz, is frequently experienced by women during their fertile years. Vollman, in his treatise on the menstrual cycle, describes this intermenstrual pain as acute and peristaltic in nature which is localised in the right or left lower abdominal quadrant (Vollman, 1977). He stressed that intermenstrual pain should not be confused with more diffuse complaints of dull pain in the middle of the abdomen, a pelvic heaviness, abdominal bloating, or periodic backache. These he considers may be more related to the complex condition of premenstrual tension. The cause of mittelschmerz is unknown but may be due to muscular cramps in the uterus, tubes or large bowel (Jeffcoate, 1975).

In a recent study incorporating ultrasound observations of the ovary and plasma LH measurements, the occurrence of mittelschmerz was investigated in a group of 96 regularly ovulating women (O'Herlihy et al, 1980b). Thirty-four women (35 per cent) noticed lower abdominal pain, usually lasting six to 12 hours, during the mid-cycle period. In 27 subjects, discomfort was localised in one or other iliac fossa, which in all but two subjects corresponded to the side of the developing follicle. In the other seven subjects, the pain was central and supra-pubic. The pain occurred on the day of the LH peak in 25 (77 per cent) of the 34 subjects. The pain occurred from 24 to 48 hours before the ultrasonically determined time of ovulation. The mean ±SD follicular diameter on the day of the pain was 19.3 ± 2.2 mm. Ovulation was confirmed in each cycle by a mid-luteal phase urinary pregnanediol level of greater than 6.2 μmol/l (2 mg/24 hr). The study shows that mittelschmerz clearly precedes ovulation and it eliminates follicle rupture as a possible cause of the pain.

The importance of mittelschmerz should no longer be neglected in the detection of ovulation. In contributing to her fertility awareness it can be a valuable observation to the woman practising natural family planning. Likewise, in assessing the infertile woman, a history of intermenstrual pain may indicate she has ovulatory cycles.

PREMENSTRUAL SYMPTOMS (MOLIMINA)

Careful history taking can, in general, identify if the infertile patient who experiences relatively regular episodes of menstrual bleeding is ovulatory or not. Mittelschmerz and cervical mucorrhoea have already been discussed. Premenstrual abdominal fullness, breast tenderness, headache, mood changes oedema, and dysmenorrhoea, symptoms grouped together under the designation of premenstrual molimina, occur almost exclusively in ovulatory cycles (Scommegna & Dmowski, 1973; Magyar et al, 1978). Anovulatory bleeding usually is not associated with premenstrual symptoms and occurs unexpectedly.

ULTRASONOGRAPHY

Assessment of follicular growth and maturation by ultrasound is a new and potentially very useful technique for ovulation detection. Studies such as those of Hackelöer et al (1979) and Robertson et al (1979) using static scanners and Queenan et al (1980) with a sector scanner have shown a good correlation between hormonal parameters and ultrasound measurements in identifying the day of ovulation. O'Herlihy et al (1980a) showed that follicular dimensions based on the volume of aspirated fluid obtained at laparoscopy correlated well with ultrasound measurements, confirming the value of the technique for examining preovulatory follicular development.

The diameter of preovulatory follicles has a wide range precluding any prediction of the day of ovulation from a single ultrasound examination. Serial measurements are necessary around the estimated time of ovulation to monitor follicular growth and to identify ovulation from the morphologic changes from follicle to corpus luteum. Queenan et al (1980) report that with a sector scanner accurate information could be obtained in less than 10 minutes per patient. They found a mean follicle diameter of

0.8 mm with a range of 6 to 13 mm at five days before peak follicle size. Follicular growth subsequently was exponential to reach a mean maximum diameter of 21.1 mm with a range of 14 to 29 mm. They noted that the follicle often became slightly ovoid in shape when it reached a diameter of 14 mm. The changes associated with follicular rupture they found to be variable but could be described under the following four categories: (1) The follicle disappeared and no distinguishable corpus luteum could be seen; (2) An irregular cyst could be seen which gradually decreased in size over five or six days; (3) The follicle appeared to 'fill in' with ultrasonic echoes and either remained the same size or increased in diameter. This structure was usually distinguishable for up to six days after ovulation; (4) The follicle collapsed and two to three days later was replaced by a corpus luteum cyst which grew slowly (Queenan et al, 1980).

Ultrasound provides a rapid non-invasive technique for visualising the dynamic changes in ovarian morphology associated with ovulation. It has an important future in the management of infertility. It will play an increasing role in the monitoring of patients who are taking drugs to stimulate ovulation, to assess response and particularly to identify the possibility of multiple ovulation. Other applications are in determining the most appropriate time for artificial insemination and in timing the collection of oocytes for in vitro fertilisation.

CONCLUSION

From the considerable research efforts in human reproductive physiology seen in recent years, significant advances have taken place in the detection of ovulation.

Radioimmunoassay has made measurement of plasma progesterone a simple and readily available test, replacing the endometrial biopsy and vaginal cytology as the preferred laboratory method for documenting ovulation.

The most notable advance has been the development of teaching methods for instructing women in self-recognition of cervical mucus symptoms. The fertile period of the menstrual cycle and the time of ovulation can be reliably identified from these symptoms. By themselves (the Ovulation Method) or in association with temperature charting (the Sympto-thermal Method), cervical mucus symptoms are the basis of natural family planning, the modern approach to family planning using periodic abstinence. Their role in the investigation and management of the infertile couple has yet to be defined. However, they can be valuable in timing blood or urine collections for LH or progesterone determinations and for timing intercourse close to ovulation.

The future should see ultrasound becoming increasingly important in its application in the infertility clinic. Dip-stick tests for urinary pregnanediol and rapid electronic thermometers will simplify home recognition of ovulation and the luteal phase of the cycle particularly for family planning purposes.

REFERENCES

Adams M, Lenton E, Singleton G, Cooke I D 1976 Hormonal profiles in defective ovulation. British Journal of Obstetrics and Gynaecology 83: 331–332
Ball M 1976 A prospective field trial of the 'ovulation method' of avoiding conception. European Journal of Obstetrics, Gynecology and Reproductive Biology 6(2): 63–66
Barrett S A, Brown J B 1970 An evaluation of the method of Cox for the rapid analysis of pregnanediol in urine by gas-liquid chromatography. Journal of Endocrinology 47: 471–480.

Ben-Aryeh H, Filmar S, Gutman D, Szargel R, Paldi E 1976 Salivary phosphate as an indicator of ovulation. American Journal of Obstetrics and Gynecology 125: 871–874

Billings E L, Billings J J, Brown J B, Burger H G 1972 Symptoms and hormonal changes accompanying ovulation. The Lancet 1: 282–284

Billings E L, Billings J J, Catarinich M 1977 Atlas of the ovulation method. The mucus patterns of fertility and infertility, 3rd edn. Advocate Press, Melbourne

Billings E, Westmore A 1980 The Billings method. Anne O'Donovan Ltd, Melbourne

Birnberg C H, Kurzrok R, Laufer A 1958 Simple test for determining ovulation time. Journal of the American Medical Association 166: 1174–1175

Black W P, Martin B T, Whyte W G 1972 Plasma progesterone concentrations as an index of ovulation and corpus luteum function in normal and gonadotrophin-stimulated menstrual cycles. The Journal of Obstetrics and Gynaecology of the British Commonwealth 79: 363–372

Black W P, Coutts J R T, Dodson K S, Rao L G S 1974 An assessment of urinary and plasma steroid estimations for monitoring treatment of anovulation with gonadotrophins. The Journal of Obstetrics and Gynaecology of the British Commonwealth 81: 667–675

Boyer K G, France J T 1976 Alkaline phosphatase, arylsulphatase and β-glucuronidase in saliva of cyclic women. International Journal of Fertility 21: 43–48

Brown J B, Evans J H, Adey F D, Taft H P, Townsend L 1969 Factors involved in the induction of fertile ovulation with human gonadotrophins. The Journal of Obstetrics and Gynaecology of the British Commonwealth 76: 289–307

Brown J B, Beischer N 1972 Current status of oestrogen assays in gynecology and early pregnancy. Obstetrical and Gynecological Survey 27: 205–235

Burger H G, Catt K J, Brown J B 1968 Relationship between plasma luteinizing hormone and urinary estrogen excretion during the menstrual cycle. Journal of Clinical Endocrinology and Metabolism 28: 1508–1512

Cockle S M, Harkness R A 1978 Changes in salivary peroxidase and polymorphonuclear neutrophil leucocyte enzyme activities during the menstrual cycle. British Journal of Obstetrics and Gynaecology 85: 776–782

Collins W P, Collins P O, Kilpatrick M J, Manning P A, Pike J M, Tyler J P P 1979 The concentrations of urinary oestrone-3-glucuronide, LH and pregnanediol-3-α-glucuronide as indices of ovarian function. Acta Endocrinologica 90: 336–348

Cooke I D, Morgan C A, Parry T E 1972 Correlation of endometrial biopsy and plasma progesterone levels in infertile women. The Journal of Obstetrics and Gynaecology of the British Commonwealth 79: 647–650

Cox R I 1963 Gas chromatography in the analysis of urinary pregnanediol. Journal of Chromatography 12: 242–245

Davis R H, Balin H 1973 Saliva glucose: A useful criterion for determining the time of fertility in women. American Journal of Obstetrics and Gynecology 115: 287–288

Diczfalusy E, Landgren B M 1977 Hormonal changes in the menstrual cycle. In: Diczfalusy E (ed) Regulation of human fertility. Scriptor, Copenhagen, pp 21–71

Elstein M, Moghissi K S, Borth R (eds) 1973 Cervical mucus in human reproduction: World Health Organisation Colloquium. Scriptor, Copenhagen

Evans J J, Stewart C R, Merrick A Y 1980 Oestradiol in saliva during the menstrual cycle. British Journal of Obstetrics and Gynaecology 87: 624–626

Ferin J, Thomas K, Johansson E D B 1973 Ovulation detection. In: Hafez E S E, Evans T N (eds) Human reproduction, conception and contraception. Harper and Row, New York, ch 11, p 260

Fink G 1977 Hypothalamic pituitary ovarian axis. In: Stallworthy J, Bourne G (eds) Recent advances in obstetrics and gynaecology — 12. Churchill Livingstone, Edinburgh, ch 1, p 3

Flynn A M, Bertrand P V 1973 The value of a cervical score in the assessment of ovarian function. Journal of Obstetrics and Gynaecology of the British Commonwealth 80: 152–159

Flynn A M, Lynch S S 1976 Cervical mucus and identification of the fertile phase of the menstrual cycle. British Journal of Obstetrics and Gynaecology 83: 656–659

France J T, Boyer K G 1975 The detection of ovulation in humans and its application in contraception. Journal of Reproduction and Fertility. Suppl. 22: 107–120

Guerrero R 1974 Association of the type and time of insemination within the menstrual cycle with the human sex ratio at birth. The New England Journal of Medicine 291: 1056–1059

Hackelöer B J, Fleming R, Robinson H P, Adam A H, Coutts J R T 1979 Correlation of ultrasonic and endocrinologic assessment of human follicular development. American Journal of Obstetrics and Gynecology 135: 122–128

Hafez E S E 1980 Male and female inhibin. Archives of Andrology 5: 131–158

Hardy N R, Lewis L, Little V, Swyer G I M 1970 Use of a spot test for chloride in cervical mucus for self-detection of the fertile phase in women. Journal of Reproduction and Fertility 21: 143–152

Hilgers T W, Abraham G E, Cavanagh D 1978 Natural family planning. I. The peak symptom and estimated time of ovulation. Obstetrics and Gynecology 52: 575–582

Hilgers T W, Prebil A M 1979 The ovulation method — vulvar observations as an index of fertility/infertility. Obstetrics and Gynecology 53: 12–22

Hilgers T W, Bailey A J 1980 Natural family planning. II. Basal body temperature and estimated time of ovulation. Obstetrics and Gynecology 55: 333–339

Insler V, Melmed H, Eden E, Serr D, Lunenfeld B 1970 In: Bettendorf G, Insler V (eds) Clinical application of human gonadotrophins. Proceedings of a workshop conference. Hamburg 1970. Georg Thieme Verlag, Stuttgart, p 87

Insler V, Bettendorf G (eds) 1977 The uterine cervix in reproduction. Georg Thieme Publishers, Stuttgart

Jeffcoate T N A 1975 Principles of gynaecology, 4th edn. Butterworth, London, p 544

Johansson E D B, Wilde L, Gemzell C 1971 Luteinizing hormone (LH) and progesterone in plasma and LH and oestrogens in urine during 42 normal menstrual cycles. Acta Endocrinologica 68: 502–512

Johansson E D B, Larsson-Cohn U, Gemzell C 1972 Monophasic basal body temperature in ovulatory menstrual cycles. American Journal of Obstetrics and Gynecology 113: 933–937

Keefe E F 1962 Self-observation of the cervix to distinguish days of possible fertility. Bulletin of the Sloane Hospital for Women VIII: 129–136

Kippley J, Kippley S 1979 The art of natural family planning, 2nd edn. The Couple to Couple League, International, Inc., Cincinatti

Klaus H, Goebel J M, Muraski B, Egizio M T, Weitzel D, Taylor R S, Fagan M U, Ek K, Hobday K 1979 Use-effectiveness and client satisfaction in six centres teaching the Billings' ovulation method. Contraception 19: 613–629

Klopper A I, Michie E A, Brown J B 1955 A method for the determination of urinary pregnanediol. Journal of Endocrinology 12: 209–219

Knaus H 1933 Die periodische Frucht- und Unfruchtbarkeit des Weibes. Zentralblatt der Gynäkologie 57: 1393–1408

Landgren B M, Undén A L, Diczfalusy E 1980 Hormonal profile of the cycle in 68 normally menstruating women. Acta Endocrinologica 94: 89–98

Lenton E A, Weston G A, Cooke, I D 1977 Problems in using basal body temperature recordings in an infertility clinic. British Medical Journal 1: 803–805

Lundy L E, Lee S G, Levy W, Woodruff J D, Wu C H, Abdalla M 1974 The ovulatory cycle. A histologic, thermal, steroid and gonadotrophin correlation. Obstetrics and Gynecology 44: 14–25

McGarrigle H H G, Radwanska E, Little V, Swyer G I M 1974 The monitoring of gonadotrophin therapy by plasma oestradiol and progesterone determinations. The Journal of Obstetrics and Gynaecology of the British Commonwealth 81: 657–666

McIntosh, J A E, Matthews C D, Crocker J M, Broom T J, Cox L W 1980 Predicting the luteinizing hormone surge: relationship between the duration of the follicular and luteal phases and the length of the human menstrual cycle. Fertility and Sterility 34: 125–130

McSweeney D J, Sbarra A J 1964 A new cervical test for hormone appraisal. American Journal of Obstetrics and Gynecology 88: 705–709

Magyar D M, Boyers S P, Marshall J R, Abraham G E 1978 Regular menstrual cycles and premenstrual molimina as indicators of ovulation. Obstetrics and Gynecology 53: 411–414

Marshall J 1963 Thermal changes in the normal menstrual cycle. British Medical Journal 1: 102–104

Marshall J 1968 A field trial of the basal body temperature method of regulating births. Lancet 2: 8–10

Marshall J 1975 The prevalence of mucous discharge as a symptom of ovulation. Journal of Biosocial Science 7: 49–55

Metcalf M G 1968 Gas chromatography of urinary pregnanediol. Analytical Biochemistry 25: 510–522

Metcalf M G 1973 Use of small samples of urine to follow ovarian and placental changes in progesterone secretion. American Journal of Obstetrics and Gynecology 117: 1041–1045

Metcalf M G, Livesey J H 1979 Use of small samples of urine to monitor gonadotrophins in menopausal women. Clinica Chimica Acta 94: 287–293

Moghissi K S, Syner F N, Evans T N 1972 A composite picture of the menstrual cycle. American Journal of Obstetrics and Gynecology 114: 405–418

Moghissi K S 1973 Sperm migration through the human cervix. In: Blandau R J, Moghissi K (eds) The biology of the cervix. The University of Chicago Press, Chicago, ch 16, p 306

Moghissi K S 1976 Accuracy of basal body temperature for ovulation detection. Fertility and Sterility 27: 1415–1421

Moghissi K S, Syner F N, Borin B 1976 Cyclic changes of cervical mucus enzymes related to the time of ovulation. 1. Alkaline phosphatase. American Journal of Obstetrics and Gynecology 125: 1044–1048

Morris N M, Underwood L E, Easterling W Jr 1976 Temporal relationship between basal body temperature nadir and luteinizing hormone surge in normal woman. Fertility and sterility 27: 780–783

Ogino K 1930 Ovulationstermin und Konzeptionstermin. Zentralblatt de Gynäkologie 54: 464–479

O'Herlihy C, De Crespigny L, Ch, Lopata A, Johnston I, Hoult I, Robinson H 1980a Preovulatory
follicular size: A comparison of ultrasound and laparoscopic measurements. Fertility and Sterility
34: 24–26
O'Herlihy C, Robinson H P, De Crespigny L J Ch 1980b Mittelschmerz is a preovulatory symptom. British
Medical Journal 280: 986
Oster G, Yang S 1972 Cyclic variation of sialic acid content in saliva. American Journal of Obstetrics and
Gynecology 114: 190–193
Pauerstein C J, Eddy C A, Croxatto H D, Hess R, Siler-Khodr T M, Croxatto H B 1978 Temporal
relationships of oestrogen, progesterone and luteinizing hormone levels to ovulation in women and
infrahuman primates. American Journal of Obstetrics and Gynecology 130: 876–886
Queenan J T, O'Brien G D, Bains L M, Simpson J, Collins W P, Campbell S 1980 Ultrasound scanning of
ovaries to detect ovulation in women. Fertility and Sterility 34: 99–105
Robertson R D, Picker R H, Wilson P C, Saunders D M 1979 Assessment of ovulation by ultrasound and
plasma estradiol determinations. Obstetrics and Gynecology 54: 686–690
Rosado A, Delgado N M, Velazquez A, Aznar R, Martinez-Manautou J 1977 Cyclic changes in salivary
activity of N-acetyl-β-D-glucosaminidase. A possible efficient indicator for predicting ovulation and
pregnancy. American Journal of Obstetrics and Gynecology 128: 560–565
Royston J P, Abrams R M, Higgins M P, Flynn A 1980 The adjustment of basal body temperature
measurements to allow for time of waking. British Journal of Obstetrics and Gynaecology 87: 1123–1127
Sans L J 1977 Ovulation symptoms and ovarian function in blind women. Fertility and Sterility
28: 277–278
Saxena B N, Poshyachinda V, Dusitsin N 1976 A study of the use of intermittent serum luteinizing
hormone, progesterone and oestradiol measurements for the detection of ovulation. British Journal of
Obstetrics and Gynaecology 83: 660–664
Schumacher G F B 1973 Soluble proteins in cervical mucus. In: Blandau R J, Moghissi K (eds) The biology
of the cervix. The University of Chicago Press, Chicago, ch 11, p 201
Scommegna A, Dmowski W P 1973 Dysfunctional uterine bleeding. Clinical Obstetrics and Gynecology
16: 221–254
Shaaban M M, Klopper A 1973 A study on the monitoring of gonadotrophin therapy by the assay of plasma
oestradiol and progesterone. The Journal of Obstetrics and Gynaecology of the British Commonwealth
80: 783–793
Shepard M K, Senturia Y D 1977 Comparison of serum progesterone and endometrial biopsy for
confirmation of ovulation and evaluation of luteal function. Fertility and Sterility 28: 541–548
Sherman B M, Korenman S G 1974 Measurement of plasma LH, FSH, estradiol and progesterone in
disorders of the human menstrual cycle: The short luteal phase. Journal of Clinical Endocrinology and
Metabolism 38: 89–93
Shindler J S, Haworth K, Axon A, Bardsley W G, Tindall V R, Laing I 1977 A study of peroxidase levels in
human cervical mucus as an index of ovulation. Journal of Reproduction and Fertility 51: 413–417
Skerlavay M, Epstein J A, Sobrero A J 1968 Cervical mucus amylase levels in normal menstrual cycles.
Fertility and Sterility 19: 726–730
Smith D C, Hunter W B, Spadoni L R 1970 Alkaline phosphatase concentration in cervical mucus.
Fertility and Sterility 21: 549–554
Southan S L, Gonzaga F P 1965 Systemic changes during the menstrual cycle. American Journal of
Obstetrics and Gynaecology 91: 142–165
Speroff L, Vande Wiele R L 1971 Regulation of the human menstrual cycle. American Journal of
Obstetrics and Gynecology 109: 234–247
Stanczyk F Z, Miyakawa I, Goebelsmann U 1980 Direct radioimmunoassay of urinary estrogen and
pregnanediol glucuronides during the menstrual cycle. American Journal of Obstetrics and Gynecology
137: 443–450
Trounson A, Herreros M, Burger H, Clarke I 1980 Precise detection of ovulation using a rapid (3 hour)
radio-immunoassay of urinary LH. Proceedings of the Endocrine Society of Australia 23: 73
Vollman R F 1977 The menstrual cycle. Vol 7 of Major Problems in Obstetrics and Gynecology. W B
Saunders, Philadelphia
Weed, J C, Carrera A E 1970 Glucose content of cervical mucus. Fertility and Sterility 21: 866–872
Weissman M C, Foliaki L, Billings E L, Billings J J 1972 A trial of the ovulation method of family planning
in Tonga. The Lancet 2: 813–816
Weid G L 1968 Evaluation of endocrinologic condition by exfoliative cytology. In: Gold J J (ed) Textbook
of gynecologic endocrinology. Hoeber Medical Division, Harper and Row, New York, ch 8, p 133
World Health Organisation 1967 Technical Report Series No 360. Biology of fertility control by periodic
abstinence. Report of a WHO Scientific Group
World Health Organisation Special Programme of Research, Development and Research Training in Human
Reproduction. Ninth Annual Report 1980 p 79

World Health Organisation, Task Force on Methods for the Determination of the Fertile Period, Special
Programme of Research, Development and Research Training in Human Reproduction 1981. A
prospective multicentre trial of the ovulation method of natural family planning: the teaching phase.
Fertility and Sterility 36: 152–158
Yen S S C 1978 The human menstrual cycle (integrative function of the hypothalamic-pituitary-ovarian-
endometrial axis). In: Yen S S C, Jaffe R B (eds) Reproductive endocrinology, physiology,
pathophysiology and clinical management. Saunders, Philadelphia, ch 7, p 126
Yussman M A, Taymor M L 1970 Serum levels of follicle stimulating hormone and luteinizing hormone
and of plasma progesterone related to ovulation by corpus luteum biopsy. Journal of Clinical
Endocrinology and Metabolism 30: 396–399

11. The management of dysovulatory infertility

Simon R. Henderson

INTRODUCTION

The term, ovulatory dysfunction, as used in this chapter, is defined as embracing absent ovulation (anovulation), infrequent ovulation (oligo-ovulation), abnormal follicular phase, and abnormal luteal phase. Any one of these entities alone, or in combination with one another, can lead to infertility. Ovulatory dysfunction is a common cause of infertility and in countries that have a relatively low incidence of tubal inflammatory disease, it is the commonest cause (Evans & Townsend, 1976). The most recent advances in the diagnoses of dysovulation in its various guises and its subsequent treatment are due to a better understanding of the neuro-endocrinology of the normal reproductive menstrual cycle (Yen, 1978).

The various modalities for inducing ovulation have changed little over the past five to 10 years; however, the appreciation of the abnormal luteal phase, the infertile ovulatory menstrual cycle, eumenorrhoea and hyperprolactinaemia, and the amenorrhoea/oligomenorrhoea/galactorrhoea/hyperprolactinaemia syndrome have led to a much greater chance of pregnancy for many infertile women. This chapter will discuss the concept of the fertile menstrual cycle, the assessment of women with dysovulatory infertility, and the management and treatment of these women.

THE FERTILE MENSTRUAL CYCLE

A fertile menstrual cycle is defined as one which, when occurring in a woman with normal tubal, uterine, and vaginal anatomy, would have resulted in conception had sexual intercourse with a fertile partner taken place at the correct times. A fertile menstrual cycle must have a normal follicular phase, normal ovulation, and a normal luteal phase in order for fertilisation of the ovum and nidation of the blastocyst to take place.

A variety of cycle abnormalities can occur, for instance, a very abnormal follicular phase can result in little or no follicular growth and will usually be associated with amenorrhoea. A moderately abnormal follicular phase can lead to sufficient follicular development and enough gonadal steroids to produce a proliferative endometrium, but insufficient development to allow ovulation. This often leads to shortened cycles, with either excessive or scant menses (dysfunctional uterine bleeding). A slightly abnormal follicular phase might be associated with sufficient follicular oestradiol output to trigger an LH surge, but this surge might be subnormal, and as the follicle is poorly matured, a luteinised follicle may result. This is seen, biochemically, as serum progesterone levels in the subovulatory range (1 to 4 ng/ml). Sometimes a slightly abnormal follicular phase results in ovulation and, very occasionally, conception; but the resulting corpus luteum and luteal phase is often abnormal;

nidation seldom occurs, but if so, a very early abortion may result because of insufficient hormonal support of the endometrium. Ovulation sometimes does not occur, in spite of a normal follicular phase. This may be due to inability of the hypothalamo-pituitary axis to recognise and respond to the rising blood oestradiol levels with an LH surge. This sometimes happens in the perimenarcheal period, and is seen either as dysfunctional uterine bleeding or sometimes oligomenorrhoea (Apter et al, 1978). The concept that ovulation is an all or nothing event is still valid, but ovulation of a premature or postmature or abnormal ovum is unlikely to lead to conception, and if it does, nidation and intrauterine growth will almost certainly not take place.

Methods for evaluating the menstrual cycle

The obvious question now is: 'How can we find out if a certain woman with regular monthly menstrual cycles is having reasonably consecutive fertile menstrual cycles?' The answer is, by evaluating the patient's menstrual cycle with cervical mucus symptoms, basal body temperature (BBT) charts, properly timed post coital tests and serum progesterone levels (see also Ch. 10, p. 215).

The cervical score (Insler et al, 1972) gives us a reasonable semi-quantitative bioassay of oestrogen production in the follicular phase, when performed one to three days before or at the time of ovulation. The cervical score, when coupled with a microscopic score (Table 11.1) results in a post-coital test which is practical, reasonably objective and accurate between observers. This test, therefore, provides a clinical assessment of the unopposed oestrogen effect on the cervix, of the ability of the mucus to harbour motile sperm, and of the sperm's ability to penetrate and maintain motility in that particular mucus.

The serum progesterone levels, if obtained between the starting day of the next menses (M) minus five days and M–11 days should tell us whether ovulation has occurred (if the serum progesterone is 4 or more ng/ml) and if the luteal phase is adequate (serum progesterone 10 or more ng/ml). The temperature rise on the BBT chart and the length of time the temperature stays elevated should provide a guide as to when ovulation has occurred, and the length of the luteal phase. The temperature should be elevated for 12 or more days for the luteal phase to be considered normal. According to Moghissi (1976) approximately 20 per cent of women will have normal ovulation and normal luteal phases, but have no temperature rise, as progesterone has no thermogenic effect in such women (see Ch. 10, p. 224). Occasionally a woman may have an adequate serum progesterone level (10 ng/ml or more) and yet the duration of temperature elevation is short (less than 12 days). Such luteal phases can sometimes be seen in infertile women and demonstrate the need for, not only progesterone, but also, probably, other corporal luteal hormones to be secreted in sufficient quantities for a sufficient length of time.

These methods of evaluating the luteal phase are not uniformly accepted, especially by those who continue to use endometrial biopsies as their final arbiter of luteal phase normality (Jones, 1976). Jones and coworkers consider that the best way to evaluate the luteal phase is to perform an endometrial biopsy two days prior to the onset of menses, or Day 26 of a 28-day cycle. Their definition of a normal luteal phase is one in which the histological date, using the histological criteria of Noyes et al (1950), of the timed biopsy agrees with the date of the cycle as calculated by the onset of the menses

Table 11.1   The post-coital test: The post-coital test is a practical way of assessing cervical oestrogenization and the male component. The cervical score is taken from Insler et al (1972)

Patient Name _______________________________________   Date _______________________

LMP _______________________________________   Day of Cycle _______________

Time & Date of Last Intercourse ____

Treatment ____

CERVICAL SCORE

	0	1	2	3	Patient Score
Amount of mucus	none	scant	dribble	cascade	_______
Spinnbarkeit	none	1–3 cm	4–7 cm	×8 cm	_______
Ferning	none	linear	partial	complete	_______
Cervical os	closed	—	partially open	gaping	_______

Cervical Score

MICROSCOPE SCORE

	0	1	2	3	Patient Score
Cellularity (Cells/HPF)	Dense	20–40	10–20	0–10	_______
Total Sperm (/HPF)	None	0–5	6–20	>20	_______
Motile Sperm (/HPF)	None	0–5	6–20	>20	_______
Sperm Progression	None	Caught by Tails	Slow Linear	Fast Linear	_______

Microscope Score _______________________________

Total Post-Coital Test Score (Cervix Score + Microscope Score) _______________________

and by the time of ovulation, which, in turn, is estimated from the temperature rise on the BBT chart. The rationale of this approach is that the endometrial biopsy is a bioassay which reflects the histological response of the endometrium to all the ovarian hormones. However, when these histological criteria were described, there were no radioimmunoassays, and, therefore, it cannot be certain that some subjects, having abnormal hormonal cycles, were not included in setting up these criteria. Endometrial biopsies, therefore, have disadvantages; and these have been realised when correlations with serum progesterones have been attempted (Cooke et al, 1972; Shephard and Senturia, 1977). Disagreement also occurs between different observers as to the precise histological date of a particular endometrium; such subjectivity detracts from any value that dating the endometrium might have. The present trend is away from endometrial biopsies, which are invasive, painful, and expensive to have evaluated by a gynaecological pathologist, and which have the rare dangers of disturbing an early pregnancy or inducing a tubal infection. The only obvious advantages of an endometrial biopsy are to rule out endometrial hyperplasia, tuberculous endometritis, and the very rare case of endometrial non-response to progesterone and probable lack of appropriate receptors (Keller et al, 1979).

The use of timed serum progesterone levels between M-5 and M-11 is now more common and although these assays are expensive, they are a quarter of the cost of an endometrial biopsy and twice as convenient. Abraham et al (1974), consider three serum progesterone values between M-5 and M-11 give more information about the luteal phase than endometrial biopsy, and they suggest that the sum of these three levels should be 15 ng/ml or more for the luteal phase to be normal. However, Swyer et al (1975) consider that if the value of a single serum progesterone assay performed on Day 22 of a 28-day cycle, or M-7, is 10 ng/ml or more, then the luteal phase is normal. The rationale for this is that in their studies all patients who became pregnant during a particular treatment cycle had serum progesterones of 10 ng/ml or more (Swyer et al, 1975). The author has found this latter approach to be very practical and has used it for the last seven years.

There is also both direct and indirect evidence that 'normograms' for serum progesterone in the second half of the cycle are abnormally low, because they include values of women who, although they had normal menstrual cycles with regard to duration, LH surge, and ovulation, were almost certainly having an abnormal luteal phase in the particular cycle during which daily progesterone levels were being obtained. Indirect evidence for inclusion of abnormal data can be found on reviewing the 95 per cent confidence limits for serum progesterone values seven days before the onset of menses. These values, according to Keletzky et al (1975), vary between 3 ng and 35 ng/ml, with a mean of 10 ng/ml. Such a range is extremely wide for physiological variation, and suggests the inclusion of abnormal data. Direct evidence can be found in the data of Abraham et al (1974), in which the patients used for the 'normogram' can be separated into two groups, using a luteal phase index (see Table 11.2). These two groups can be displayed graphically (Figs. 11.1 and 11.2), and show that the patients with possibly abnormal luteal phases also have short luteal phases. There is also a good correlation between the serum progesterone levels and the length

Table 11.2   The luteal phase index (LPI) was used to analyse the raw data of Abraham et al (1974). Patients could be divided into two distinct groups (Group I & II) with significantly different LPI values (T value = 6.32, p = < 0.001)

	LPI = No. of days serum progesterone < 5 ng/ml × peak serum progesterone level	
	Group I N = 18	Group II N = 12
LPI	230–403	56–189

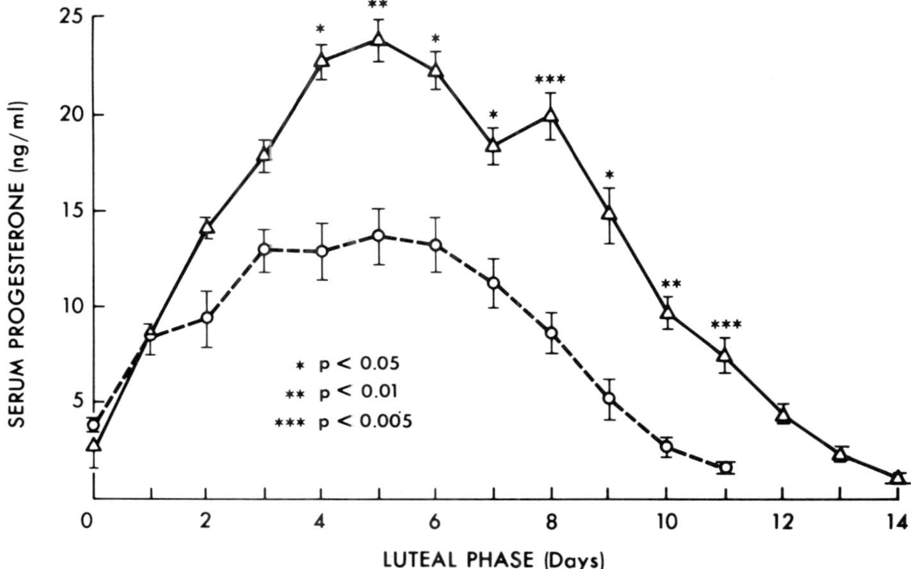

Fig. 11.1   Mean daily serum progesterone levels ($\pm$ SEM) in Group I Δ–Δ (18 patients) and Group II
$\bigcirc$–$\bigcirc$ (12 patients) during the luteal phase. Raw data used was obtained from Abraham et al (1974).

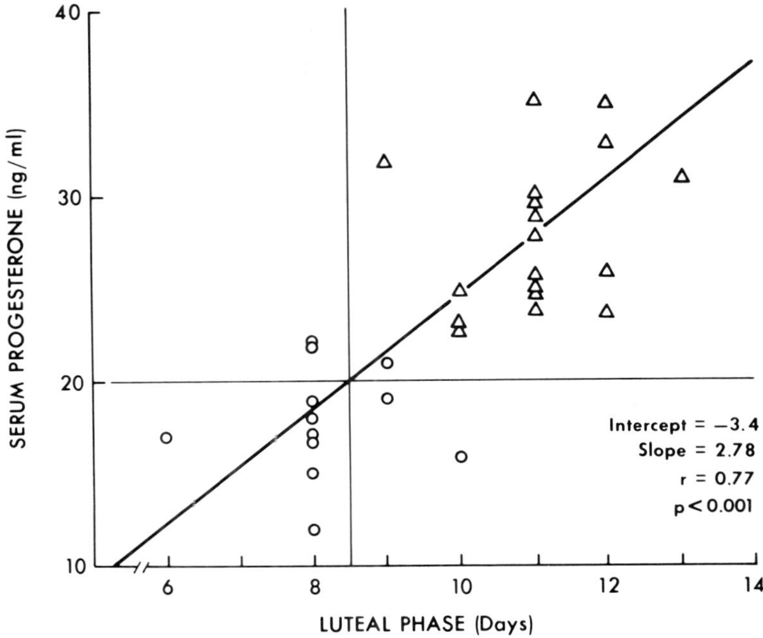

Fig. 11.2   Positive correlation between serum progesterone levels (ng/ml) and Day of the luteal phase in
Group I (Δ, 18 patients) and Group II ($\bigcirc$, 12 patients).

of the luteal phase in the patients considered by the luteal phase index to have adequate luteal phases (Fig. 11.2).

An appreciation of the abnormal luteal phase may explain the large discrepancy between the ovulation rates and pregnancy rates of various different treatment regimens for dysovulatory infertility.

Initial assessment of the couple

The aim of the initial assessment of a woman with dysovulatory infertility is to determine whether a specific medical contraindication to pregnancy or a neuroendocrinopathy exists, and if so, to correct, if possible such problems before augmentation of ovulation. A full history is essential from both partners, which should include prenatal exposure to hormones, past and present exposure to medications, toxic substances, radiation, tobacco, alcohol, marijuana, and other drugs. A full examination of the female partner is necessary, and also of the male partner if the post-coital test shows less than 20 motile sperms per high power field (HPF) or the semen analysis is less than 20 million normally formed motile sperm per ml.

If there is any suggestion on complete physical examination of an endocrinopathy appropriate biochemical testing should be carried out. Patients with amenorrhoea of six months or longer should have a LH, FSH, prolactin (PRL), dehydroepiandosterone sulphate (DHEA-S), thyroxine (T4) levels, triiodothyronine uptake (T3U), and thyroid stimulating hormone (TSH) levels, in order to rule out ovarian, pituitary, adrenal or thyroid dysfunction. Patients with hirsutism should also have a testosterone (T) and androstenedione (A) drawn. If the LH and FSH values are more than 100 mIU/ml and 50 mIU/ml, respectively, ovarian failure is highly suspect and should be confirmed by repeating the gonadotrophin levels and obtaining a serum oestradiol level of less than 20 pg/ml. If the serum oestradiol is in the 30 to 60 pg/ml range, a diagnosis of resistant ovary syndrome (Jones & Moraes-Ruehsen, 1969) is possible. The importance of making the distinction between resistant ovary syndrome and ovarian failure is that the resistant ovary contains follicles, whereas, the ovary in a patient with ovarian failure does not. Pregnancy has been reported following treatment of resistance ovary syndrome with exogenous gonadotrophin (Polansky & dePapp, 1976). Once ovarian failure is confirmed, any attempt to induce ovulation is useless. A chromosome analysis is warranted if the patient has primary amenorrhoea or is less than 25 years old, as Turner's syndrome either full, partial, or mosaic, is possible and can be associated with congenital heart disease and coarctation of the aorta. If a Y chromosome appears in a Turner's mosaic, then a full search for gonadal tissue should be made and, if found, excised, so as to prevent subsequent development of dysgenetic ridge tumours.

If LH levels are more than 20 mIU/ml and are three or more times the FSH level, the polycystic ovarian disease is strongly suggested, and this is usually associated with either an increased testosterone or androstenedione, or both. Increased serum levels of DHEA-S (more than 3.4 μg/ml) can be found in polycystic ovarian disease and indicate an adrenal component, possibly even Cushing's Disease or a hydroxylase deficiency. In this situation, a dexamethazone suppression test should be carried out, to rule out Cushing's Disease and plasma 17α hydroxyprogesterone and desoxycortisol levels should be performed. Patients with less than six periods in a year, and those patients with galactorrhoea, in spite of regular periods, should have a serum PRL and, if amenorrhoeic for more than 36 days, a progesterone withdrawal test, consisting of medroxyprogesterone (Provera) 10 mg for five days orally or 25 mg progesterone in oil intramuscularly. Uterine bleeding within 10 days of stopping Provera or having the injection is a positive test and suggests reasonable levels of oestrogen (usually more than 40 pg/ml of total serum oestrogens) which further alludes to adequate levels of LH and FSH. Any question of an early pregnancy can be easily and accurately tested for by performing a serum HCG assay.

Prolactin levels between 20 to 50 ng/ml should be repeated and, if still elevated, or if the initial value is over 50, hypocyloidal polytomography or computerised axial tomography (CAT) should be performed to determine whether the patient has a micro or macro prolactin secreting pituitary tumour. Those patients with oligomenorrhoea, defined as menses occurring more than 34 days apart, and those patients with cycles less than 26 days apart, with or without dysfunctional uterine bleeding, need not keep BBT charts or have serum progesterone levels to evaluate whether they are anovulatory or ovulatory. This is because oligomenorrhoeic infertile women, even if they are ovulating, will nearly always need induction/augmentation of ovulation in order to increase the frequency of ovulation; and those patients with short cycles usually have anovulation or inadequate follicular and luteal phases and, therefore, also need augmentation/induction of ovulation.

The initial examination of the patient with regular 26 to 32 day periods should, if possible, be performed between 13 and 17 days prior to the onset of next menses, and within 24 hours of the last intercourse, so that a post-coital test can be performed. This test gives some insight into the quality of the follicular phase and into the sperm count of the male. Other routine investigations should include a complete blood count, urinalysis, and erythrocyte sedimentation rate (ESR), serum progesterone seven days before date of expected next period, rubella titre, and semen analysis. Toxoplasmosis and cytomegalic virus titres should probably also be obtained in areas where the incidence of these diseases is high.

It is usually not necessary to evaluate the tubes, ovaries, and uterus in a woman with demonstrable anovulation and usually not in a woman with an abnormal luteal phase, as these abnormalities are usually the cause of her infertility. There are, of course, exceptions to this generalisation, for instance, a woman with a history and physical findings of chronic salpingitis or endometriosis should probably have a hystero-salipingogram or hysteroscopy and then a diagnostic laparoscopy and hydrochromo-tubation. A useful clue to chronic salpingitis is an ESR of more than 20 mm/hr. Tubal evaluation for women with demonstrable dysovulation should be reserved for lack of conception after treatment that results in five to six cycles with good ovulations, post-coital tests and normal luteal phases. Lastly, couples should be given a likely scenario of further investigation and treatment at the first visit.

TREATMENT OF DYSOVULATORY INFERTILITY

The aim of treatment of dysovulatory infertility is to achieve pregnancy as soon as possible, using the safest available modality. A clear explanation of the treatment decided upon, its risks and the usual protocol should be given to the patient prior to starting the treatment.

Clomiphene (Clomid)

Clomiphene is exceptionally safe and the drug of first choice for stimulating the secretion of LH and FSH and, thus, initiating follicular growth and maturation. It is ironical that this drug was initially evaluated as a contraceptive agent. Clomiphene does not directly induce ovulation but starts a sequence of neuro-endocrine events which are similar to the normal menstrual cycle. Clomiphene is an orally active, weak, synthetic oestrogen, which acts by competing with endogenous oestrogens for, and preventing replenishment of, the cytoplasmic oestrogen receptors in the hypothalamus (Clarke et al, 1974) thereby decreasing the negative feedback of the circulating endogenous oestrogens (Vandenberg & Yen, 1973) and allowing the release of gonadotrophin releasing hormone (GnRH) into the hypothalamopituitary portal system. GnRH in turn stimulates the release of LH and FSH which is responsible for follicular growth and maturation in the ovary.

Clomiphene is usually given as Clomid or racemic mixture of two isomers, cis- and trans-clomiphene citrate. It is not a steroid and is structurally related to diethylstilboestrol (DES). It is usually given as a five-day course, starting either two or five days after the start of spontaneous menses or after bleeding induced by progesterone treatment and withdrawal. An appreciable increase in blood LH and FSH is usually observed on Days 3, 4 and 5 of clomiphene treatment, and oestradiol levels start to increase slowly a day or two later. The oestradiol levels continue to increase thereafter and LH and FSH levels fall slightly due to the negative feedback on the hypothalamus and pituitary. A more rapid rise of blood oestradiol is observed five to 10 days after stopping clomiphene, indicating follicular maturation. If the hypothalamo-pituitary axis is capable of recognising the oestrogen surge, and its eventual positive feedback effect, then the combination of increased GnRH release and vastly increased pituitary responsiveness to GnRH results in a LH surge, which, in turn, is responsible for ovulation.

Most clomiphene protocols call for increasing dosages up to 250 mg/day for five days, or even eight days, until ovulation and a normal luteal phase has been achieved, and then maintained at this particular dosage for five to six months (Rust et al, 1974; Evans & Townsend, 1976). Large doses and longer courses of clomiphene seldom result in ovulation when this is not being achieved by the regimen outlined above. Patients should keep BBT charts and a pelvic examination and post coital test should be performed six to eight days after stopping clomiphene, to rule out ovarian cyst formation and to evaluate the oestrogen effect on the cervix, and the sperm penetrability of the mucus. Ovarian cyst formation is a relatively rare event occurring in 1 to 6 per cent of women and less than 2 per cent of clomiphene cycles. If a cyst does form, a one- to two-month delay of further treatment is usually followed by spontaneous regression and does not preclude further courses of clomiphene. Other side effects are also rare and consist of hot flushes in 5 to 10 per cent, tiredness in 4 to 6 per cent, and visual symptoms in 1 to 3 per cent of women. Visual symptoms, usch as blurring of vision, have not been connected with structural changes in the lens, but probably should be taken seriously, and alternative methods of inducing ovulation considered. There is no evidence to date, that clomiphene given inadvertently to women in pregnancy causes abnormalities of the reproductive tract in either mother or fetus, as has been shown in rats by McCormack & Clark (1979); however, as clomiphene is structurally related to DES, it should be avoided in early pregnancy. In situations where a patient may have an early pregnancy, i.e. abnormal menstruation or amenorrhoea, then a serum-β HCG is extremely useful. There is some suggestion that the spontaneous abortion rate may be higher (26 per cent) than normal (15 to 20 per cent) and that the chance of twins is about twice normal (13 per cent). However, there is no evidence of an increased rate of multiple pregnancy other than twins or an increase in fetal abnormality (Adashi et al, 1979).

A serum progesterone should be performed as close to seven days prior to the expected next menses as possible; this usually works out to be Day 21 of the cycle, when clomiphene has been started on Day 2. It is important to increase the clomiphene dosage cycle by cycle, until the patient has both an ovulatory level of serum progesterone (4 or more ng/ml) and an adequate luteal phase (10 or more ng/ml). The patient who responds best to clomiphene in terms of ovulation and pregnancy is usually the one with good endogenous levels of oestrogen prior to treatment and with normal or slightly elevated gonadotrophin levels. Such patients nearly always have withdrawal bleeding after progesterone treatment. Excessive body weight is negatively correlated to ovulation and pregnancy rates; and Shephard et al (1979) found that the average weight of patients who did not respond to clomiphene was significantly higher (mean 203 lb) that the patients who did respond (154 lb). Patients should be made aware of this if they are overweight. Likewise women who are below ideal body weight have also more difficulty conceiving on clomiphene.

Patients with low endogenous levels of oestrogen and gonadotrophins seldom have withdrawal bleeding with progesterone, and only 5 to 10 per cent respond to clomiphene with ovulation.

Clomiphene and corticosteroid
There are a small group of patients with polycystic ovarian disease who have elevated levels of dexamethazone suppressible DHEA-S and who do not ovulate on clomiphene alone or on clomiphene and HCG. They have been found to ovulate on clomiphene when dexamethazone 0.5 mg is given daily, starting two weeks prior to clomiphene (Lobo et al, 1981). The rationale for this treatment is that androgens can interfere with follicular maturation and the adrenal source of excessive androgens can be eliminated by adrenal suppression with corticosteroids such as dexamethazone and prednisone.

Clomiphene and oestrogen
On reviewing the literature, there appears to be two main reasons for adding oestrogens to the clomiphene regimen. The most common reason is that some investigators find a 10 to 25 per cent incidence of poor preovulatory cervical mucus in patients taking clomiphene who appear to ovulate by BBT chart changes, endometrial biopsies or by serum progesterone estimations. This observation is accredited to the antioestrogenic effect of clomiphene. In the author's experience, this is a rare occurrence (less than 5 per cent of cycles) and is usually a reflection of a poor follicular phase; if serum oestradiol levels are performed, these are usually less than 300 pg/ml. Also, serum progesterones are usually less than 10 ng/ml between M-5 and M-11, indicating poor luteal phases. If clomiphene is given earlier in the cycle, Day two to six rather than Day five to nine, a prolonged antioestrogen effect on the cervix should not be seen. In those rare instances where a patient does appear to have

abnormal preovulatory mucus, in spite of normal follicular phases, ovulations, and luteal phases, the mucus can sometimes be improved with 0.625–1.25 mg of Premarin (conjugated equine oestrogens), or its equivalent, a day for 5 days from Day 10 to 15 of the cycle.

A second reason given for treating with clomiphene and oestrogen is to improve the ovulation rates. Canales et al, 1978, reported that giving oestradiol benzoate 1 mg, IM, after five days of clomiphene 100 mg a day, resulted in ovulation in 13 patients who had not previously responded to clomiphene with ovulation, but who did produce an LH and FSH surge 72 hours after oestrachol benzoate 1 mg i.m. Of these 13 patients, 10 became pregnant. These observations have yet to be confirmed and such treatment is not in common practice.

Clomiphene and HCG

The addition of HCG to clomiphene regimens usually receives but passing mention and mixed reviews in the literature, but it is probably the single most valuable therapeutic addition to clomiphene therapy. It is particularly valuable in the woman who is having a good follicular phase on clomiphene treatment, but who is either not ovulating or who is ovulating, but having a poor luteal phase. Some of these women have low endogenous oestrogen and gonadotrophins on initial evaluation; and most of these women do not respond to an adequate preovulatory surge of oestradiol with a large enough LH surge to result in ovulation. HCG 10 000 or 5000 IU is usually given empirically on Day 14 or 15 of the cycle, or seven to 10 days after stopping clomiphene (Drake et al, 1979) and sometimes repeated seven days later (Swyer et al, 1975). However, I am unaware of any report describing the use of urinary or serum oestrogen levels to determine when the follicle is mature and, therefore, when to give HCG in a clomiphene treatment cycle. The rationale for giving HCG when the follicle is mature is so as not to induce luteinisation of the follicle, which can happen if HCG is given too early, or to prevent ovulation of a post-mature ovum when HCG is given too late

The author gives such patients clomiphene 200 mg a day for five days, starting M+2, and then draws serum oestradiol levels on Day 11 to 13 of the cycle and sees the patient for a post coital test on Day 12 to 14 of the cycle. If the last oestradiol level is more than 300 pG/ml and the post coital test good, then 5000 IU of HCG is given i.m. If the oestradiol level is less than 300 pg/ml, then a further level is drawn the following day (Day 13 to 15 of the cycle) and, if necessary, on Day 15 to 17 of the cycle. In this situation, HCG is delayed until estradiol levels indicate follicular maturation (more than 300 pg/ml). A second injection of 5000 IU of HCG is given five to seven days after the first injection, in order to support the corpus luteum. A serum progesterone is performed seven days after the first HCG injection, and if this is more than 4 and less than 10 ng/ml, or if the BBT rise is less than 12 days, then HCG 2500 IU is given twice weekly for two weeks after the first injection of HCG in the next cycle. Occasionally, 2500 IU of HCG is given twice weekly for six weeks following ovulation, as a further support of the corpus leuteum, when it appears possible that the patient is conceiving, but having a very early abortion. If the serum oestradiol levels do not exceed 300 pg/ml during this monitoned clomiphene regime, then the patient is considered a clomiphene failure and is evaluated for gonadotrophin treatment.

Placebo effect

It is most important to appreciate the placebo component of any method used for inducing ovulation. When placebo tablets were given to women with secondary amenorrhoea and oligomenorrhoea in an identical manner to clomiphene, ovulation and pregnancy rates of 40 to 42 per cent and 19 to 17 per cent, respectively, have resulted (Evans & Townsend, 1976; Connaughton et al, 1974). Such a placebo effect might, to some extent, explain the occurrence of ovulation following a variety of medications and even after just the preliminary fertility evaluation (Rakoff et al, 1973). An example of a rather unlikely drug inducing ovulation is the report of 11 out of 12 women ovulating when treated with phenobarbital (Csaba et al, 1974).

Oestrogen, progesterone and combined hormones

A variety of oestrogen treatment regimes have been tried to induce ovulation following the demonstration by Van de Wiele et al (1970) that oestrogen therapy results in an increase in LH. However, the resulting pregnancy rates of 19 to 20 per cent are not significantly greater than the placebo rates already described (Rakoff, 1979). Synthetic oestrogens, such as Epimestrol, Cylofenil, although useful for regulating mild menstrual cycle abnormalities, have not been shown to be of any value for inducing ovulation.

Progesterone derivatives have also been reported to induce ovulation in Germany and Switzerland (Lunenfeld & Insler, 1978a). However, as a rule, progestins are not advocated for inducing ovulation, but rather for inducing a withdrawal bleed prior to the use of clomiphene or gonadotrophins.

Human gonadotrophins

Patients who fail to achieve good follicular development and maturation on clomiphene treatment are candidates for gonadotrophin treatment. However, before such treatment is started, the patient should have an evaluation of her internal genitalia, preferably by hysterosalpingography or hysteroscopy and laparoscopy. If only one of these is to be performed, laparoscopy is the most informative (Templeton & Kerr, 1977; Corson, 1979).

In most countries, gonadotrophins are available as Pergonal or human menopausal gonadotrophins (HMG). This preparation contains 75 IU of both LH and FSH per ampoule and is expensive, being approximately $20, or £11 sterling. The source of gonadotrophin in Pergonal is human post-menopausal urine, and the extraction process is difficult which accounts for its expense. In some countries, such as Australia, there are national pituitary hormone agencies, which make available human pituitary gonadotrophins (HPG) to specialists and infertility clinics.

Ovulation rates following HMG and HCG, or HPG and HCG, treatments have been excellent (70 to 95 per cent), but unfortunately pregnancy rates have been much lower (25 to 65 per cent). This may be due to lack of appreciation of abnormal luteal phases, or to reporting and patient selection problems. Dor et al (1980) found that the cumulative pregnancy rate in patients, who did not have withdrawal bleeding to progesterone and probably had low serum gonadotrophin and oestrogen levels (Group 1), was 91.2 per cent after six cycles of treatment. But the cumulative pregnancy rate for patients who did withdraw to progesterone (Group 2) was 50 per cent after 12 treatment cycles. They also found that patients in Group 1, who were 35 or older, had a cumulative conception rate of 60.1 per cent, but Group 2 patients in this age group had conception rates of only 10.2 per cent. Only one out of 14 of their patients who were over 40 conceived.

The history, development, monitoring and complications of HPG and HCG and HMG and HCG treatment regimes has already been well reviewed (Gemzell, 1977; Lunenfeld & Insler, 1978b; Wu, 1978; Schenker & Weinstein, 1978). In addition to ovarian hyperstimulation (0.1 to 18 per cent, Schenker & Weinstein, 1978), multiple pregnancy (6 to 66 per cent; Schenker et al, 1981), and slightly increased spontaneous abortion rates, unexpectedly high ectopic rates (3.1 per cent) have been reported with HPG and HCG (McBain et al, 1980). There is also evidence that the proportion of girl babies resulting from induction of ovulation with either HMG and HCG or clomiphene is much increased from a normal boy/girl ratio of 1:0.5 to 1:1.3 (James, 1980).

TREATMENT WITH HUMAN GONADOTROPHINS

Treatment with clomiphene, except for perhaps when oestrogen monitoring is required, falls well within the ability of the general obstetrician/gynaecologist who is not frequently called away from his office or clinic for deliveries and emergencies. However, treatment with human gonadotrophins should be in the hands of experienced specialists who are managing at least 20 patients a year with gonadotrophins. Three or more patients should be scheduled together for each treatment cycle, as it is clearly inefficient to gear up the clinic for daily patient visits and the clinical radioimmunoassay laboratory to process rapid serum or urinary assays for just one patient per treatment cycle.

There are two main groups of regimes for HMG and HCG treatment. The first, and the most commonly used in the majority of large centres, involves a variation in both dose and duration of HMG therapy (Lunenfeld & Insler, 1978b), and the second, which employs a non-variable schedule (Marshall & Wider, 1971; Ellis & Williamson, 1975).

The variable dosage regime calls for daily urinary or serum oestrogen levels, daily injections of HMG, frequent pelvic exams, cervical scores, and ultrasound examinations. HMG is started at one to two ampoules a day and increase every three to five days, unless oestrogen levels start to rise. The aim is to achieve adequate follicular maturation without overstimulation. Ideally, total urinary and serum oestrogen levels should rise gradually to 100 to 200 µg/24 hrs, and 300 to 1000 pg/ml, respectively, within eight to 14 days of the start of HMG therapy. These levels indicate follicular maturation, if they have been maintained from three to five days. Once oestrogen levels start to increase, daily HMG dosage is maintained; and when the range described above is reached, then a further day or two of HMG is given. This is followed by an injection of 5000 or 10 000 IU of HCG, a day or two after the last HMG injection, and the patient is advised to have intercourse that night and for the next two to three days. One week after the HCG injection, a serum progesterone should be obtained, to confirm ovulation and a normal luteal phase. Such a laborious intensive and expensive regime can be modified somewhat by obtaining oestrogen levels only every two to four days, with a local physician administering the daily Pergonal. Such a regime, although often much more convenient for the patient, involves some inspired guesswork by an experienced specialist, if hyperstimulation and multiple pregnancy are to be avoided. The inherent risk of abnormal luteal phases in these cycles, encourages one to give a second injection of 5000 IU of HCG five to seven days after the first, or ovulating, injection of HCG. In some instances, even this may be insufficient to support the corpus luteum, and 2500 IU of HCG can then be given every three to four days; this may be required for up to six weeks, if the patient appears to be having recurrent early abortions. In order to decrease the chance of ovarian hyperstimulation, it is wise to withhold HCG and advise abstinence when urinary and serum total oestrogens are more than 250 μg/24 hrs and 1000 pg/ml, respectively. However, Schenker & Weinstein (1978) suggest that HCG be withheld, if serum oestrogen levels are more than 800 pg/ml.

A practical fixed dosage regime involves giving the same dose of Pergonal on Day one, three and five of the treatment cycle. If patients have endogenous total serum oestrogens of less than 30 pg/ml, 5 ampoules of Pergonal are given a day in the first cycle, and if 30 pg/ml or more, then 3 ampoules a day. Total serum oestrogens are performed on Days five and eight, and the patient is evaluated on Day eight or nine for an injection of 5000 or 10 000 IU of HCG, with a pelvic examination and postcoital test. If the levels of oestrogen are not in the ideal range, a further oestrogen level is obtained on Day 10, and the patient evaluated for HCG on Day 11 or 12. If ideal levels are still not obtained, the next course is begun on Day one to five of the next cycle if she has a period. If no period occurs, a serum-β-HCG pregnancy test is performed, and if negative, Provera (medroxyprogesterone) 10 mg is given orally for five days. If no withdrawal bleeding occurs, the next treatment cycle is started seven to ten days after the last Provera tablet. Subsequent HCG injections are given to support the luteal phase routinely, as described under the variable dosage section.

A more recent modality for evaluating follicular growth and maturation is both compound B scan and realtime ultrasound (Hackeloer et al, 1979; Robertson et al, 1979; O'Herlihy et al, 1980) (see also Ch. 10, p. 234). This is still in an investigational stage, however follicular diameters of 2 to 2.5 cm seem to correlate well with peak serum oestradiol levels and occur the day before or the day of ovulation. In 68 per cent of cycles, the maximum follicular size was reached on the day of the LH peak and in 32 per cent on the day after the LH peak. Although realtime ultrasound has been reported effective in monitoring follicular development (O'Herlihy et al, 1980), such machines may not be capable of achieving the required definition to measure follicular size accurately. However, O'Herlihy et al (1981) describe the use of ultrasound in patients undergoing induction/augmentation of ovulation in an in vitro fertilisation programme and use it to determine when to start intensive LH monitoring. In some clinics, frequent ultrasound is being used to monitor the early growth of the follicle to about 1.5 cm and then daily oestrogen are measured. However, other investigators have not found ultrasound monitoring to be so useful (Seibel et al, 1981); there may also be difficulties in measuring follicles in patients who are receiving HMG, as these ovaries can have as many as six large follicles with diameters of more than 1.5 cm (Edwards et al, 1980).

March et al (1976) have reported that pretreatment with clomiphene for five days followed by HMG and HCG result in pregnancies which are achieved with fewer numbers of ampoules and in a shorter period of time than when HMG and HCG are given alone. However, such results were only obtained in those patients who have normal FSH and oestradiol levels.

Bromocriptine

Bromocriptine is a dopamine agonist and its main mode of action appears to be as a prolactin inhibitory factor working at the pituitary level to inhibit the release of prolactin. As dopamine is also an important neurotransmitter in the brain, bromocriptine may also influence generation of GnRH and other releasing hormones. Bromocriptine has not yet been designated as a drug for use in infertility by the US Drug Administration. However, more than 600 babies have been born to mothers who took bromocriptine during early pregnancy, and the incidence of congenital malformations and spontaneous abortions in these pregnancies did not exceed that reported for the population at large. Animal studies, so far, confirm these findings.

The indication, par excellence, for bromocriptine treatment are those patients with amenorrhoea, oligomenorrhoea, or abnormal luteal phases and hyperprolactinaemia, with or without galactorrhoea, but without a demonstrable pituitary tumour. These patients are given bromocriptine 2.5 mg twice daily and prolactin levels fall in 90 to 98 per cent of patients, with normal reproductive cycles usually resulting within two to three months of treatment. Reported pregnancy rates have been good (60 to 75 per cent) and treatment is stopped as soon as the patient misses her period or has a positive pregnancy test (Thorner et al, 1979). Those patients with pituitary macro-adenomata (more than 1 cm in diameter) who want to get pregnant, should have prior microsurgical removal of these tumours or radiotherapy if neuromicrosurgery is not available, because such patients have a five to 20 per cent chance of experiencing rapid expansion of the tumour in pregnancy, causing headaches and mild to severe bitemporal hemianopia. Such events may require either conservative close monitoring of visual fields and symptoms or treatment during pregnancy with bromocriptine or neurosurgery. Management of those patients with hyperprolactinaemia and micro-adenomata who want to get pregnant varies from centre to centre, some preferring neurosurgical removal prior to pregnancy, and others, bromocriptine treatment. As rapid expansion of the pituitary tumour in this group of patients is less common (approximately five per cent), it is reasonable to treat with bromocriptine without prior pituitary surgery. There is also some evidence that bromocriptine treatment can result in regression of the tumour with radiological improvement (Hancock et al, 1980).

Some investigators have advocated giving bromocriptine to normoprolactinaemic infertile women (Lenton et al, 1977) and patients with abnormal luteal phases (Seppala et al, 1976). Although pregnancies have been reported, other studies have not confirmed a use for bromocriptine in these situations (Pepperell et al, 1977; Saunders et al, 1979).

Further possibilities in combination treatment may include bromocriptine and clomiphene in normoprolactinaemic patients not responding to clomiphene alone. Initial studies by Koike et al, 1981, suggest that 61 per cent of patients ovulated on this regime, but the pregnancy rate was only 13 per cent.

Side effects are observed in approximately half the patients who take bromocriptine; these are usually nausea, headache and constipation. Occasional fainting episodes have been reported. To minimise side effects start with one tablet a night for three to four days and then increase to two tablets a day.

Danazol (Danocrine)

Danazol is an isoxazol derivative of 17 α-ethinyl-testosterone and is usually used for the treatment of endometriosis, as it induces a state of relative gonadal hormone acyclicity and absence of menstruation by preventing midcycle gonadotrophic surges (Dmowski & Cohen, 1975). However, Greenblatt et al (1974) described a 40 per cent pregnancy rate following the administration of 200 mg of danazol of day for 100 days to 27 women with unexplained infertility. This study did not have a placebo treated control group but a more recent study by van Dijk et al (1979) had a control group and reported that using the same regimen, five out of 21 (24 per cent) patients conceived in the first six months following treatment, whereas none of the 19 placebo treated patients conceived. These studies, if confirmed, would suggest that a course of danazol might be of value in a patient in whom no cause of infertility can be found after a complete infertility workup.

Gonadotrophin releasing hormone (GnRH)

In the early 1970s, shortly after the characterisation and synthesis of GnRH, there was considerable optimism that GnRH would be a more effective and a safe alternative to HMG for women who failed to ovulate with clomiphene. Initial reports in which frequent large doses of subcutaneous GnRH were used appeared promising (Zarate et al, 1974. Henderson, et al, 1976). However, a review of eight reports revealed that 45 per cent of 182 anovulatory patients who received GnRH ovulated and only 20 per cent became pregnant. This is no better than can be achieved with placebo treatment. It was also considered that orally active long-acting potent analogues of GnRH would be of value. However, these appear to be antigonadotrophic and potentially more useful as contraceptive agents. It is now well established that GnRH to exert its maximum gonadotrophin-releasing effect has to be given in two-hourly intravenous doses. The recent development of special automatic syringes which deliver predetermined volumes at intervals, and which can be worn by the patient on a special belt make such treatment technically possible (Auto-Syringe, Hookset, New Hampshire 03104, USA). However, for the time being, GnRH treatment for dysovulatory infertility is still in the research stage.

SUMMARY AND CONCLUSIONS

Recent advances in reproductive neuroendocrinology have provided a firm basis on which modern treatment of dysovulatory infertility can be laid. The concept of the fertile menstrual cycle and the normal luteal phase should result in pregnancy rates which do not lag far behind ovulation rates when clomiphene or HMG (HPG) and HCG treatment are given. In this context, additional support of the corpus luteum by exogenous HCG may result in improved viable pregnancy rates. Ovulation rates with clomiphene are currently 60 to 75 per cent, with pregnancy occurring in 25 to 32 per cent of patients. HMG and HCG treatment usually results in ovulation in 90 to 98 per cent of cases and pregnancy in 35 to 45 per cent.

Identification of patients with hyperprolactinaemia, and their subsequent treatment with bromocriptine, has led to a further increase in pregnancy rates. Appreciation of androgen interference with follicular development and the elimination of excessive adrenal androgens with exogenous corticosteroids, such as prednisone and dexamethazone in patients taking clomiphene have resulted in more pregnancies.

Second generation drugs for inducing augmentation of ovulation have been slow in coming. GnRH, when given parenterally and intermittently, can induce ovulation, but only placebo pregnancy and ovulation rates have been achieved. Unfortunately, the highest potent long-acting GnRH analogues are antigonadotrophic. Third generation methods await an increase in our knowledge of basic reproductive neuroendocrinology and, particularly, the relationships between the hypothalamus and the higher centres of the brain. Perhaps then we can look forward to physical, psychological, and biochemical methods for augmenting pulsatile hypothalamic GnRH output.

REFERENCES

Abraham G E, Maroulis G B, Marshall J R 1974 Evaluation of ovulation and corpus luteum function using measurements of plasma progesterone. Obstetrics and Gynecology 44: 522–525

Adashi E Y, Rock J A, Sapp K C, Martin E J, Wentz A C, Jones G S 1979 Gestational outcome of clomiphene-related conceptions. Fertility and Sterility 31: 620–626

Apter D, Viinikka L, Vihko R 1978 Hormonal pattern of adolescent menstrual cycles. Journal of Clinical Endocrinology and Metabolism 47: 944–954

Canales E S, Cabezas A, Vazquez-Matute L, Zarate A 1978 Induction of ovulation with clomiphene and estradiol benzoate in an ovulatory woman refractory to clomiphene alone. Fertility and Sterility 29: 496–499

Clarke J H, Peek E J Jr, Anderson J N 1974 Oestrogen receptors and antagonism of steroid hormone action. Nature 251: 446–448

Connaughton J F Jr, Garcia C-R, Wallach E E 1974 Induction of ovulation with cisclomiphene and a placebo. Obstetrics and Gynecology 43: 697–701

Cooke I D, Morgan C A, Parry T E 1972 Correlation of endometrial biopsy and plasma progesterone levels in infertile women. Journal of Obstetrics and Gynaecology of the British Commonwealth 79: 647–650

Corson S L 1979 Use of the laparoscope in the infertile patient. Fertility and Sterility 32: 359–369

Csaba I, Nagy P, Szabo I, Bucs G, Varga V 1974 Induction of ovulation with phenobarbital in anovulatory states. A preliminary report. Fertility and Sterility 25: 865–871

Dmowski W P, Cohen M R 1975 Treatment of endometriosis with an antigonadotropin, danazol. Obstetrics and Gynecology 46: 147–154

Dor J, Itzkowic D J, Mashiach S, Lunenfeld B, Serr D M 1980 Cumulative conception rates following gonadotropin therapy. American Journal of Obstetrics and Gynecology 136: 102–105

Drake T S, Treadway D R, Buchanan G C 1978 Continued clinical experience with increasing dosage regimen of clomiphene citrate administration. Fertility and Sterility 30: 274–277

Edwards R G, Steptoe P C, Baillie J 1980 Observation on preovulatory human ovarian follicles and their aspirates. British Journal of Obstetrics and Gynecology 87: 769–779

Ellis J D, Williamson J G 1975 Factors influencing the pregnancy and complication rates with human menopausal gonadotrophin therapy. British Journal of Obstetrics and Gynaecology 82: 52–57

Evans J, Townsend L 1976 The induction of ovulation. American Journal of Obstetrics and Gynecology 125: 321–327

Gemzell C A 1977 Induction of ovulation with human gonadotropins. Journal of Reproductive Medicine 18: 155–158

Greenblatt R B, Borenstein R, Hernandez-Ayup S 1974 Experiences with danazol (an anti-gonadotropin) in the treatment of infertility. American Journal of Obstetrics and Gynecology 118: 783–787

Hackeloer B J, Fleming R, Robinson H P, Adam A H, Coutts J R 1979 Correlation of ultrasonic and endocrinologic assessment of human follicular development. American Journal of Obstetrics and Gynecology 135: 122–128

Hancock K W, Scott J S, Lamb J T, Gibson R M, Chapman C 1980 Conservative management of pituitary prolactinomas; evidence for bromocriptine-induced regression. British Journal of Obstetrics and Gynaecology 87: 523–529

Henderson S R, Bonnar J, Moore A, MacKinnon P C B 1976 Luteinizing hormone-releasing hormone for induction of follicular maturation and ovulation in women with infertility and amenorrhea. Fertility and Sterility 27: 621–627

Insler V, Melmed H, Eichenbrenner I, Serr D M, Lunenfeld B 1972 The cervical score- and simple semiquantitative method for monitoring the menstrual cycle. International Journal of Gynecology and Obstetrics 10: 223–228

James W H 1980 Gonadotrophin and the human sex ratio. British Medical Journal 281: 711–712

Jones G S 1976 The luteal phase defect. Fertility and Sterility 27: 351–356

Jones G S, Moraes-Ruehsen M de 1969 A new syndrome of amenorrhea in association with hypergonadotropism and apparently normal ovarian follicular apparatus. American Journal of Obstetrics and Gynecology 104: 597–600

Keletzky O A, Nakamura R M, Thorneycroft I H, Mishell D R Jr 1975 Log normal distribution of gonadotropins and ovarian steroid values in the normal menstrual cycle. American Journal of Obstetrics and Gynecology 121: 688–694

Keller D M, Wiest W G, Askin F B, Johnson L W, Strickler R C 1979 Pseudo corpus luteum insufficiency: A local defect of progesterone action on endometrial stroma. Journal of Clinical Endocrinology and Metabolism 48: 127–132

Koike K, et al 1981 Induction of ovulation in patients with normoprolactinemic amenorrhea by combined therapy with bromocriptine and clomiphene. Fertility and Sterility 35: 138–141

Lenton E A, Sobowale O S, Cooke I D 1977 Prolactin concentrations in ovulatory but infertile women: treatment with bromocriptine. British Medical Journal 2: 1179–1181

Lobo R A, Paul W, Kletzky O A, March C 1981 Ovulatory and anovulatory hormonal profiles in women treated with high-dose clomiphene citrate with and without the addition of dexamethazone. Fertility and Sterility 35: 248 Abstract

Lunenfeld B, Insler V 1978a Infertility, diagnosis and treatment of functional infertility. Grosse Verlag, Berlin, p 26–28

Lunenfeld B, Insler V 1978b Infertility, diagnosis and treatment of functional infertility. Grosse Verlag, Berlin, p 61–89

March C M, Tredway D R, Mishell D R Jr 1976 Effect of clomiphene citrate upon amount and duration of human menopausal gonadotropin therapy. American Journal of Obstetrics and Gynecology 125: 699–704

Marshall J R, Wider J A 1971 Results of human menopausal gonadotropins (HMG) therapy for anovulatory infertility using a nonvariable treatment schedule: Comparison with previous reports. Fertility and Sterility 22: 19–25

McBain J C, Evans J H, Pepperell R J, Robinson H P, Smith M A 1980 An unexpectedly high rate of ectopic pregnancy following the induction of ovulation with human pituitary and chorionic gonadotrophin. British Journal of Obstetrics and Gynaecology 87: 5–9

McCormack S, Clark H 1979 Clomid administration to pregnant rats causes abnormalities of the reproductive tract in offspring and mothers. Science 40: 629–631

Moghissi K S 1976 Accuracy of basal body temperature for ovulation detection. Fertility and Sterility 27: 1415–1421

Noyes R W, Hertig A T, Rock J 1950 Dating the endometrial biopsy. Fertility and Sterility 1: 3–25

O'Herlihy C, de Crespigny L J Ch, Robinson H P 1980 Monitoring ovarian follicular development with real time ultrasound. British Journal of Obstetrics and Gynaecology 87: 613–618

O'Herlihy C, de Crespigny L Ch, Robinson H, Hoult I 1981 The role of ultrasound in an in vitro fertilization program. Fertility and Sterility 35: 235 (Abstract Supplement)

Pepperell R J et al 1977 Serum prolactin levels and the value of bromocriptine in the treatment of anovulatory infertility. British Journal of Obstetrics and Gynaecology 84: 58–66

Polansky S, de Papp E W 1976 Pregnancy associated with hypergonadotropic hypogonadism. Obstetrics and Gynecology 47: 47s–51s

Rakoff A E 1979 Ovulatory failure: clinical aspects. In: Wallach E E, Kempers R D (eds) Modern trends in infertility and conception control, Vol I. Williams and Wilkins, Baltimore, Sect. II, ch 8, p 157–176

Rakoff A E, Plaster E L, Goldfarb A F 1973 Comparison of various therapies for treatment of anovulation. In: Rosenberg E (ed) Gonadotropin in female infertility, Excerpta Medica, Amsterdam, p 125–128

Robertson R D, Picker R H, Wilson P C, Saunders D M 1979 Assessment of ovulation by ultrasound and plasma estradiol determinations. Obstetrics and Gynecology 54: 686–691

Rust L A, Israel R, Mishell D R Jr 1974 An individualized graduated therapeutic regimen for clomiphene citrate. American Journal of Obstetrics and Gynecology 120: 785–790

Saunders D M, Hunter J C, Haase H R, Wilson G R 1979 Treatment of luteal phase inadequacy with bromocriptine. Obstetrics and Gynecology 53: 287–289

Schenker J G, Yakoni S, Granat M 1981 Multiple pregnancies following induction of ovulation. Fertility and Sterility 35: 105–123

Schenker J G, Weinstein D 1978 Ovarian hyperstimulation syndrome: A current survey. Fertility and Sterility 30: 255–268

Seibel M M, McArdle C, Thompson I E, Berger M J, Taymor M L 1981 The role of ultrasound in ovulation induction: A critical appraisal. Fertility and Sterility 35: 260 (Abstract Supplement)

Seppala M, Hirvonen E, Ranta T 1976 Hyperprolactinaemia and luteal insufficiency. Lancet 1: 229–230

Shephard M K, Balmaceda J P, Leija C 1979 Relationship of weight to successful induction of ovulation with clomiphene citrate. Fertility and Sterility 32: 641–645

Shephard M K, Senturia Y D 1977 Comparison of serum progesterone and endometrial biopsy for confirmation of ovulation and evaluation of luteal function. Fertility and Sterility 28: 541–548

Swyer G I M, Radwanska E, McGarrigle H H G 1975 Plasma oestradiol and progesterone estimation for the monitoring of induction of ovulation with clomiphene and chorionic gonadotrophin. British Journal of Obstetrics and Gynaecology 82: 794–804

Templeton A A, Kerr M G 1977 An assessment of laparoscopy as the primary investigation in the subfertile female. British Journal of Obstetrics and Gynaecology 84: 760–762

Thorner M O et al 1979 Pregnancy in patients presenting with hyperprolactinaemia. British Medical Journal 2: 771–774

Vande Wiele R L et al 1970 Mechanisms regulating the menstrual cycle in women. Recent Progress in Hormone Research 26: 63–103

Vandenberg G, Yen S S C 1973 Effect of anti-estrogenic action of clomiphene during the menstrual cycle: Evidence for a change in the feedback sensitivity. Journal of Clinical Endocrinology and Metabolism 37: 356–365

van Dijk J G, Frolich M, Brand E C, van Hall 1979 The treatment of unexplained infertility with danazol. Fertility and Sterility 31: 481–485

Wu C H 1978 Monitoring of ovulation induction. Fertility and Sterility 30: 617–630

Yen S S C 1978 The human menstrual cycle. Integrative function of the hypothalamic-pituitary-ovarian-endometrial axis. In: Yen S S C, Jaffe R B (eds) Reproductive endocrinology. Physiology, pathophysiology, and clinical management. Saunders, Philadelphia, ch 7, p 126–151

Zarate A, Canales E S, Soria J, Gonzalez A, Schally A V, Kastin A J 1974 Further observations on the therapy of anovulatory infertility with synthetic luteinizing hormone releasing hormone. Fertility and Sterility 25: 3–10

12. In vitro fertilisation and embryo transfer

Carl Wood   Alan Trounson

INDICATIONS

Tubal infertility — alternatives

In the human, in vitro fertilisation (IVF) and embryo transfer (ET) have been developed in order to overcome the problem of tubal infertility. The motivation for the development was a consequence of the limitations of other methods of treatment.

Hydrotubation and tubal surgery are the main therapies, but their effect is restricted to the correction of mechanical defects in the tube. The overall success rate of tubal surgery is only about 30 per cent (Siegler, 1960; Cohen et al, 1972), and even in the most favourable circumstance, only a 75 per cent success rate can be achieved. Surgery has little or no chance of success in many patients with severe tubal disease (Gommel, 1977). The development of microsurgery has improved the technique, but improvement in pregnancy rate has been less certain, perhaps in the order of 10 per cent (Siegler & Perez, 1975; Winston, 1977). Replacing the tube by a graft has been attempted, but so far, without success. While microvascular techniques are available which give a reasonable chance of technical success, the problems associated with finding suitable histo-compatible donors and the hazards of anti-immune therapy are current barriers to further progress in tubal transplantation. A silastic artificial fallopian tube has been developed, but the one surgical attempt to use it failed (Wood et al, 1971). A device which can replace both anatomical and physiological functions of the tube has not been made.

Attempts to overcome tubal infertility by transposing the ovary to the uterus, as in Estes' operation (Estes & Heitmeyer, 1934), have been occasionally successful, but the risk of ovarian damage and uterine rupture, should pregnancy occur, have deterred surgeons from performing the operation. Analogous to uterine implantation of ovaries is the transfer of a mature oocyte from the ovarian follicle to the uterine cavity, insemination occurring subsequent to previous coitus or by the coincident transfer of washed sperm with the oocyte. Experience of oocyte to uterine transfer by Steptoe & Edwards (personal communication) and our own group in a small number of patients did not meet with success, but more recently Shettles et al, 1980, have reported two pregnancies in seven patients. However, the technique used to obtain mature oocytes, the failure to identify oocyte in the follicular aspirates, the volume of fluid (5 to 10 ml) transferred to the uterine cavity and the possible influence of coincident tubal surgery would argue strongly against the success of this procedure. Pregnancies resulting from the transfer of single cell fertilised eggs in the monkey directly to the uterus (Marston, 1979) suggests that uterine transfer of the oocyte should be further explored.

More certain ways of achieving parenthood are by adoption or use of a surrogate mother, although most couples prefer to have a child from their own genetic pool. In many western countries, adoption is restricted by lack of babies and waiting lists may be as long as five years. When adopted babies are scarce, new barriers are introduced to exclude potential adoptive parents. Few pregnancies using surrogate mothers have been reported. Psychological problems consequent to the mother giving up the child may be serious and until the circumstances can be defined under which women can become surrogate mothers without encountering psychological harm, the method will not be popular. Social, legal and financial aspects of the surrogate system also require consideration and resolution.

Most of the patients having IVF and ET have failed to conceive after reconstructive tubal surgery, have been unsuitable for tubal surgery because of severely damaged or absent tubes, and either do not wish to or are unable to adopt a child.

Idiopathic infertility

Patients in whom the cause of infertility is unknown after adequate investigation (idiopathic) are suitable for IVF and ET. Views on what constitutes adequate investigation vary, but most authors agree that assessment of temperature charts, plasma progesterone and prolactin levels, laparoscopy, hydrotubation, curettage, post-coital test and semen analysis are required. One possible reason for the occurrence of infertility in the presence of normal investigations is that undetected abnormalities of the sperm or oocyte may lead to the failure of, or abnormal fertilisation, or abnormal embryonic development. This is supported by the observation that IVF is more often successful in patients with tubal disease than in patients with idiopathic infertility (Lopata et al, 1980a, Trouson et al, 1980a).

In our current research programmes we aim to obtain more than one mature oocyte so that a test for the normality of fertilisation and early embryonic development can be established (Table 12.1). In this test, oocytes are placed with both the husband's sperm and sperm of a donor of known fertility. Failure of fertilisation with husband's sperm and success with donor sperm may indicate that the husband has undetected sperm abnormalities. At the present time we are still evaluating the diagnostic value of this test but it is apparent that there are abnormalities of oocytes (Trounson et al, 1980a) and sperm (Sathananthan & Trounson, unpublished data) that mitigate against normal fertilisation. We have also detected irregularities of granulosa cells and oocytes in follicular aspirates and found evidence for the retention of oocytes in the follicle following ovulation. Normal fertilisation and pregnancy after embryo transfer can be achieved in these patients (Wood et al, 1981b) which suggests that there may be other factors preventing the interaction of sperm and oocytes in vivo in at least a proportion of these patients.

Abnormality of spermatozoa

The procedure has been suggested as a method of treating oligospermia or male infertility involving other sperm defects. The assumption has been made that as IVF requires only a small number of sperm, less than one million, then it should be an ideal system for achieving pregnancy in men with sperm concentrations less than 20 million per ml. Insufficient experience of IVF and ET using oligospermic semen has accrued although in few cases (two of 15) fertilisation has been achieved in semen of concentrations less than 10 million per ml. At present the question cannot be answered with any surety. Low sperm concentrations are often associated with other

Table 12.1   The use of IVF for diagnostic assessment of idiopathic infertility

| Group | Semen tested | | | Comments on diagnosis |
	Husband	Donor		
1.	Fertilised	Fertilised	— Pregnancy after ET:	Infertility is not due to abnormality of the gametes but due to some unidentified factor inhibiting the association of gametes (immunological or chemical interference to sperm or oocyte transport, failure of the release of oocytes from the follicle or physical abnormalities preventing oocyte entry into the oviduct, such as the absence of fimbrial cilia).
			— Not pregnant after ET:	Infertility may be due to unidentified chromosomal or uterine abnormality preventing embryo development or implantation or due to failure of technique.
2.	No fertilisation	Fertilised	—	Infertility due to abnormality of husband's sperm. Recommend A.I.D.
3.	No fertilisation	No fertilisation	—	Infertility due to abnormality of the oocyte or to a technical failure of IVF.
4.	Fertilised	No fertilisation	—	This should not occur and would be due to attempted donor IVF with immature or abnormal oocytes. If it did occur the same comment would apply to this group as the first group.

defects in sperm, such as low motility and anatomical defects and the quality of the sperm from such patients may be insufficient to achieve normal fertilisation and embryo development.

SELECTION OF PATIENTS

Emotional and physical condition

The patient needs to be emotionally and physically capable of proceeding through pregnancy, birth and rearing the child. Some of the couples seeking IVF and ET have serious emotional problems. Depression may result from feeling inadequate as a result of being infertile, or from pressures to sustain a marriage by achieving fertility. Referral to a psychiatrist may be necessary before a decision concerning the use of IVF and ET can be made. Suicide may be precipitated by a failed attempt at IVF and ET in a patient who is chronically depressed. Warning of an unstable state of mind may occur as the result of the patient's inability to realise or accept the low rate of success of the procedure. Other emotional reactions to infertility are common and need not debar the couple from attempting IVF and ET. Mild depression, anxiety, anger and jealousy of other fertile couples occur and represent different psychological reactions to the couple's frustration in not being able to conceive. Recognition of emotional states can assist the couple to adjust to their infertility, and very often the couple's emotional state improves during the experience of IVF and ET. Talking to other couples in the research programme is also helpful.

Reproductive efficiency declines with increasing age, and until the success rate of IVF and ET improves, patients over 40 years of age have been excluded from our programme.

Fertility assessment

When selecting patients with infertility resulting from tubal disease, it is important to ensure that other fertility systems are normal. Regular ovulation is ensured by examining at least three temperature charts for biphasic changes. The adequacy of corpus luteum function is assessed by plasma progesterone measurements in the mid-luteal phase and hyperprolactinaemia is excluded by several prolactin assays. If anovulation or hyperprolactinaemia is present, these abnormalities are corrected by ovulation induction or antiprolactin therapy prior to accepting the patient for IVF and ET.

Semen analysis

Semen analysis is carried out on two occasions. If either of the samples are abnormal, then at the time of a satisfactory collection, a portion of the semen is frozen. This specimen may be used instead of the husband's semen for insemination at the time of IVF. In patients with blocked tubes if the husband's semen is habitually unsatisfactory, donor semen is offered.

Pelvic status

The ovaries have to be accessible to laparoscopic inspection, in order that an oocyte be aspirated and this is checked by preliminary laparoscopy. The slight risk of laparoscopy has led to the suggestion that preliminary laparoscopy to determine access to the ovaries is unnecessary and this should be determined at the time of a definitive attempt at IVF. The reasons for preferring laparoscopy prior to IVF are that if the ovaries are inaccessible, other investigations are avoided, the extra cost and staff time associated with IVF are saved, and the patient suffers less disappointment.

When the ovaries are inaccessible to inspection by laparoscopy, patients have requested surgery (adhesolysis) to remedy this. The possibility of IVF and ET should be considered at the time of tubal surgery, particularly if the tubal disease is severe and the operation is unlikely to be successful. The ovaries should be left in a position favourable for subsequent oocyte pickup. The risk of adhesions covering the ovary after surgery may be reduced by careful surgical technique such as, absolute haemostasis using point diathermy, the use of fine non-absorbable suture material, reperitonealisation of rough surfaces, care not to abrade the peritoneum, irrigation of the pelvic peritoneal cavity after surgery with Hartmann's solution or Dextran and parenteral antibiotics and corticoids.

The possibility of an embryo being flushed into a tubal remnant at the time of embryo transfer led Steptoe & Edwards (1976) to the recommendation that surgical blockage of the tubes should be carried out prior to IVF. They reported an ectopic pregnancy after IVF and ET. The advantage of preliminary surgical blockage of the tubes has to be weighed against the disadvantage of blocking tubes which may still be patent, providing the patient with a chance of achieving pregnancy normally. The technique of uterine transfer can be modified to reduce the risk of flushing an embryo into the tube by the site of placement of the transfer catheter and the volume of fluid injected.

Apart from pelvic adhesions, the existence of active pelvic disease is a contraindication to IVF and ET. Endometriosis and pelvic infection should be quiescent prior to an attempt at oocyte pick-up.

Ideal couple
It is not possible to define an ideal couple for IVF and ET. Youth has the advantage of ensuring adequate time for repeated attempts at the procedure, the likelihood of a high state of natural fertility, apart from the tubal problem, and a low risk of fetal malformation. Previous childbearing has the advantages of ensuring that fertility other than the tubal abnormality is likely and embryo transfer is easier as the cervical canal is generally easier to pass with transfer catheters after birth of a baby. Giving preference to parous patients may be considered unethical if they have a live child. Educated couples more easily understand IVF and ET and the possible reasons for success and failure. Nevertheless, the procedure can be explained in simple terms, so that the less educated and/or less intelligent couples can understand and give informed consent. Farmers or biology students find IVF and ET easy to comprehend. No specific personality type is suitable for the procedure, but those who cope best are usually realistic, understanding the relatively low success rate, yet wishing to leave no avenue unexplored in trying to resolve their infertility.

Patient preference
Patients with tubal infertility unresolved by surgery form the majority of patients having IVF and ET. The attitude of patients to alternative methods of treatment varies. Information concerning the possible success of repeat tubal surgery or

microsurgery, as well as the low success rate of IVF and ET, are presented. A rigid policy is not presented, so that some patients pursue IVF and ET whilst others pursue further surgery before attempting IVF and ET. An increasing number of patients are selecting IVF and ET as a method of investigation of their infertility. Those that fail to achieve fertilisation, either because of defects in either the husband's spermatozoa or the oocyte, are satisfied that a cause has been isolated. On the other hand, the patients with idiopathic infertility who succeed in developing an embryo are encouraged to pursue IVF and ET as a method of treatment. The production of a normal oocyte and development of an embryo, even if pregnancy does not follow, may enhance self-esteem.

Costs

At the present time the facilities and cost of IVF and ET are not met by the Government Health Service. The couples join a private health insurance fund or save specifically for IVF and ET costs. Health insurance is preferable as $1000 (Aust.) of the estimated $1500 (Aust.) cost per treatment can be recovered from insurance funds. Improvement in success rate of IVF and ET may enlist Government support and increase rebates from private medical insurance funds.

PRETREATMENT INVESTIGATION

Special clinic

The patients are seen at a special clinic as this facilitates the exchange of information between the couple and those involved in IVF and ET and the organisation of the procedure. The clinic is attended by the gynaecologists, the scientist who does the IVF, the sister who organises the service, and a member of the patient's support association.

Genital tract

Embryo transfer requires the passage of a catheter into the upper part of the uterine cavity, but short of the fundus to avoid bleeding or stimulating uterine activity. Uterine length is determined either by ultrasonography or by the passage of a uterine sound. A trial uterine transfer is carried out in patients who have not given birth, as the internal cervical os may be very narrow and tortuous particularly during the luteal phase of the cycle. The preliminary trial of uterine transfer enables the selection of the most suitable catheter and if difficulty is encountered, then antispasmodic and/or epidural anaesthesia may be organised more easily for the actual embryo transfer.

Vaginal and cervical smears are taken, and if pathogenic bacteria are present, they are treated by appropriate antibiotics. At the time of embryo transfer, the catheter may collect pathogenic bacteria from the vagina or cervix and carry them into the uterus.

Psychological state

Discussion with other couples who are in the programme and transmission of information concerning the procedure by the IVF team reduces anxiety. The trial run of ET also informs and reassures the patient concerning this procedure. After failure, the couples are seen at the special clinic and the reasons for failure explained. The reaction of the couple to each attempt at IVF and ET determines whether they continue. The decision may be influenced by progress in the research, of which the couple are informed.

Semen analysis (see Selection of patients, p. 262)
Semen analysis is required within a month of IVF and ET because of the possibility of an unfavourable change in semen, count or motility, or the occurrence of infection. Leucocytes in the semen indicate infection in the male genital tract and appropriate antibiotics are given. Urological referral may be necessary. The presence of pathogenic bacteria in the absence of leucocytes is most often due to contamination of the specimen by skin flora. At the time of IVF, the husband is advised to wash both hands and penis prior to masturbation, as pathogenic bacteria may contaminate the culture system. Antiseptics should not be used, as the chemicals may be toxic to sperm and oocytes. If the husband has difficulty providing semen samples by masturbation, then arrangements are made so that the wife can assist the husband at the time of IVF and, if this fails, a frozen semen sample is used.

Endocrine system
Normal genital endocrine function is ensured by examining several temperature charts and measuring the plasma progesterone and prolactin levels.

Consent form
The couple are asked to sign a consent form which includes a statement that the risks of the procedure have been explained, that success is not guaranteed, the possibility of fetal malformation has been discussed and that fetal diagnostic tests will be carried out in an endeavour to detect fetal malformation.

TREATMENT CYCLE

Organisation
The patients telephone the sister co-ordinating the IVF service on the first day of the menses to determine whether they will be accepted for treatment. It is not possible to book patients months ahead of schedule as the number of patients treated each week is limited by staff and hospital facilities and the onset of menstruation cannot be accurately predicted.

Drug schedule
Patients may have IVF in a normal menstrual cycle or in a cycle stimulated by Clomid (see Trounson et al, 1981a). All the patients in our service have Clomid therapy, 150 mg per day, on Day 5 to 9 of the cycle (first day of menstruation = Day 1). Ultrasound is carried out during the follicular phase (Day 10, 11 or 12) to determine whether follicular growth is occurring at a normal rate. If follicular growth is normal, then 4000 IU of HCG is given on Day 13 or 14 of the cycle and laparoscopy is performed 35 to 36 hours later. If follicular growth is faster or slower than normal the time of HCG injection is varied accordingly. Premature injection of HCG produces abnormal oocyte maturation (see Trounson et al, 1981b). When the patients are admitted to hospital urinary LH excretion rate is measured twice daily in three hourly

urine samples by the Higonovis kit assay (Mochida, Japan) or radioimmunoassay (Trounson et al, 1980b). If the endogenous LH surge occurs before the time of HCG injection, the time of laparoscopy is rescheduled for 25 to 27 hours after the start of the LH rise.

Genital tract

Vaginal and cervical smears are repeated in the follicular phase to exclude vaginitis or the presence of pathogenic bacteria which may be introduced into the uterus at the time of embryo transfer. Appropriate therapy is given, but if the infection does not resolve, IVF and ET are deferred to the subsequent cycle.

The cervical mucus is also examined by microscopy to assess the degree of oestrogen activity (Trounson et al, 1979) and this may be used to determine the time of HCG injection in patients where no follicle is visible by ultrasound.

Admission to hospital

The day of admission to hospital is dependent on a number of factors: the previous length of the menstrual cycle and the expected day of ovulation; follicular size determined by ultrasound; the cervical mucus score; and previous experience of treating the patient for IVF. Urinary oestrogen excretion is useful in the natural cycle, but after Clomid the level of oestrogen is dependent upon the number of mature follicles and the range of oestrogen levels for various numbers of mature follicles is not precisely known.

Treatment in hospital

HCG is given by single injection. Whether this produces optimum maturation of the follicle is uncertain. Endogenous LH has an episodic release pattern and intermittent injection or infusion of HCG may produce more predictable oocyte maturation. About one hour before the laparoscopy, an ultrasonic examination may be carried out to determine whether ovulation has already occurred and the presence and number of follicles in each ovary. Knowledge of the site of the follicles can assist the surgeon, particularly if adhesions partly obscure the ovaries. If HCG is not given, detection of the rise in endogenous LH can be difficult because of the baseline LH excretion and the variable rate of rise. The onset of the rise can be taken as: the first visible rise above baseline; the first sample which is greater than two standard deviations above the mean baseline level of LH; or at a point half way in time between the baseline and the first rise in LH determined by either method. In the current programme, the rise has been taken as the mid-point in time of the first of at least three consecutive urine samples greater than two standard deviations above the mean of the previous baseline samples. Sometimes the LH rise is not high and it may be difficult to distinguish this from a preliminary peak of LH which occurs before the definitive rise of LH. A small LH peak may represent an inadequate release of LH and be associated with incomplete development of a mature oocyte and follicle. In this circumstance, the patient is best discharged from hospital.

RETRIEVAL OF MATURE OOCYTES

IVF depends upon the collection of mature oocytes which, in turn, depends upon accurate timing of surgery in relation to oocyte development, surgical access to the ovaries and a satisfactory technique for oocyte collection. A preliminary laparoscopy is carried out to ensure that the ovary is accessible, as even when the adhesolysis has been performed at the time of infertility surgery in order to facilitate subsequent oocyte pick-up, adhesions may recur.

Laparoscopy technique

The procedure of laparoscopy is modified in several ways (Wood et al, 1981a). Carbon dioxide is used to induce the pneumoperitoneum. This gas is readily soluble and is less likely to cause serious sequelae should gas embolus occur. It has previously been thought that carbon dioxide may be harmful to the oocyte by inducing acidosis within the follicular fluid. As pregnancies have now occurred in association with the use of carbon dioxide, it may be concluded that either the acidosis is so temporary as not to harm the oocyte, or alternatively, acidosis does not occur, due to the buffering capacity of the follicular fluid.

Access to the ovary

Surgical access to the ovaries is assisted by adequate volume of gas in the peritoneal cavity, extra head down tilt of the patient on the operating table and manipulation of the ligament of the ovary. The key to gaining access to the ovary is to pick up and manipulate the ligament of the ovary as close as possible to the ovary (Fig. 12.1). By

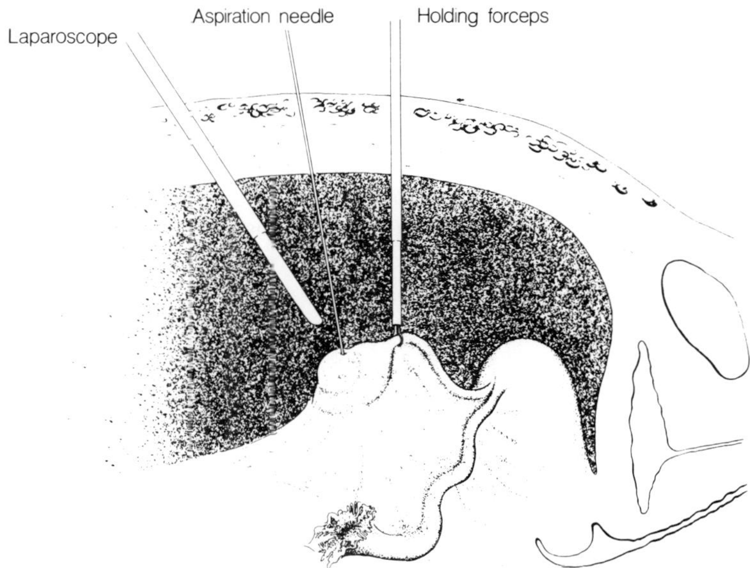

Fig. 12.1 Laparoscopy and exposure of the ovary.

pulling and rotating on the ligament, all surfaces of the ovary can be examined. Occasionally, the uterus has to be elevated in order to gain access to the ovary and, in these circumstances, the uterus is pushed gently upwards in the mid-line.

Aspiration instrument

A special instrument has been designed for oocyte collection (Fig. 12.2) (Renou et al, 1981). A stainless steel needle of 23 cm length was lined by a 19 gauge Teflon tubing giving the needle lumen an internal diamter of 1.7 mm. The Teflon tube of 52 cm is continuous, lining and passing beyond the needle through a sterile silicone rubber bung, thereby delivering follicular aspirates direct to the collecting tube. Previously, stainless steel needles of internal diameter of 2.2 mm and 1.4 mm have been used. Both these needles were joined to the collecting tube by a series of connections. Comparison of the three needles showed the Teflon protected needle to be the most efficient, although the reduction in needle diameter from 2.2 to 1.4 mm also showed a marked improvement in oocyte recovery rate.

Steptoe & Edwards (1970) and Edwards et al (1980), have reported oocyte recovery rates of 33 and 66 per cent. Lopata et al (1974), reported recovery rates of 21 to 46 per cent. The Teflon protected instrument has been adopted for routine use of oocyte collection in both controlled and spontaneous ovulating patients, and the results have remained similar to that reported by Renou et al (1981) (more than 96 per cent recovery rate).

Aspiration of the follicle

If the needle has entered the mature follicle, the fluid will either be straw coloured or slightly blood-stained. Watery fluid usually indicates that the needle is in a cyst. The aspirate in the collecting tube is watched carefully, and if a small opaque mass, which may contain the oocyte and cumulus, is seen, aspiration is stopped and the tube is sent immediately to the laboratory. Reducing follicle aspiration to a minimum reduces the possible disturbance of follicular physiology. The cells of the follicle may be damaged either by deep needle puncture or by excessive aspiration. The aspirating tube is kept warm during passage to the laboratory. If blood appears in the aspirate, then aspiration is stopped, so that the clear fluid already in the collecting tube is not contaminated with blood. Oocytes are detected more easily in clear fluid. If blood is being aspirated, the heparin in culture medium is added either to the collecting tube or the follicle. If the oocyte is not found, the follicle is flushed. This is done by injecting culture medium by a syringe attached to the aspirating system. Sufficient fluid is injected to distend the follicle back to its original size and shape. If the follicle is already ruptured at the time of laparoscopy, the follicle and pouch of Douglas are washed and aspirated in an endeavour to recover the oocyte. It is unknown whether oocytes recovered in this way can develop to normal fetuses.

Difficulties may occur during oocyte aspiration. Obesity and pelvic adhesions increase the difficulty of gaining access to the ovaries. However, neither have prevented successful IVF and ET. Delay in collecting the oocyte of up to 50 minutes after induction of anaesthesia has also been associated with pregnancy. The prolonged use of general anaesthesia and intraperitoneal carbon dioxide are not necessarily harmful to the oocyte. Embryos have developed after oocytes were recovered following difficult dissection in a blood clot when the oocyte was physically deformed.

FERTILISATION CULTURE

Quality control procedures

The use of model systems for the development of new procedures and for the control

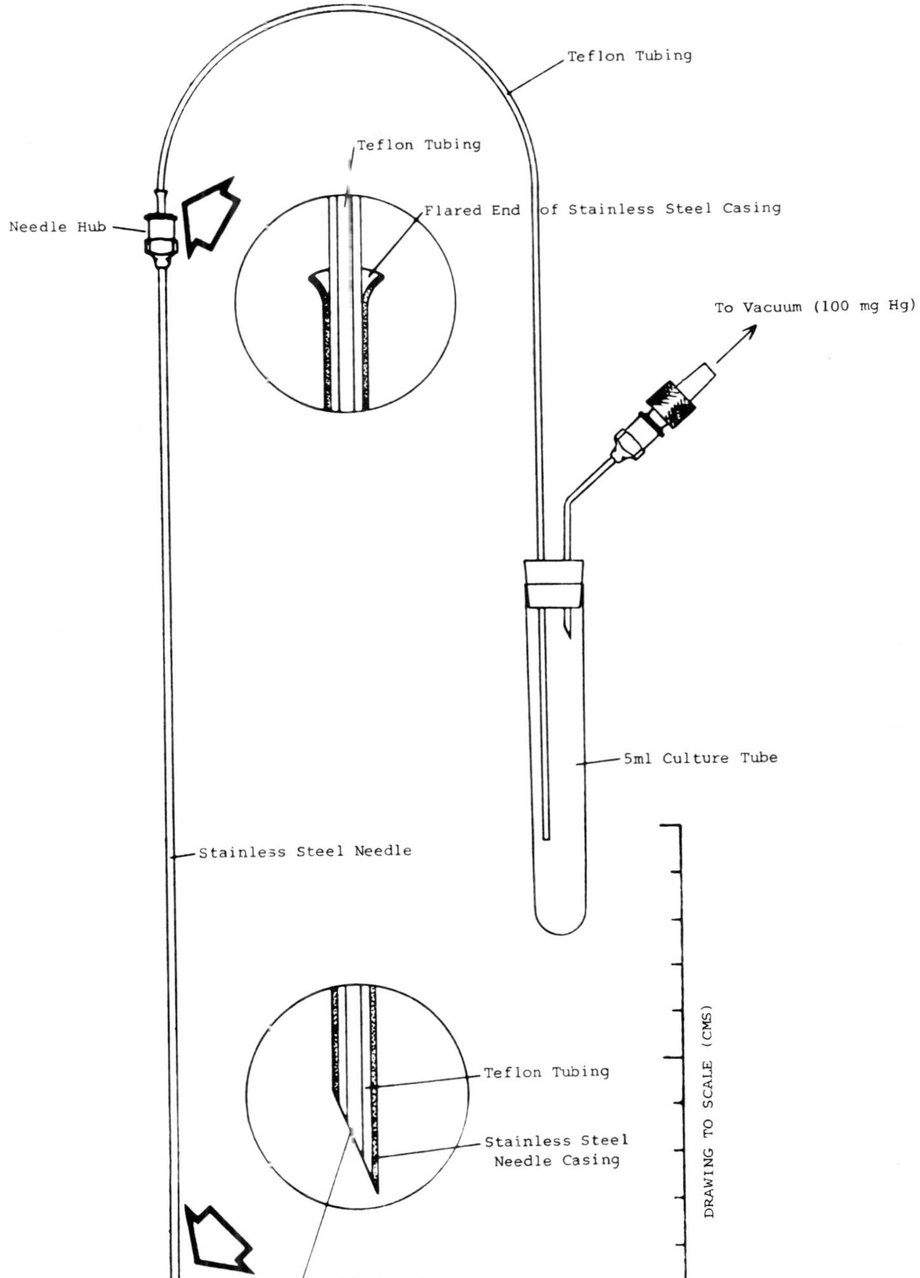

Fig. 12.2   Renou's instruments. A special instrument designed for oocyte recovery. (From Renou P, Trounson A O, Wood C, Leeton J F 1981 The collection of human oocytes for in vitro fertilization I: an instrument for maximizing oocyte recovery rate. Fertility and Sterility 35:409. Reproduced with the permission of the publisher, The American Fertility Society.)

of established techniques cannot be over-emphasised. We have used the development of mouse embryos from the one-cell or two-cell stage to the hatched blastocyst stage as the model system and is based on the methods reported by Hoppe & Pitts (1973).

For the introduction of new instruments, procedures and chemicals, replicated and controlled experiments are carried out with mouse embryos. New introductions to the IVF technique require that mouse embryos, exposed to these procedures, develop at the same rate as those in routine culture (more than 90 per cent exposed blastocysts). Examples to illustrate the necessity of checking methods with such a model are:

1. Prior to 1979, human embryos were cultured in droplets of culture medium under light-weight paraffin oil. Experiments reported by Mohr & Trounson (1980) showed that this particular oil inhibited the cleavage of mouse embryos and, furthermore, toxic effects of the oil on mouse embryos could be determined within 12 hours of the fluorescein diacetate viability test. Other paraffin oils were also shown to inhibit mouse embryo cleavage, and it was decided to use Falcon tissue culture tubes without oil for fertilisation and culture of human embryos; a procedure that had been found to result in high rates of fertilisation and development of mouse embryos (Hoppe & Pitts, 1973; Mohr & Trounson, 1980). Removal of this oil from the cultures and the introduction of tissue culture tubes led to a dramatic increase in the development of normal embryos (Trounson et al, 1980a) and pregnancies after embryo transfer (Lopata et al, 1980b; Trounson et al, 1981a).

2. Nylon intravenous catheters had been used to transfer human embryos to the patients' uterine cavity prior to 1980. However, when two-cell mouse embryos were drawn into these catheters and kept at 37°C for one hour, further cleavage was completely inhibited. Using the same procedures, two other types of transfer catheters were found to have no effect on the continued cleavage of mouse embryos. The toxic effect of these catheters led to their immediate withdrawal from the ET procedure and the introduction of non-toxic teflon catheters.

Regular testing of culture medium in the incubators used for human IVF was introduced to control conditions that tend to drift without notice. These include incubation temperature, gas composition and humidity. All culture medium is prepared in a special laboratory for this purpose. Five-times glass distilled water is used for preparation of culture medium and all glassware for embryo culture is soaked for 24 hours in 2 per cent tissue culture detergent (7X, Flow Laboratories, UK), boiled in this solution, washed in once or twice glass distilled water and rinsed in two- and three-times glass distilled water. The osmolarity and pH of the culture medium is always checked after preparation and is discarded if not within 8 m osmoles of the known osmolarity for that medium. This ensures against weighing mistakes. If the medium supports the development of one- or two-cell mouse embryos to hatched blastocysts, it is accepted for human embryo culture. Culture medium is prepared fresh every seven days.

Oocyte identification

Follicular fluid aspirates are collected in sequentially labelled 5 ml Falcon tissue culture tubes kept at 35°C (Renou et al, 1981). The oocyte and cumulus mass can be usually identified in aspirates and are transferred to small tissue culture petrie dishes (Kayline, Australia) to confirm the presence of an oocyte in the cumulus liquor. The oocyte is transferred immediately to 1 ml culture medium in a 5 ml Falcon tube,

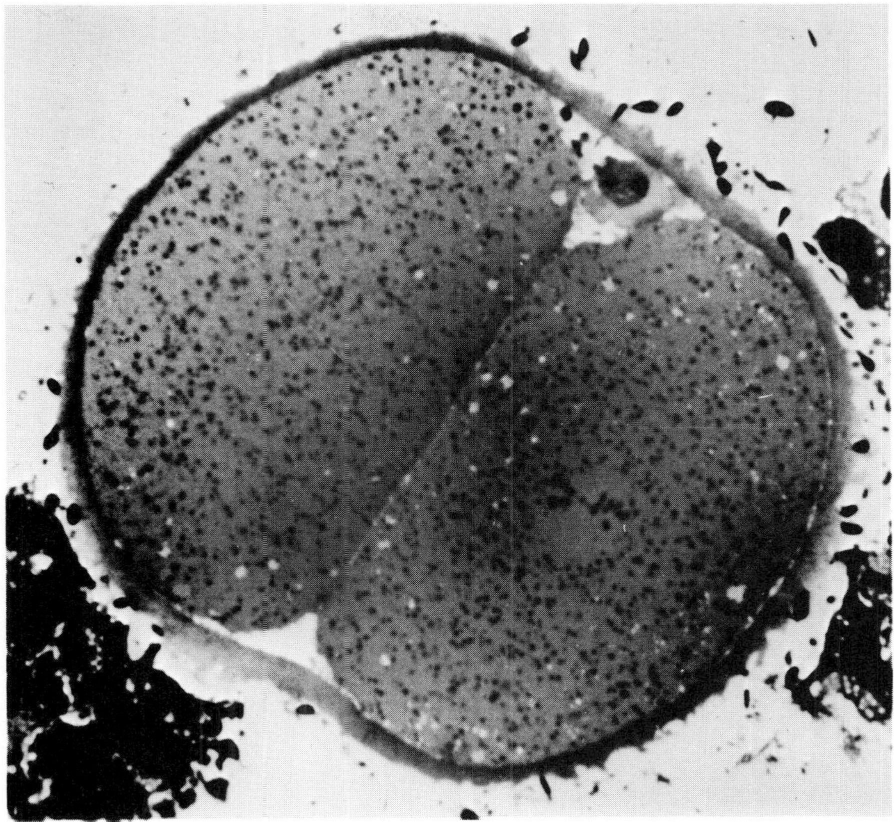

Fig. 12.3a Two-cell embryo. Shortly after first cleavage division. Condensed chromosomes are visible in the right cell. -1 μm section; Toluidine Blue $\times$ 1050.

preincubated for at least four hours at 37°C in a humidified atmosphere at 5 per cent CO_2, 5 per cent O_2 and 90 per cent N_2. In erythrocyte contaminated follicular aspirates, the contents of the tubes are examined in petri dishes and the oocytes washed in clear follicular fluid or culture medium before transfer to the culture tube. It is essential to examine all follicular aspirates completely because it is not infrequent to find more than one oocyte in an aspirate of one follicle or even one tube. Presumably a follicle adjacent to the one visible by the laparoscopicist has been punctured in these cases. All oocytes with activated cumulus (dispersed cumulus cells in liquor) are inseminated but those with tightly packed cumulus cells, typical of immature oocytes, and atretic oocytes are not inseminated. Naked oocytes without cumulus are examined carefully and if the first polar body is present, these are inseminated. On occasion these oocytes fertilise and develop to normal embryos. If blood clots within the follicle during aspiration, oocytes can become entrapped within the fibrin clot. The oocyte can be dissected free with fine (26 gauge) needles. Extreme care is required not to damage the zona pellucida during dissection. Fibrin remaining on the oocyte has the tendency to adhere to all surfaces. These oocytes are usually fertilised and develop normally if undamaged.

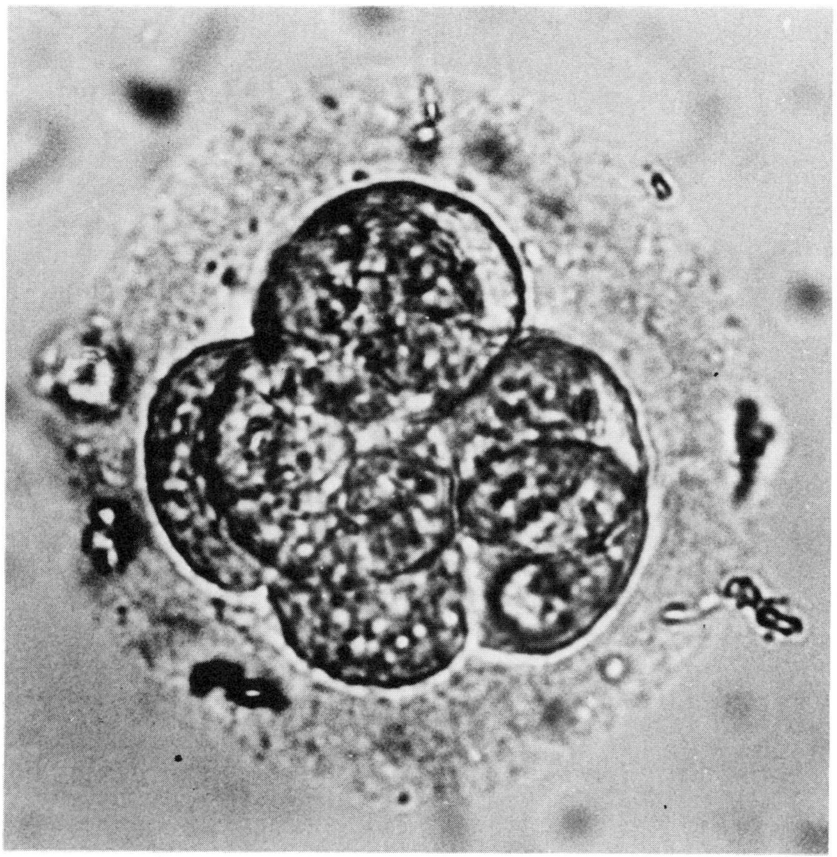

Fig. 12.3b Eight-cell embryo. — Whole mount; phase contrast × 900. (Magnifications refer to submitted prints.)

Insemination and culture

This has been dealt with in detail by Trounson et al (1981b). The optimum procedure is to delay insemination until five to five-and-a-half hours after oocyte collection. The husband is asked to provide a semen sample one-and-a-half to two hours before insemination, in a room close to the laboratory. The sample is examined immediately to determine sperm concentration and motility. Depending on the findings, 0.5 to 4 ml (usually 0.5 to 1.0 ml) semen is added to a 5 or 10 ml Falcon tissue culture tube and diluted with 3 to 5 ml of culture medium (equilibrated for three to 12 hours previously at 37°C). Viscous semen samples are liquified and mixed by continual pipetting, and any large debris removed. The mixture is centrifuged for 10 minutes at 500 g. The supernatant is removed and the sperm pellet resuspended in 3 ml culture medium. The tube is recentrifuged for five minutes and the supernatant discarded. Usually 1 to 2 ml of culture medium is added carefully to the tube so as not to disturb the sperm pellet and the tube incubated at 37°C for 20 to 60 minutes at 37°C. The cloudy supernatant is carefully removed and this is used for insemination. Using this method, a very high proportion of motile sperm is obtained. The motility and concentration of sperm are determined and 1 to 8 $\times$ 10^5 motile sperm in 10 to 20 μl are added to each tube containing an oocyte. The tube containing sperm and the oocyte is returned to the incubator. The tubes are capped but not sealed to allow equilibration with the gas phase.

The oocytes remain with sperm for 12 to 21 hours. At this time pronuclei are clearly visible, providing adhering cumulus cells are removed. This is achieved by gentle pipetting in finely drawn glass pipettes and small petrie dishes containing culture medium with 15 per cent heat inactivated serum. Serum is collected from the patient one to two days before laparoscopy. Oocytes with two pronuclei are transferred to 1 ml of serum enriched medium in a 5 ml Falcon culture tube and returned to the incubator. Various culture media have been used in human IVF successfully to obtain fertilisation and embryonic development. A procedure based on modified Tyrodes medium for insemination of oocytes, followed by Hams F10 with serum from the patient for embryo growth developed by Edwards et al (1970) has been commonly used (Lopata et al, 1978; Edwards et al, 1980). Medium used for fertilisation and embryo development of mouse embryos (Hoppe & Pitts, 1973) is also successful in the human (Trounson et al, 1980a) and this was the first time a single culture medium was used for both fertilisation and culture. A modified procedure for fertilisation and culture in Hams F10 was reported by Lopata et al (1980b) and Trounson et al (1981a, b) to obtain successful pregnancies. Fertilisation and cleavage may also be obtained in other simplified embryo culture medium (Trounson & Whittingham, unpublished data).

There would be a strong preference for the use of a single relatively simple medium for both insemination and culture because this could be prepared in the laboratory from chemical stocks that are completely controlled. Assessment of these simple media is continuing in our laboratory.

Low oxygen concentration (5 per cent O_2) in the gas phase for embryo culture is frequently reported in animals and is common to all published reports in the human. However, it is not essential for either animal (Whittingham, 1979) or human embryo development (Trounson, unpublished data).

EMBRYO TRANSFER

Developmental stage of the embryo

The first successful pregnancies in the human resulted from the transfer of eight-cell and 16-cell embryos fertilised in vitro (Edwards et al, 1980; Lopata et al, 1980b). Although it is not made clear in their publications, apparently most of the embryos transferred by Edwards and Steptoe before the successful transfers were more advanced than eight-cell, mostly morulae and blastocysts (Edwards et al, 1970, 1980; Edwards & Steptoe, 1979). In our own studies we have given consideration to two major factors. The first is the possibility that embryo viability decreased with increasing time in culture in vitro. The extent to which this affects embryo viability will depend on how well the culture conditions mimic conditions in vivo. Sub-optimal culture conditions may allow apparently normal embryo cleavage, but on close examination by high-power light or electron microscopy, considerable abnormalities of cell structure and functions may be seen. This was a common observation in human embryos before the culture procedures were improved. It is likely that detrimental effects on biochemical function of embryos also occur which reduce embryo viability. This would mean that embryos should be transferred to the patient as soon as possible so that the time in culture can be kept to a minimum. The second factor we have considered is the detrimental effect on embryo survival of transfer of embryos to the uterus within the first few days of ovulation. This has been best demonstrated in the

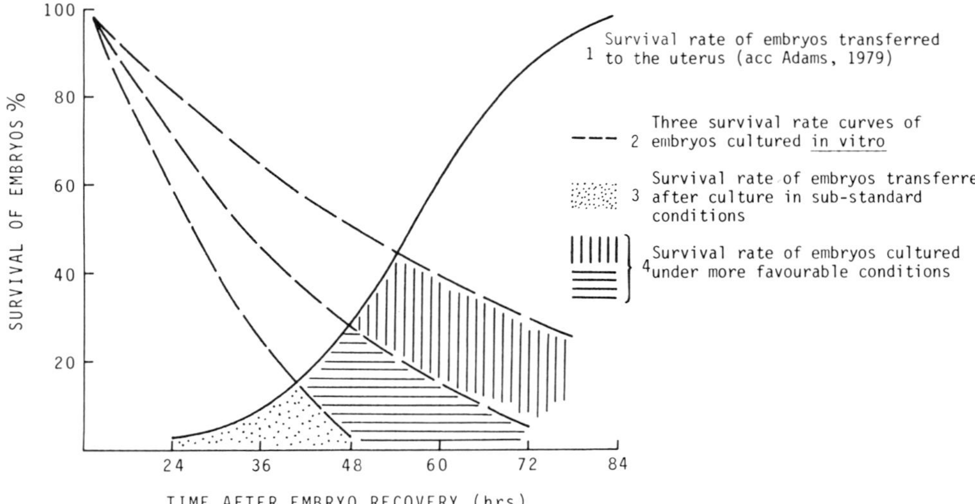

Fig. 12.4   Interaction between embryo viability and uterine receptivity.

rabbit (see Adams, 1979) but has also been reported in other species (Moore & Shelton, 1964). However, Marston (1979) obtained pregnancies by transfer of one- and two-cell embryos to the uterus in monkeys which may suggest that the situation in primates is different. When both factors are considered together, curves of embryo viability during culture will intersect an embryo survival rate curve for uterine transfers (Fig. 12.4). We are endeavouring to determine the stage for maximum embryo survival rate and this will probably occur somewhere between the two-cell and eight-cell stage as predicted. At the present time, normal pregnancies have been obtained with two-cell, four-cell and eight-cell embryos (Fig. 12.3) (Trounson et al, 1981b; Wood et al, 1981b). Even though early pregnancy has been established following transfer of morulae and blastocysts, successful term pregnancies have been confined to embryos transferred up to the 16-cell stage of development (Table 12.2). The conclusions of Edwards et al (1980) that transfer of 16-cell stage embryos result in maximum pregnancy rate is not supported by our data.

The number of embryos transferred

In animals that normally have only one offspring such as the sheep and cow, transfer of single embryos directly from a donor to recipient results in pregnancy rates of between 55 to 75 per cent. The transfer of two embryos in the sheep increases the percentage of pregnant recipients. However, there is little increase with more

Table 12.2 Cell stage of embryos transferred and pregnancies obtained

Cell stage of embryos transferred	Number of patients	Number of pregnancies (full-term babies)	Reference
2-cell	3	1 (1)	Trounson et al (1981)
4-cell	27	5 (4)	Trounson et al (1981)
6 to 7-cell	6	0	Edwards et al (1980)
8-cell	17	2 (1)	Edwards et al (1980)
8-cell	8	0	Lopata et al (1978)
8-cell	21	1 (1)	Trounson et al (1981)
8 to 16-cell	19	2 (1)	Lopata et al (1980)
16-cell to morula	9	2 (1)	Edwards et al (1980)
8-cell to blastocyst	77	3 (0)	Edwards et al (1980)

embryos transferred (Lawson, 1977). There is apparently a percentage (15 to 25 per cent) of recipients that fail to establish pregnancy, which in the case of transfer involving two or more embryos, would be unlikely to be due to non-viable embryos. This may be an abnormality in the recipient in that particular cycle or be due to defects in the embryo transfer technique. It is difficult to separate the effect of embryo viability and that of the recipient, but if the following assumptions are made, the effect of single and twin embryo transfers on pregnancy rate may be computed (Fig. 12.5).

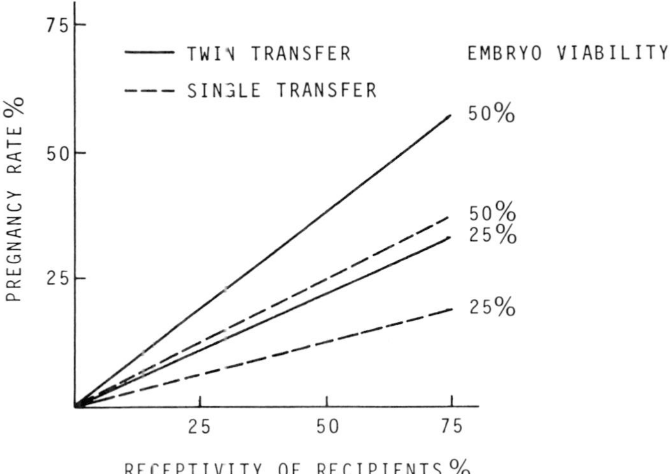

Fig. 12.5 Pregnancy rate and transfer of single and twin embryos.

1. Embryo viability is constant for each embryo assessed as morphologically normal.
2. A constant proportion of recipients will fail to establish pregnancy even if viable embryos are transferred to them.

Neither assumption is likely to be true because, as argued earlier, embryo viability will depend on the stage of cleavage and variation in the quality or maturity of the oocyte obtained from the donor. Transfer technique, the time of transfer and receptivity of the recipients will also vary. However, given these reservations it can be demonstrated that pregnancy rate should be substantially increased by twin transfers (Fig. 12.5) and that some idea of the relative contributions of embryo viability and recipient fertility (including transfer technique) may be gauged by the results of twin and single embryo transfers. In our initial series (Trounson et al, 1981b) we obtained an 8 per cent pregnancy rate for single embryo transfers, compared with a 31 per cent pregnancy rate for twin embryo transfers. This confirmed our hypothesis of increased pregnancy rate with twin embryo transfers, although the difference is greater than predicted. This could be due to the relatively small sample size in this study or some inherent advantage of recipients with multiple follicles and corpora lutea.

Route of transfer

Embryo transfer is conducted through the cervical canal. This route has the advantages of being simple, rapid and requiring no anaesthesia. It has the disadvantages of sometimes displacing blood or mucus into the uterine cavity, which may trap the embryo and prevent implantation and also create an exit track through the cervical mucus via which the embryo may pass. In the cow, transuterine ET is more successful than transcervical ET (Rowson, 1976). The reasons for this are varied; infection of the uterus with vaginal flora during the luteal phase; expulsion of embryos due to uterine contractions; placement of the embryo closer to the cervix than after transuterine transfer and trauma to the uterus with catheters rigid enough to pass through the cervix. As demonstrated by Trounson et al (1978) pregnancy rate increases with the age of embryo transferred. This may argue in favour of transfer of more advanced embryos. Uterine transfer has the advantage of leaving the cervical mucus intact, but has the disadvantage of requiring aneasthesia and the introduction of blood into the uterine cavity, which may disturb embryo development or implantation. Development of the uterine transfundal technique may be worthwhile, either to establish a better method than the transcervical technique, or as an alternative when transcervical transfer is difficult or fails.

Catheters

The simplest method of uterine transfer employs a single fine catheter (Fig. 12.6). The narrower the diameter of the catheter, the more likely it will traverse a narrow internal cervical os and the less likely cervical mucus will be carried into the uterine cavity. On the other hand, narrow catheters have less rigidity and, therefore, are less easily directed through the cervical canal and there is more difficulty in overcoming a mechanical barrier at the internal cervical os.

The adhesive property of the tube is important. Teflon has the advantage of a low surface adhesive property, so that mucus and blood are less likely to adhere to the catheter and be carried into the uterine cavity, where they may inhibit expulsion of the embryo from the catheter, or entrap the embryo after expulsion. Another technique of in vitro transfer employs two tubes. A wide bore catheter acts as a cannula. The cannula is rigid and can be used to overcome a mechanical barrier at the internal cervical os. Because of the size of the cannula, it is more likely to cause bleeding and also to carry mucus and blood into the uterine cavity. A fine catheter containing the embryo is passed through the cannula. Another method is to use a metal cannula (Lopata et al, 1980b) which almost guarantees passage through the internal cervical os, but is likely to cause haemorrhage because of its rigid nature. A

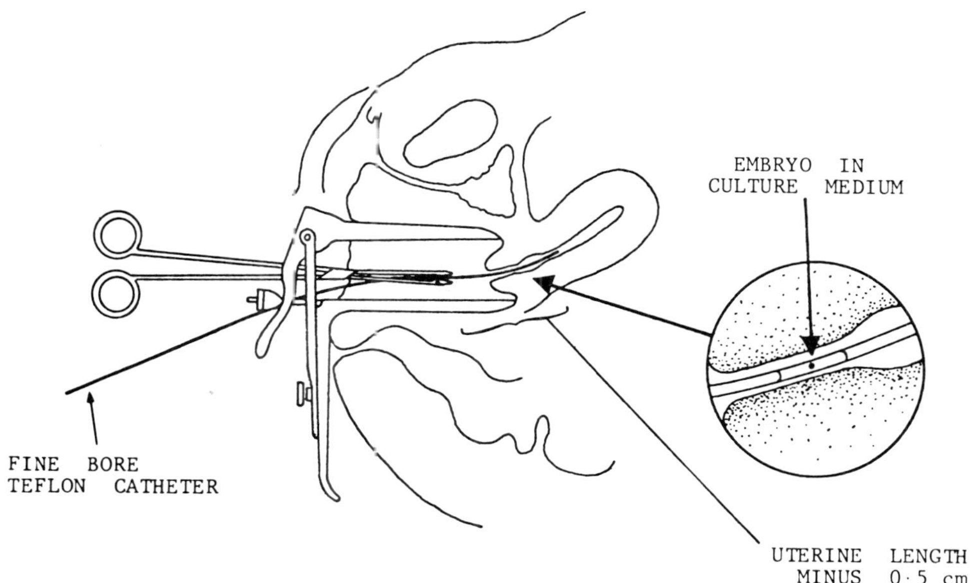

Fig. 12.6   Single catheter embryo transfer technique.

fine catheter containing the embryo is passed through the metal cannula. Because the success of IVF and ET is low, it is not possible to compare the success rates of various catheters.

Technique of transcervical transfer

The two important principles of technique are to avoid introduction of foreign material into the uterus, vaginal contents, cervical mucus and blood, and to avoid stimulating uterine activity.

The patient is premedicated with a sedative or hypnotic and the procedure is done in the operating theatre to ensure asepsis and good lighting. The lithotomy or left lateral position is used with a head down tilt, so that the fundus of the uterus is always below the level of the cervix. Usually, the procedure is painless, so anaesthesia is not required. Sometimes the catheter will not pass easily through the internal os, particularly in the non-parous patient. Epidural anaesthesia may facilitate passage of the catheter, by reducing either spasm of the vagina and cervix or pain. A bivalve speculum is used as this speculum exposes the opening of the cervical canal effectively, excludes vaginal skin from touching the cannula, and slightly dilates the lower end of the cervical canal. The cervix and upper vagina are cleared of mucus in order to prevent the catheter carrying this material into the uterus. Mefenamic acid may be used to inhibit uterine activity, but it is unknown whether this drug may influence conception. In nulligravidae, uterine transfer is practised prior to the treatment cycle. The trial transfer has the advantages of reducing the patient's anxiety at the time of the definitive procedure and also determining whether any difficulty may occur when the catheter is passed through the internal os. If a catheter does not pass the internal os, cervical dilatation is carried out one month before IVF and ET.

The length of the uterine cavity is determined by previous passage of an uterine sound or by ultrasonic measurement. The catheter is picked up with sponge forceps at a distance $\frac{1}{2}$ cm less than the uterine length from the end of the catheter.

This enables the catheter to be placed in a position just short of the top of the fundus of the uterus when the forceps reach the external cervical opening. The position of the uterus is rechecked and this assists in determining the direction of the passage of the catheter. The embryo is placed in 10 to 50 μl of culture medium in the catheter with air between the culture medium and the tip of the catheter. The catheter is passed slowly along the cervical canal, the slowness of passage perhaps helping the catheter to find its way through an irregular canal and also making the catheter more flexible as it is warmed by the body. If the slightest obstruction occurs, the catheter is retracted and gently moved forward again in a different direction. Rotating the cannula may facilitate a change in direction. When the catheter is in the upper portion of the uterus, the embryo is injected. After the embryo is injected, the catheter is removed slowly after a delay of one minute. The slow withdrawal of the catheter may diminish the risk of culture fluid passing along the track of the catheter. If there has been difficulty in passage of the catheter, it may be advisable to wait two or three minutes before injecting the embryo, in order that uterine contractions stimulated by passage of the catheter cease. After withdrawal, the catheter is examined under the microscope to check that the culture medium and embryo have been expelled.

Difficulties

Difficulties may occur at the time of uterine transfer. Vaginal and cervical spasm may be overcome by verbal relaxation techniques, narcotics, or epidural anaesthesia. Obstruction at the internal os may be overcome by using a catheter of either finer or larger bore diameter, by repeated gentle attempts with the same catheter, or by more forceful attempts under local anaesthesia. When repeated attempts have failed, a metal catheter may be used, but this may cause bleeding. Excessive blood at the time of ET probably reduces embryo survival. If bleeding is marked, the embryo can be replaced in the culture medium and ET attempted some hours later. Sometimes the embryo is not expelled from the catheter due to a block of mucus or blood. The embryo is recovered from the blocked catheter and ET is attempted again. If ET is impossible, the embryo may be preserved by freezing and ET attempted in another cycle after thawing the embryo. Freeze-thawing of human embryos has not yet been established as successful, although preliminary studies show that human embryos may survive the procedures (Trounson & Mohr, unpublished data).

Successful Embryo Transfer

In all the pregnancies following IVF and ET, the ET has been performed quickly and without difficulty (Steptoe et al, 1980; Wood et al, 1981b). In two of nine patients who became pregnant, the catheter contained mucus or blood which had partly blocked the catheter (Wood et al, 1981b). In two other patients, a brown discharge occurred within 24 hours of the transfer. Blood appearing at the time of transfer may be due either to bleeding from the endometrial cavity or from the cervical canal. The former is more likely to cause failure.

The overall results in our clinic between June and October, 1980 are shown in Table 12.3.

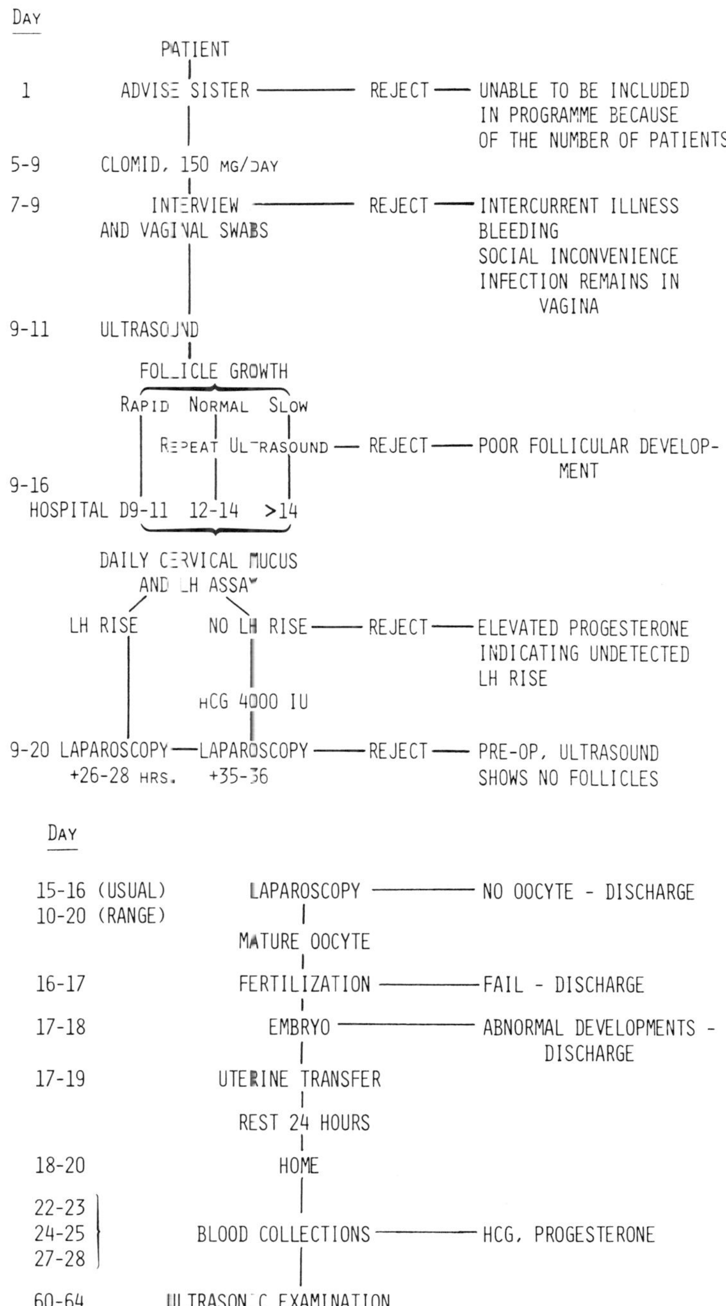

Fig. 12.7   Summary of IVF and ET procedures.

Table 12.3   Pregnancy in patients having laparoscopy in relation to cause of infertility

Cause of infertility	Number of patients having laparoscopy	Number of pregnancies 9 weeks or more
Tubal	58	5
Idiopathic	29	3
Male	16	1*

*Donor semen

Two of the pregnancies aborted at eight and 10 weeks and the remainder are between 19 and 33 weeks. One patient has a twin pregnancy. The ongoing pregnancies have normal fetuses as determined by ultrasound.

Post-ET care

The patient rests in hospital for 24 hours after ET. At home the patient limits activity for three or four days. Diminished physical activity is not essential for normal conception. Uncertainty concerning the behaviour of embryos subsequent to trans-cervical uterine transfer led us to advise patients to behave cautiously until after the possible date of implantation. Subsequently, no special precautions are taken. Seven, ten and fourteen days after laparoscopy, βHCG and progesterone plasma estimations are carried out in order to determine whether embryo implantation has occurred.

MANAGEMENT OF PREGNANCY

If the patient becomes pregnant, serial plasma HCG and progesterone levels are measured weekly for the first 12 weeks of pregnancy, and subsequently plasma progesterone is measured monthly. Plasma oestriol is measured weekly from the 26th week to assess feto-placental function.

Acknowledgements

We wish to thank the Ford Foundation and the N.H. & M.R.C. for research support and St Andrew's Hospital and Queen Victoria Medical Centre, Associate Professor J. F. Leeton and the members of the Department of Obstetrics and Gynaecology for assistance and support in the project.

REFERENCES

Adams C E 1979 Consequences of accelerated ovum transport, including a re-evaluation of Estes' operation. Journal of Reproduction and Fertility 55: 239–246
Biggins J D, Whitten W K, Whittingham D G 1971 The culture of mouse embryo in vitro. In: Daniel J C (ed) Methods of mammalian embryology. Freeman, San Francisco, pp 86–116
Cohen J, Feinerman D, Palmer R, Rumeau-Rouquette C 1972 Results of a retrospective study on the outcome of tubal repair surgery in sterility. Acta Europea Fertilitatis 3: 321–327
Edwards R G, Steptoe P C 1977 The relevance of the frozen storage of human embryos in clinical practice. In: The freezing of mammalian embryos. Ciba Foundation Symposium 52: 235–243
Edwards R G, Steptoe P C, Purdy J M 1980 Establishment of full-term human pregnancies using cleaving embryos grown in vitro. British Journal of Obstetrics and Gynaecology 87: 737–756
Estes W L Jr, Heitmeyer P L 1934 Incidence of pregnancy following ovarian implantation. American Journal of Surgery 24: 563–581

Fletcher J 1971 Ethical aspects of genetic controls: designed genetic changes in man. New England Journal of Medicine 285: 776–783

Gomel V 1977 Tubal reanastomosis by microsurgery. Fertility and Sterility 28: 59–65

Hoppe P C, Pitts S 1973 Fertilization in vitro and development of mouse ova. Biological Reproduction 8: 420–426

Lawson R A S, Rowson L E A, Moor R M, Teruit H R 1975 Experiments on egg transfer in the cow and ewe: dependence on conception rate on the transfer procedure and stage of the oestrous cycle. Journal of Reproduction and Fertility 45: 101–107

Lawson R A S 1977 Research applications of embryo transfer in sheep and goats. In: Betteridge K J (ed) Embryo transfer in farm animals. Canada Department of Agriculture, Monograph 16, Ottawa, Canada, pp 72–78

Lopata A, Johnston W I H, Leeton J F, Muchnick D, Talbot J Mc, Wood C 1974 Collection of human oocytes at laparoscopy and laparotomy. Fertility and Sterility 25: 1030–1038

Lopata A, Brown J B, Leeton J F, Talbot J Mc, Wood C 1978 In vitro fertilization of preovulatory oocytes and embryo transfer in infertile patients treated with clomiphene and human chorionic gonadotrophin. Fertility and Sterility 30: 27–35

Lopata A, Johnston W I H, Leeton J F, McBain J C 1980a Use of in vitro fertilization in the infertile couple. In: Pepperell R J, Hudson B, Wood C (eds) The infertile couple. Churchill Livingstone, Edinburgh, pp 209–228

Lopata A, Johnston W I H, Hoult I J, Speirs A I 1980b Pregnancy following intrauterine implantation of an embryo obtained by in vitro fertilization of a preovulatory egg. Fertility and Sterility 33: 117–120

MacQuarie J (ed) 1967 A dictionary of christian ethics. Westminster Press, Philadelphia, P.A.

Marston J H 1979 Personal communication to C E Adams, in Adams 1979 Consequences of accelerated ovum transplant, including a revaluation of Estes' operations. Journal of Reproduction and Fertility 55: 239–246

Mohr L R, Trounson A O 1980 The use of fluorescein diacetate to assess embryo viability in the mouse. Journal of Reproduction and Fertility 58: 189–196

Moore N W, Shelton J N 1964 Egg transfer in sheep. Effect of degree of synchronization between donor and recipient, age of egg, and site of transfer on the survival of transferred eggs 7: 145–152

Renou P, Trounson A O, Wood C, Leeton J F 1981 The collection of human oocytes for in vitro fertilization I: an instrument for maximizing oocyte recovery rate. Fertility and Sterility 35: 409–412

Shettles B 1980 Embryo transfer and instrumental insemination world conference. 24th to 27th September, 1980. Kiel, West Germany

Siegler A M 1960 Tubal plastic surgery, the past, the present and the future. Obstetrical and Gynaecological Survey 15: 680–701

Siegler A M, Perez R J 1975 Reconstruction of fallopian tubes in previously sterilized patients. Fertility and Sterility 26: 383–392

Steptoe P C, Edwards R G 1970 Laparoscopic recovery of preovulatory human oocytes after priming of ovaries with gonadotrophins 1: 683–689

Steptoe P C, Edwards R G, Purdy J M 1971 Human blastocysts grown in culture. Nature (Lond.) 229: 132–133

Steptoe P C, Edwards R G 1976 Re-implantation of a human embryo with subsequent tubal pregnancy. Lancet 1: 880–882

Steptoe P C, Edwards R G, Purdy J M 1980 Clinical aspects of pregnancies established with cleaving embryos grown in vitro. British Journal of Obstetrics and Gynaecology 87: 757–768

Trounson A O, Rowson L E A, Willadsen S M 1978 Non-surgical transfer of bovine embryos. Veterinary Record 102: 74–75

Trounson A O, Mahadevan M, Wood J, Leeton J 1979 Studies on the deep-freezing and artificial insemination of human semen. In: Richardson D, Joyce D, Symonds M (eds) Frozen human semen. Royal College of Obstetricians and Gynaecologists, London, pp 173–186

Trounson A O, Leeton J F, Wood C, Webb J, Kovacs G 1980a The investigation of idiopathic infertility by in vitro fertilization. Fertility and Sterility 34: 431–438

Trounson A O, Herreros M, Burger H, Clarke I 1980b The precise detection of ovulation using a rapid radioimmunoassay of urinary LH. Proceedings of the Endocrinology Society of Australia 23: 73

Trounson A O, Leeton J F, Wood C, Webb J, Wood J 1981a Pregnancies in humans by fertilization in vitro and embryo transfer in the controlled ovulatory cycle. Science 212: 681–682

Trounson A O, Mohr L R, Wood C, Leeton J F 1981b In vitro fertilization, culture and transfer of human embryos: effect of delayed insemination. Journal of Reproduction and Fertility (in press)

Whittingham D G 1979 In vitro fertilization, embryo transfer and storage. British Medical Bulletin 35: 105–111

Winston R M L 1977 Microsurgical tubocornual anastomosis for reversal of sterilisation. Lancet 1: 284–285

Wood C, Leeton J, Taylor R 1971 A preliminary design and trial of an artificial human tube. Fertility and Sterility 22: 446–450

Wood C, Leeton J, Talbot J Mc, Trounson A O 1981a The technique for collecting mature human oocytes for in vitro fertilization. British Journal of Obstetrics and Gynaecology 88: 756–760

Wood C, Trounson A O, Leeton J, Talbot J Mc, Buttery B, Webb J, Wood J, Jessup D 1981b A clinical assessment of nine pregnancies obtained by in vitro fertilization and embryo transfer. Fertility and Sterility 35: 502–508

13. Sexual dysfunction in gynaecological and obstetrical practice

Alan D. G. Brown

The study of sexuality as a vital human function has been largely neglected until recent decades. Sexual dysfunction causes much personal anguish and marital disharmony and it requires the same investigation and treatment as any other disordered bodily system. Gynaecologists are increasingly consulted about sexual dysfunction because of more open and healthy attitudes to sexuality in society and the particular relationship which they have with their patients. Whether or not gynaecologists have an interest in or an aptitude for treating sexual dysfunction it is essential that they are able to recognise and discuss sexual problems.

The busy gynaecological clinic rarely provides the privacy or time to explore sexual problems in any detail. The gynaecological history should normally include enquiry on sexual function. When a patient volunteers a problem, often with trepidation and embarassment, her first needs are sympathetic listening and acceptance of her difficulty. In a short time simple education and advice may be given based on the principles of counselling described later. Patients are often reassured to read about these disorders and to learn that others are affected similarly, therefore a reading list is useful (see p. 306). The simple disorders will often be alleviated by these measures, but if on review the problem persists, more detailed counselling by the gynaecologist is necessary or referral for psychosexual therapy. The dysfunctional woman may state the problem directly or give clues during the interview — whatever the presenting complaint, so the gynaecologist must be aware of these disorders and deal with them sympathetically otherwise the patient may never summon up the courage to discuss the problem again.

FEMALE SEXUAL ANATOMY AND PHYSIOLOGY

A comprehensive review of the physiology of female sexuality has been carried out by Levin (1980). The important anatomical and physiological features are outlined here as they help in the understanding of sexual dysfunction.

Pelvic vascularity and musculature

During sexual stimulation vasocongestion occurs throughout the genital tract which may be caused by increased arterial flow to and reduced drainage from the tissues. The mechanisms involved are not understood but the vessels of the vagina and erectile tissue (in the vestibular bulbs and clitoris) have smooth muscle protruberances called intima pads or 'polsters' which when contracted reduce blood flow. Danesino & Martella (1976) suggested that erectile tissue engorgement results from polster activity so that relaxation of the arterial ones and contraction of those in the arteriovenous anastomoses and venous drainage cause increased inflow and reduced outflow respectively. The neural control of the vessels is not known but the widely held view that vasodilatation results from autonomic cholinergic activity has been challenged by Levin & Wagner (1980) and Wagner & Levin (1980), who suggested that other neurotransmitters may be involved.

The pelvic muscles primarily involved in female sexual activity may be grouped as follows.

Bulbospongiosus and ischiocavernosus. Bulbospongiosus are thin muscles covering the vestibular bulbs at the vaginal introitus where they act as a sphincter. Bulbospongiosus and ischiocavernosus are inserted into the pubic arch and clitoris so that on contraction they pull down the latter thus compressing its venous drainage and thereby facilitating clitoral erection.

Pubococcygeus and iliococcygeus. These form the levator ani muscle. The medial fibres of pubococcygeus, as they pass posteriorly, are attached to the vagina and are called pubovaginalis muscle. Because of this attachment it has been suggested that pubococcygeus contributes to the sensations experienced during coitus (Kegel, 1952; Kline-Graber & Graber, 1975); also stimulation of this muscle using a vaginal faradic electrode to treat urinary incontinent women has produced increased coital satisfaction (Scott & Hsueh, 1979).

Other muscles. The vaginal wall contains smooth muscle which runs longitudinally and the superficial and deep transverse perinei muscles are only indirectly involved in sexual activity as their main action is to help stabilise the central tendon of the perineum.

The resting vagina contracts intermittently and Levin (1980) suggests that this may be related to the maintenance of tissue circulation and expulsion of menstrual and other fluid. Masters & Johnson (1966) and Gillan & Brindley (1979) observed that orgasm is accompanied by clonic contractions of the distal vagina which the former authors called the 'orgasmic platform': up to ten contractions have been noted, the number depending on orgasmic intensity. The interval between contractions initially is 0.6 to 0.8 seconds and this lengthens as contraction strength diminishes. Gillan & Brindley observed also that there was a sustained pelvic floor contraction which is equivalent to that caused by the male's bulbocavernosus reflex.

Spastic contraction of the introital muscles results in an inability to penetrate the vagina. This condition, called vaginismus, is due to a phobic anxiety to vaginal penetration (Duddle, 1977). Its causes and management are described later.

Genital secretions

The lower genital tract is constantly bathed in secretions, two major sources of which are the cervix and vagina. The vaginal epithelium has no glands but it is covered by fluid containing epithelial cells, bacteria and organic and inorganic solutes; this fluid is present irrespective of whether the uterus and/or ovaries are present (Perl, Milles & Shimozato, 1959). Vaginal fluid has variable ionic concentrations and Levin & Wagner (1978) observed that when plasma is applied to the vagina in vivo that Na^+ is reabsorbed against an electrochemical gradient while its K^+ concentration is increased significantly; they conclude that these changes are effected by a vaginal epithelial transport mechanism and may be necessary for optimal sperm function. The normal vaginal pH of between 4 and 5 is unfavourable for sperm activity but the male ejaculate contains buffers which neutralise the acidity resulting in a pH of 7 (Fox et al, 1973).

During sexual arousal Masters & Johnson (1966) observed vaginal lubrication within 10 to 30 seconds which they described as a 'sweating' phenomenon and they considered that this resulted from dilatation of the venous plexus surrounding the vagina. Studies by Levin & Wager (1977) and Wagner & Levin (1978) suggest that this fluid is a plasma transudate modified by the vagina's reabsorptive activity which passes through 'pore' pathways seen on scanning electron microscopy by Ludwig & Metzer (1976).

Sexual response

Masters & Johnson (1966) described four progressive phases of sexual arousal which are similar in men and women. These are: excitement; plateau; orgasm; resolution. The *excitement phase* develops from any source of stimulation and during it sexual tenson or arousal is increased; its length depends on the stimulus but generally it is prolonged compared with the next two phases. During the *plateau phase* sexual tension increases to a level from which orgasm may result; the length depends on the effectiveness of the stimulus and on individual characteristics. *Orgasm* is the few seconds of involuntary climax during which there is relief of tension accompanied by an overwhelming sensation of pleasure. The subjective awareness of orgasm is within the pelvis but the whole body is involved to a variable degreee. *Resolution* may follow the plateau or orgasmic phase and during it there is an involuntary reversal of the process with continued loss of tension. During this phase women have the potential for further orgasms but men have an absolute refractory period when further stimulation is ineffectual; the length of this refractory period depends on age and other factors.

In women these four phases are manifested by changes in the genitalia and elsewhere so that, for example, during the excitement and plateau phases the labia thicken, the clitoris enlarges, the vagina lubricates and expands and the uterus becomes elevated. The breasts show nipple erection and enlargement and there is skin flushing particularly of the chest and face. Other effects include such cardiovascular changes as transient tachycardia and hypertension.

Kaplan (1974) recognised the descriptive value of Masters & Johnson's four stages but she proposed an alternative classification which described a *biphasic response* in both sexes. She considered that there are two distinct and relatively independent components which are:

1. Vasocongestive reaction which produces penile erection or vaginal lubrication and swelling.
2. Reflex clonic muscular contractions and orgasm.

Kaplan's rationale was based on the knowledge that erection/lubrication is mediated by autonomic parasympathetic innervation whereas orgasm/ejaculation is primarily a sympathetic function. She noted that the two phases are affected differently by such factors as trauma, drugs and age. Also the biphasic response concept recognises that impaired erection/lubrication and ejaculation/orgasm are different problems which have separate psychopathological mechanisms and respond to different treatments.

Orgasm

Orgasm is the climax of sexual excitement and is part of sexual development. The phenomenon is difficult to explain, particularly to women (about 10 per cent) who have never experienced it. Javert's pictorial representation is shown in Figure 13.1.

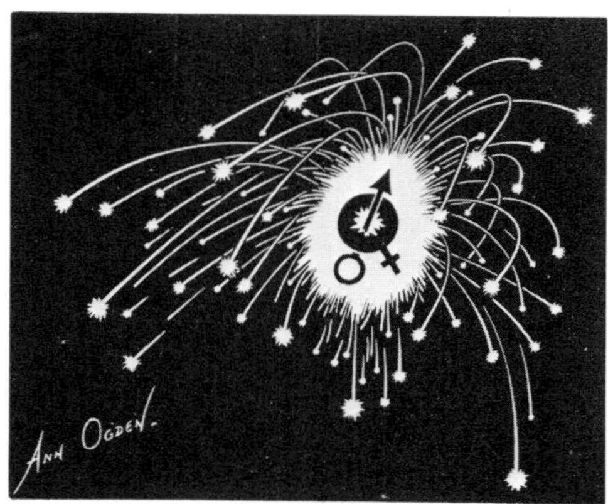

Fig. 13.1 Coitus to orgasm. (Javert, 1957. Reproduced by kind permission of the McGraw-Hill Book Co.)

An early concept was proposed by the Freudean psychoanalytical school which assumed that the clitoris and vagina were the major erogenous zones. During sexual development the clitoris was important in infancy but after puberty the vagina became predominant. Thus they considered that clitoral-induced orgasm represented infantile sexuality which was associated with neuroticism, whereas orgasm following coitus indicated normal development.

Masters & Johnson (1966) suggested that only one type of female orgasm occurred irrespective of how it was produced and this depended on direct or indirect clitoral stimulation. Kaplan (1974) considered that female orgasm had both clitoral and vaginal components as the evidence suggested that orgasm required clitoral stimulation whereas vaginal sensation, although pleasurable, was a minor triggering mechanism; also, direct clitoral manipulation was a greater stimulus than coitus which caused pubic pressure and traction on the clitoral hood.

Singer (1973) suggested that three types of orgasm occur. *Vulval orgasm* is characterised by contractions of the orgasmic platform and is produced by a variety of stimuli such as clitoral manipulation or coitus. *Uterine orgasm* affected breathing so that a period of apnoea was followed by explosive exhalation at orgasm. This phenomenon depended on coitus alone and resulted from contact between the penis and cervix and adjacent structures. *Blended orgasm* had elements of the other two.

The purpose of orgasm is not understood and Fox (1978) suggested that the positive and negative pressures which result in the vagina and uterus respectively may facilitate sperm transport and hence fertilisation; this may be an important factor in infertile couples. Orgasm in both sexes has many similarities, for example in the male it is triggered by penile stimulation and ejaculation results also in rhythmic muscle contractions. The differences are that the female has neither ejaculation nor a refractory period, however, her orgasm is more easily inhibited as orgasmic dysfunction is commoner than retarded ejaculation. Kaplan observed that the female response is more variable, possibly due to psychological and cultural influences, whereas the male particularly when young is more affected by physical disorders.

Effect of ageing
Kinsey et al (1953) found that in unmarried persons aged up to 55 years, men's sexual activity declined slowly from puberty whereas women's interest continued steadily. In married couples coital frequency declined progressively and this was thought to be related to the ageing husband; this observation was confirmed by Pfeiffer et al (1972). Activity is related also to the availability of a regular partner. Newman & Nichols (1960) showed that in 250 women aged 60 to 93 years, 54 per cent of those still married and seven per cent of the single-divorced-widowed group were sexually active.

Hällström (1980) studied 800 Swedish women aged 38 to 54 years who were not taking oral contraception and who had not had either hysterectomy or ovarian ablation. The findings were that with advancing age there was a marked reduction in sexual interest, orgasmic capacity and coital frequency, also that declining interest is a cause rather than a result of infrequent coitus. Furthermore, during the perimenopausal years reduced activity is due significantly to climacteric changes and not to ageing. Sexuality is affected by psycho-social as well as biological factors. Hällström noted that higher social class was related significantly to normal sexual activity and the probable causes included better education, living standards and communication and greater freedom to express individuality. Previous observations that mental depression diminished sexual interest more commonly than other mental illnesses was also confirmed. Thus studies suggest that female sexual interest remains fairly constant until the climacteric when it declines and many factors are involved.

CLASSIFICATION OF SEXUAL DISORDERS

The concept of a biphasic nature of sexual response (Kaplan, 1974) allows a simple method of classifying male and female disorders (Table 13.1). This in turn helps the understanding of sexual physiology and the management of dysfunction. Vaginismus is classified separately as both phases of response are usually normal.

Table 13.1 Classification of sexual disorders

Phase	Disorder	
	Male	Female
Vasocongestive	Erectile dysfunction (impotence)	General sexual dysfunction
Orgasmic	Premature or retarded ejaculation	Orgasmic dysfunction
	(primary or secondary)	
		Vaginismus

INCIDENCE OF SEXUAL DYSFUNCTION

Sexual dysfunction is common but the overall incidence is difficult to assess because of factors such as patient and doctor reluctance to discuss the problem, criteria for definition, the limited resources available in many areas and national variation. In general practice in the United States and United Kingdom 15 and about 6 per cent respectively of all patient contacts were considered to be related to sexual problems (Burnap & Golden, 1967; Begg et al, 1976). In a British family planning clinic Begg & colleagues (1976) found that 12.5 per cent of 622 women felt they had a disorder and the majority requested treatment.

Werner (1975) studied American college students by questionnaire and noted that 5 per cent had signs of dysfunction and 50 per cent required education. Dysfunction occurs usually either in the man or woman but Kaplan (1974) and Masters & Johnson (1970) found that both partners had problems in 25 and 44 per cent of couples respectively. The relative incidences of disorders in three British clinics are shown in Table 13.2. Discrepancies between clinics are difficult to explain

Table 13.2 Incidences of sexual disorders in three British clinics

Author/s	Duddle (1975)	Bancroft and Coles (1976)	Cooper (1979)
Site of clinic (Number of patients)	Family planning centre (220)	University department of psychiatry (200)	Alternating between teaching hospital gynaecological and psychiatric clinics (215)
Disorder	Per cent of patients		
Female			
General Sexual Dysfunction	} 51	32	} 24[1]
Orgasmic Dysfunction		9	
Abdominal/Pelvic Pain	1		9
Vaginismus	16	6	5
Male			
Erectile Dysfunction	11	21	24
Ejaculatory Disorders	5	16	9
Dyspareunia			4
General			
Sexual Deviation		12	5
Subfertility	3		5
Predominant Marital Problem	5		
Mental Illness (one partner)	4		
Sexual Dissonance[2]			11
Geriatric			2
Miscellaneous	4	5	2

[1] Defined as reduced, absent or dissatisfied sexual response.
[2] Defined as discordance between respective needs of partners.

as the usual source of referral was the general practitioner; however, the definition of disorders and the different sites for the clinic may be responsible.

FEMALE DISORDERS

Until recently the general term frigidity was used to describe inhibited female sexuality ranging from lack of responsiveness to orgasmic dysfunction. The term is no longer appropriate as it does not recognise that the two phases of female response may be affected separately and also because it is pejorative. Masters & Johnson (1966) described all sexually disordered women as having orgasmic dysfunction which could be either primary or situational. Kaplan (1974) considered that this description focused on orgasm without recognising the vasocongestive component and she classified most female disorders into general sexual and orgasmic dysfunctions.

General sexual dysfunction

In this condition there is a variable degree of sexual inhibition characterised by a lack of erotic feelings and reduced vasocongestion so that such vaginal changes as lubrication and expansion do not occur. These patients may or may not have orgasmic dysfunction.

Orgasmic dysfunction

Erotic sensations and vasocongestion usually occur with this disorder but orgasm is not experienced. Some women enjoy the arousal phase alone without wishing to proceed to climax and it may be argued that they are not dysfunctional; however, the publicity which is given to female orgasm may cause feelings of abnormality or her partner may consider that it is due to his lack of technique. Orgasmic dysfunction is commoner in women than in men. This may be related to adolescent behaviour when masturbation leading to orgasm is more frequently practiced by boys; female clitoral sensation and orgasm often starts later with the onset of heterosexual petting.

Primary orgasmic dysfunction

In this situation orgasm has never been achieved from any source of stimulation. Kinsey et al (1953) reported that about 30 per cent of women in their study had not experienced orgasm by the time they were married but after 10 years only 10 per cent remained anorgasmic; this latter figure is quoted generally as the incidence of this condition. Women with obsessional, perfectionist personalities may experience difficulty in achieving orgasm (Duddle & Brown, 1980) because always they have to be in control and will not abandon this, however fleetingly, for orgasm. Their perfectionism will result in concern because of failure to respond 'correctly'.

Secondary orgasmic dysfunction

This is present when orgasm has occurred previously but is no longer experienced and it may be accompanied by general sexual dysfunction. Sometimes it occurs early in a marriage following successful premarital activity; the lack of excitement that was associated with the guilt of pre-marital sex may be responsible. Other causes are the routine nature of married life and sex or the husband's failure to stimulate adequately his wife before coitus and ejaculation. Pregnancy and its aftermath are common predisposing factors which will be discussed later.

Vaginismus

Vaginismus is often found with normal sexual response and has therefore to be considered separately. It is a psychosomatic condition where involuntary spasm of the muscles surrounding the vaginal introitus prevents any penetration. Often both partners are able to achieve organism by other means. Phobic anxiety to vaginal penetration is the cause and only rarely is there a physical factor. Thus the classical gynaecological procedures of vaginal dilatation under anaesthesia, hymenectomy or perineotomy are rarely indicated or justified. Indeed they may aggravate the condition by causing scarring or reinforcing the patient's view that something is physically wrong. These procedures do not affect the underlying problem which usually well respond to psychosexual therapy.

Causes of female disorders

ORGANIC

The debility which accompanies disease has an effect on libido but in general Masters & Johnson (1970) noted that female sexual disorders were generally due to psychological rather than physical causes. When disease is present in the female it is usually well established before its effect, primarily on orgasm, is noted. In contrast, male sexuality is more commonly affected by physical disorders, for example secondary impotence may be an early sign of diabetes and ageing reduces ejaculatory ability and from about 30 years onwards lengthens the refractory period following orgasm (Kaplan, 1974). The effect of disease on sexual function is complicated by accompanying drug therapy which often by its sedative action further reduces response. The oral contraceptive pill may reduce libido possibly related to reduced circulating 5-hydroxytryptamine due to induced alterations in tryptophan metabolism (Hawkins & Elder, 1979).

Dyspareunia is a common gynaecological complaint which rapidly inhibits sexual arousal. When the symptom persists the increase in anxiety inhibits lubrication and discomfort is aggravated. Dyspareunia reduces the pleasure of petting and intercourse and finally the woman may reject her partner's advances construing even the simplest physical contact as a threatening sexual gesture (Duddle & Brown, 1980). Physical causes of the symptom should be looked for such as endometriosis and previous pelvic surgery such as episiotomy, hysterectomy or colporrhaphy. Treatment of a physcial cause may have to be supplemented by sexual counselling of the couple. Psychological and relationship problems may manifest themselves as dyspareunia but the diagnosis of these is more difficult.

FAILURE OF COMMUNICATION AND TECHNIQUE

It is generally accepted that male and female arousal patterns are different so that usually the man responds quickly to sexual contact, the obvious erection occurs and this may be followed soon by ejaculation. Female sexual response is more variable, with changes such as vaginal lubrication being less obvious and generally more dependent on unhurried and gentle stimulation. Also women vary more widely in their preferences for different areas to be stimulated. These different arousal patterns make it difficult for either partner to recognise the stage of excitement the other has reached, and if the male is guided by his own response he may proceed to penetration and ejaculation before his partner is ready.

These problems result from lack of communication and the woman's reluctance to indicate her requirements. It is essential, therefore, that both partners should take responsibility for their own sexual wellbeing (Kaplan, 1974). In the past cultural attitudes have dictated that the male should be sexually assertive and that the female should acquiesce to this domination. A woman may experience guilt or fear of rejection if she communicates her need for further stimulation before or during intercourse; also the man's confidence may be undermined by the implication that he is unable to arouse his partner satisfactorily. Frequently attitudes require changing so that between the couple there is open communication which results in sexual negotiation and compromise. Thus each other's needs at different times are met and when desires are unfulfilled there is no sense of rejection.

Kaplan suggests that the good male lover supplies gentle and sensitive stimulation and is not just a permanent erection; also that the couple should exercise a degree of sexual autonomy and take turns in giving and receiving pleasure. In this way they will develop an open and satisfying relationship.

MALE DISORDERS

Erectile dysfunction (impotence)

The term impotence is used commonly to describe impaired penile erection but this is inaccurate as the strict meaning is inability to copulate or reach orgasm. A more accurate description is erectile dysfunction (Kaplan, 1974). In common with the term frigidity impotence has a pejorative connotation and its use therefore, should be discouraged. Erectile dysfunction may be primary when there has never been satisfactory erection, or secondary when it has developed after normal function. The secondary disorder is commoner and in certain circumstances, such as illness or after alcohol ingestion, it may be regarded as physiological. The condition results from a failure of the erectile reflex so that vasocongestion of the penile cavernous sinuses does not occur. The circumstances in which erection is lost vary considerably, for example, maintaining it only when clothed, failure while attempting intercourse or total inability to achieve any erection under any circumstances (Kaplan, 1974). As the erectile and ejaculatory reflexes are separate it is possible for ejaculation to occur through a flaccid penis.

The aetiology may be physical or psychological. Physical causes include fatigue, debility and endocrine or neurological problems such as diabetes or multiple sclerosis. Erection may be affected by genital disease, surgery or such drug treatment as oestrogen for prostatic cancer. Psychological factors are often present and anxiety following failure of the male's all-important erectile ability is well known; this fear of 'impotence' is intense and even after one failed erection, a vicious circle may develop in which the next attempt results in failure of the vasocongestive response. The primary disorder may result from a learning failure, early oedipal or religious conflicts causing a childhood fear of sexual expression; also inhibition may develop following early sexual encounters which were interrupted for some reason.

Mental state or interpersonal relationships may be involved. Secondary depression or marital disharmony may follow erectile failure, for example, the female may suspect infidelity as the cause or fear that age is diminishing her attractiveness. The problem may be compounded by an inhibited woman who is unwilling to touch the penis and prefers to continue the asexual relationship. Conversely, endogenous depression and marital discord may cause erectile dysfunction. It is necessary therefore to establish which are the primary and secondary problems. Endogenous depression should be treated first, likewise severe relationship problems require referral for marriage counselling which may include sex therapy later.

The prognosis for the primary dysfunction is poor as the common causes of psychological and endocrine problems are difficult to treat. Often outcome depends on duration of symptoms so that when there has not been effective penetration for years the prognosis is poor.

Premature ejaculation

Premature ejaculation is a common dysfunction. It is difficult to define precisely as some authors measure the time between penetration and ejaculation (varying from one half to two minutes), while others count the number of penile thrusts before ejaculation (up to ten). Masters & Johnson (1970) defined it as a failure to control ejaculation sufficiently, following vaginal containment, 'to satisfy his partner in at least 50 per cent of their coital connections'. This condition ranges from ejaculation occurring at the sight of the partner undressing to emission after several thrusts, but Kaplan (1974) stressed that its essential feature is the absence of voluntary control of the ejaculatory reflex so that arousal is quickly followed by orgasm.

This disorder causes some degree of restricted activity for both partners. For example, in order to prevent early ejaculation the man may avoid intense arousal which may be misconstrued by his partner as indifference or rejection. Thus feelings of inadequacy and guilt may develop and result in disharmony. The primary dysfunction may be due to psychological factors such as learning failure or sexual conflict, relationship problems or simply an extreme sensitivity to erotic stimulation. The secondary disorder is more commonly due to a physical cause. Therefore a full history and examination are essential. Sometimes premature ejaculation may present as secondary erectile dysfunction due to anxiety caused by the inability to control ejaculation. The prognosis in this disorder generally is good.

Retarded ejaculation

The inability to ejaculate is uncommon but it illustrates the biphasic nature of sexual response as normal erection usually is achieved. The disorder varies from ejaculating only with masturbation to its total absence. A physical cause rarely affects ejaculation alone whereas drug therapy (e.g. hypotensives or anti-depressants) may do so. Psychological or relationship problems are other predisposing factors. The prognosis in this condition varies depending on the aetiology.

SEXUALITY IN PREGNANCY

Antenatal activity

Pregnancy is likely to have an effect on sexual activity because of the profound hormonal, physical and psychological changes which occur. Interest and activity have been shown to decline progressively towards term (Solberg et al, 1973; Perkins, 1979) particularly in the last trimester (Kumar et al, 1981) (Fig. 13.2). These last authors also found that the new levels of activity and enjoyment reflected the individual's pre-pregnancy degree of interest.

Solberg et al (1973) studied 260 variable-parity women in the immediate puerperium and found that towards term the frequency and intensity of orgasm declined in the majority, masturbation and oral-genital contact occurred less often and coital position changed from the commonly used male-superior to the side-to-side and other positions. The reasons for these changes included increasing discomfort, anxiety about the fetus and medical advice. Masters & Johnson (1966) observed that

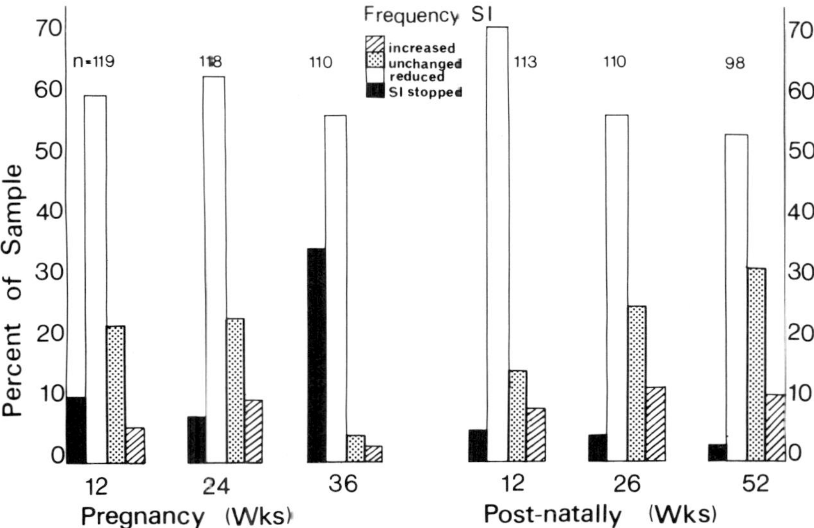

Fig. 13.2   Changes in frequency of sexual intercourse during pregnancy and after delivery. From Kumar, Brant and Robson (1981) with kind permission of the authors and the editor of the Journal of Psychosomatic Research.

husband's reasons for reduced activity was fear of injury to wife or fetus, loss of attractiveness and unknown. In these two studies medical advice to restrict coitus towards term was given in about one-third and one-half of patients and rarely was advice given on substitute sexual activity.

Effects of coitus and orgasm

Studies have shown that orgasm produces uterine contraction in the non-pregnant and pregnant uterus (Fox et al, 1970; Goodlin et al, 1972) but it is not known whether orgasm can cause abortion or premature labour. A comparison of premature and full-term babies by Goodlin et al (1971) noted increased orgasmic frequency in mothers of the premature infants, but in a better controlled series Wagner et al (1976) observed no statistical difference. The relationship of coitus to antepartum haemorrhage was studied in over 56 000 pregnancies by Naeye (1981). He found that recent coitus was associated with haemorrhage in a significant number of patients and this was independent of other factors predisposing to bleeding. Also the frequency of haemorrhage increased with coital frequency. However this study did not prove a causal relationship between the two.

The puerperium

Many factors are thought to affect female sexuality in the puerperium including the physical and hormonal readjustments and the trauma caused by episiotomy. The psychological sequelae are important, for example feelings of anxiety or inadequacy in caring for the baby or when depression results from morbidity or mortality. The husband's attitude must be considered as he may feel excluded by the new arrival. Kumar et al (1981) studied 119 primiparae during pregnancy and for one year after delivery. In the puerperium they found that persistent pain and discomfort were experienced by 40 per cent at three months and by 8 per cent at one year; also, during the year, about one quarter of the women felt that tiredness interfered with their sex lives. They noted that one year after delivery nearly 60 per cent of the women had coitus less often than before pregnancy although enjoyment had returned to normal (Fig. 13.2). After twelve months about one quarter of them enjoyed sex more than in the month before conception, particularly those who had previously not enjoyed it or who had tried to conceive for at least a year. When questioned at three months postpartum 30 per cent of women felt that sexual counselling would have been beneficial. Thus discussion between obstetrician and patient is necessary, for example avoiding coitus till the episiotomy wound has healed and the temporary use of lubricants and non-coital techniques when necessary.

Advice to couples
Coitus probably has no effect on normal pregnancy but when abnormalities such as dyspareunia, vaginal bleeding or premature rupture of the membranes have occurred intercourse should be avoided. Although orgasm causes uterine contractions no conclusive evidence shows any association with premature labour; however coitus is best temporarily avoided when habitual abortion or premature labour has occurred previously. The majority of couples will not be aware of the antenatal and postpartum effects on their sexual enjoyment and activity. The obstetrician should therefore, discuss these phenomena with the patient and give advice, for example the use of alternative coital positions towards term (Brown & Duddle, 1980) and non-coital activity.

DIAGNOSIS OF SEXUAL DYSFUNCTION

Counselling should be offered to the couple as both partners often have problems; although one person may present with a disorder the other usually contributes. A full medical and sexual history from each partner is necessary so that a diagnosis and prognosis may be given. Some therapists believe that the histories should be taken with the couple present, but it is preferable to question each person privately so that an honest account is obtained. For example, an extra-marital affair is more likely to be revealed in private and its effect on treatment and prognosis can be assessed.

An initial medical history may suggest a contributory factor and allows rapport to be established before dealing with the individual's sexuality. The history should include details of the problem as seen by the individual, frequency of sexual activity/intercourse and positions used; contraceptive practice is relevant as fear of pregnancy and religious attitudes may affect libido. The couple's emotional relationship should be explored as it will have a profound effect on sexual function. If a serious marital difficulty is discovered they should be referred initially for marriage guidance, however, relationship difficulties may emerge during treatment which have to be dealt with then.

The patient's sexual development should be noted by obtaining information on their awareness of sexuality as a child, for example, the ages of first masturbation and heterosexual activity (including intercourse), the frequency of different partners and degree of involvement, and any difficulties encountered. The sources and knowledge of sex education, attitudes towards masturbation and homosexuality and any history of sexual assault are important.

Parental attitudes to sexuality inevitably affect their children. Frequently patients describe a home background where discussion of sexuality was discouraged or never occurred and the mother and father rarely displayed affection to each other or their children. Thus relationships with parents and siblings, including episodes of incest, are important in understanding the development of dysfunction. Assessment of mental state is necessary as psychiatric illness may reduce libido; when such illness is found its treatment should take precedence but unfortunately the drugs prescribed may depress further the patient's libido (Beaumont, 1979).

PRINCIPLES OF SEXUAL COUNSELLING

Mutual responsibility
All sexual problems should be considered as shared disorders; for example the man may contribute to his partner's anorgasmia. The 'normal' partner may not accept this responsibility because of the implication that he or she is inadequate, nevertheless an emphasis on shared responsibility rather than on blame is important. The couple's co-operation may be encouraged by using co-therapists so that each partner has someone with whom to identify, but in practice this is costly, time-consuming and usually not necessary.

Education
Ignorance of human biology and effective sexual technique are widespread, particularly in dysfunctional couples. It is often necessary to describe the normal male and female sexual responses in simple terms. For example, following arousal blood pours into the genital area causing penile erection and swelling and lubrication of the labia and vagina. Whereas the changes in the penis are obvious those in the female are less so, therefore, it is necessary to wait until there is adequate lubrication so that painful intercourse does not occur. The words used to describe the anatomy may have to be varied depending on the couple's knowledge. Further information may be given using diagrams, books or educational films. Education may not relieve symptoms but it is usually a prerequisite to successful treatment (LoPiccolo & LoPiccolo, 1978).

Attitude change
A negative attitude to sexual expression may result from parental or religious influences or past experience. This is commoner in women possibly due to Western culture's double-standard morality (Christensen & Gregg, 1970). Attitude change may result from discussion and the use of suitable literature. Sometimes the male must reassure his partner that respect will grow rather than lessen if she becomes more sexual, but this may be accompanied by anxiety about his ability to cope with her increased demands.

Permission-giving
Ignorance of what is common sexual practice frequently causes anxiety and problems, therefore, permission to accept and enjoy their sexuality and to experiment with different methods of stimulation and positions are often required. Couples are helped by the knowledge that sexual expression covers a wide range of activities; normality is difficult to define but provided a particular practice is acceptable to both partners it

may be tried. Oral sexual contact for example may be acceptable to one or neither person, so reassurance that this is a common practice may be sufficient for it to be considered; however no attempt should be made to impose any practice which one partner finds unacceptable. Thus an important principle of counselling is to give the couple permission to enjoy their sexuality and to experiment and discover what is pleasurable to them. This may be reinforced by suggesting suitable literature.

Reducing performance anxiety
Anxiety about one's performance interferes with the autonomically controlled sexual responses so that vasocongestion and orgasm may not occur. This anxiety sometimes is communicated to the partner who will become affected. The couple should be discouraged from being goal-orientated, for example on coitus or orgasm, but instead they should learn to enjoy the sensations resulting from stimulation. Thus the banning of intercourse during sensate focus exercises (see later) allows the man with erectile difficulties to enjoy the kissing and fondling without worrying about an erection sufficient for intercourse.

Increasing communication
Many couples, particularly dysfunctional ones, have difficulty in communicating their sexual needs because of inhibition or sensitivity about possible criticism. Discussion between the couple and therapist is helpful as it encourages understanding. Verbal communication concerns discovering each other's likes and dislikes but also involves sharing emotional feelings (Stanley, 1981a). When problems develop confusing messages may be conveyed between the couple so that the tone of voice is not consistent with the statement made. For example, when a reply to the question 'What is the matter?' is 'Nothing' — but said in a belligerent tone, discord increases and resolution is difficult.

To prevent these double messages Stanley recommends the use of the Gestalt concept of '"I" language' (Fagen & Shepherd, 1970; Stevens, 1971). This involves the recognition of emotional feelings experienced and their expression in the first rather than the third person singular. Thus the aggressive statement 'You make me feel angry' invariably produces a defensive reply, whereas 'I feel angry' evokes concern and a desire to discuss the cause of anger. Also the couple should respond to situations by expressing their feelings rather than using intellectual observations; the response to 'I feel anxious' of 'Don't be silly' is demoralising, whereas 'I am sorry you are anxious' implies concern and favours discussion.

Non-verbal communication may be used, for example Masters & Johnson (1970) suggested guiding the partner's hand to pleasurable areas during genital touching. However, this technique must be used with care as it can be misinterpreted.

TREATMENT OF SEXUAL DYSFUNCTION

The early treatment of sexual dysfunction used analytical or behavioural techniques. Freud (1905) considered that these problems were due to neurosis which was amenable to psychoanalysis irrespective of the specific sexual difficulty. The behavioural approach used techniques such as relaxation and deconditioning to treat symptoms which were thought to have developed as a learned response. Masters &

Johnson (1970) used the latter approach but Kaplan (1974) developed the eclectic method which selects behavioural and insight directive therapy as appropriate.

A treatment programme

Treatment succeeds best when the couple are involved but if the patient has no partner such problems as premature ejaculation and vaginismus may be corrected by specific techniques (see later). Trained surrogate partners for single patients are used in the United States but for ethical reasons, rarely in the United Kingdom. The use of a therapist or co-therapists is variable but generally the results of either treatment are similar (Matthews et al, 1976). The economic and logistic advantages of a single therapist are obvious particularly when waiting lists are long, but co-therapy is helpful during training.

The first session consists of history-taking, making a provisional diagnosis and prognosis and explaining treatment including the sensate focus technique (see below). The time involved is about one hour but subsequent visits should take approximately thirty minutes. The couple should be asked to do two or three home-assignment sessions per week and the frequency of meetings with the therapist will vary; Masters & Johnson had daily meetings with the couple who had taken two weeks' holiday for intensive treatment, but in general weekly discussions are recommended as they help to maintain motivation and momentum. Because of the time-consuming nature of therapy the time of day of meetings is variable but usually it is best at the end of a clinic, surgery or working day.

A limit of six to eight sessions with the therapist should be set initially as this encourages co-operation. Also Bancroft & Coles (1976) and Cooper (1979) have shown that improvement often occurs within this number of sessions and thereafter the possibility of success is reduced.

Sensate focus

Masters & Johnson (1970) recognised that touch is a basic part of human communication and that many feelings are conveyed through it. When a couple have never experienced or have forgotten the sensual pleasure of communicating by touch, an important source of stimulation has been lost (Belliveau & Richter, 1974). Irrespective of the specific problem Masters & Johnson explained the importance of touch in expressing and receiving sexual stimuli, then the couple were asked to set aside some time in private when they are relaxed, comfortable and undressed. One partner, say the female, lies face down (thus protecting the 'sensitive' erogenous areas) while the male slowly fondles or massages the rest of her body. After some time the women turns over and the touching is repeated except for the breasts and genitals which are 'out of bounds' so that intense excitement is avoided. Intercourse also is forbidden in order to reduce anxiety concerning the need for erection, orgasm or ejaculation.

These non-demanding tasks allow each person to experience the sensations of touching. The active, or giving, partner provides pleasure, learns what is enjoyed by the other and explores their own sensations from fondling in various ways and experiencing the texture of different areas of the body. The passive, or receiving, partner should be relaxed and gently communicate verbally or otherwise the pleasant or unpleasant sensations. Bancroft & Bancroft (1978) suggest that each partner should concentrate on their own enjoyment rather than worry about pleasing the other.

When it is appropriate the couple should change places and repeat the process. The responsibility for inviting to a session and being the active partner initially should alternate so that the mutual responsibility for their sexual enjoyment is emphasised.

The sensations and problems experienced during these sessions are discussed with the therapist. The couple's initial response may vary from enjoyment and feelings of closeness, often for the first time in years, to many excuses being made for not carrying out the exercises. The reasons for these difficulties such as anxiety or ambivalence about treatment should be explored because until they are recognised and overcome progress will not be made (Duddle & Brown, 1980).

The next stage in the home sessions is to include touching either the female breasts alone or also the genitals, and the decision is made depending on the degree of inhibitions encountered. When genital contact is started it should be light and teasing so that there is no expectation of orgasm. Frequently progress over the first few sessions is rapid but the couple may become anxious or despondent if there is a temporary setback, which often occurs. Strong reassurance and encouragement are usually all that is necessary. Finally intercourse is encouraged, but often the couple progress to this before they have been given permission to do so! The female superior position (Fig. 13.3) is particularly helpful initially if she wishes to be in control, also it

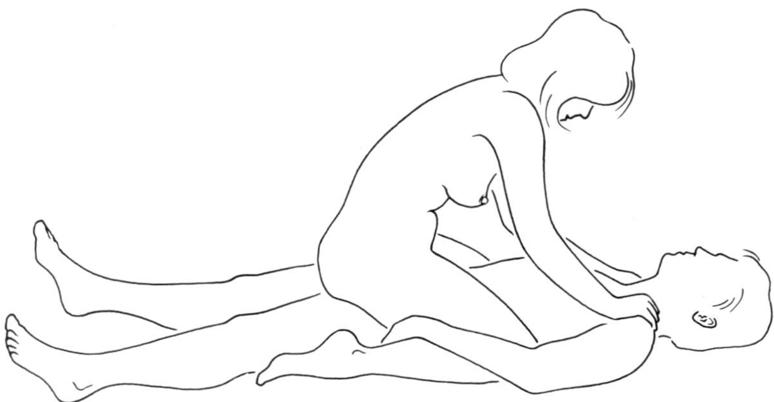

Fig. 13.3 The female superior position. This may be used in the treatment of many of the male and female disorders described in the text. After Belliveau and Richter (1974).

enables her to use the penis for stimulation in any way she likes (Duddle & Brown, 1980).

Masters & Johnson stressed that only the outline of sensate focus should be explained so that the couple could develop the technique in their own way. Thus initially some clothing may be kept on if they are particularly inhibited and a joint decision should be made concerning the place for the session (e.g. bedroom or sitting room); also whether the lights are on or off, the use of lubricating substances and a little alcohol and/or background music to help relaxation. Sometimes one or both partners misunderstand the instructions so it may be helpful to give simple written directions outlining the basic principles of the technique. A further helpful principle is that an invitation to a session of non-genital touching by one partner cannot be refused by the other, but progressing to more involved pleasuring of genitals etc depends on a mutual desire to do so.

The basis of this behavioural approach, therefore, is a gradual re-learning of sexual, or courting, behaviour which initially involves kissing, then touching first fully clothed then unclothed and finally intercourse. Sensate focus forms the basis for treatment of most dysfunctions.

FEMALE DISORDERS

Female orgasmic dysfunction

The Hite report (1976) found that almost all women who had not experienced orgasm would like to and that others were unsure about whether it had been achieved. Sexual response is under autonomic nervous control and therefore the orgasmic reflex cannot be induced at will. The patient should be discouraged from thinking about or judging her performance i.e. 'spectating', instead she should concentrate on the sensations and pleasures resulting from stimulation. Her use of fantasy is helpful and this may be supplemented by stimulation therapy using pictures, books or other erotic material (Gillan, 1979).

Masters & Johnson (1970) observed that the sensate focus technique is invaluable training for orgasmic dysfunction. During the early sessions when there is non-genital then light genital touching, the woman often discovers previously unknown areas of arousal. During these sessions the man must allow his partner to show him what she likes instead of him doing what he thinks she wants (Belliveau & Richter, 1970). Masters & Johnson found that female stimulation may be improved when the man sits supported with the women sitting between his legs and leaning backwards on him. This allows male access to a wide area for stimulation and the female can gently direct his hand at will. In this way no demands are made, the woman can express herself freely and in due course the build-up of arousal may lead to orgasm. With each new skill that is learnt the couple are reminded that all previously learned information should be used, so that always there is a gradual increase in the response to stimulation.

Masturbation is a useful method for producing orgasm and Hite (1976) observed that anorgasmia was five times more common in women who had never masturbated. The method of clitoral stimulation varies but she found that most women stimulate around the clitoral area using the hand, fingers or whatever and one site emerges as the focus of feeling, often like a burning sensation, which comes and goes; movement is adjusted so that the sensation continues and increases. Masters & Johnson found that male stimulation of the clitoris tended to start too early and was directed at the highly sensitive glans, rather than stroking the shaft which is usually more pleasurable. The woman should be reminded that when all the attention and stimulation are being directed at her, the male's need for ejaculation may be great, therefore, she should be encouraged to manipulate him to orgasm from time to time.

In due course sensate focus results in female arousal, then penile penetration should be tried to help achieve orgasm. The female superior position (Fig. 13.3) is recommended as the woman controls entry into the vagina and when this occurs there should be no movement initially so that the pleasure of vaginal dilatation is experienced. Thereafter she can rotate her pelvis on the male pubic bone thereby increasing clitoral stimulation. Hite found that only 30 per cent of women achieved orgasm regularly from intercourse alone and this agreed with other studies which showed that additional stimulation is usually necessary for orgasm.

An excellent programme for female sexual growth leading to orgasm has been developed by Heiman et al (1976). This behavioural approach recognises the problems that many women have in accepting their sexuality and in touching their own bodies. They describe exercises for the woman to do in private. She should be relaxed, for example by having a leisurely bath, then using mirrors she slowly examines her whole body and thinks about the feelings which result. Negative images should be changed to positive ones so that if she describes her genitals as ugly and wrinkled, instead she should compare their shape to parts of a flower or shell. Later she explores her body using oil or powder and experiences the sensations and pleasures which result; this progresses to clitoral stimulation which may be continued at length. The use of a vibrator during touching is described and often orgasm occurs. A series of muscle exercises are detailed which help relaxation. This book is recommended as a useful guide for the therapist and patient.

The results of treating orgasmic dysfunction are generally good. Masters & Johnson achieved about an 80 per cent success rate which was maintained for at least five years in the great majority of women. Riley & Riley (1978) compared the combined use of sensate focus, masturbation and a vibrator with sensate focus alone in two groups of anorgasmic women and the success rates were 90 and 53 per cent respectively.

Vaginismus

Vaginismus is a common cause of non-consummation of marriage but before this diagnosis is made the male disorders of premature ejaculation and erectile dysfunction should be considered as they may have a similar effect. If possible, any genital abnormality should be excluded by performing gently a one-finger pelvic examination; however, in severe cases this is impossible because of adductor muscle spasm preventing access to the introitus. Vaginismus is a psychosomatic condition and its treatment therefore involves both counselling and correction of the somatic problem of muscle spasm. The patient requires a sympathetic listener to whom she can voice her fears and fantasies particularly about intercourse so that she feels the problem is understood, also rational explanations may be given when possible. Assurance is necessary that as far as an examination has allowed she is anatomically normal, and an explanation, using diagrams, of the mechanism of muscle spasm will help to dispel misunderstandings concerning the nature of the problem. These patients face a series of hurdles at every stage of treatment, therefore constant encouragement and praise are necessary.

The somatic component of therapy involves deconditioning involuntary contraction of the vaginal introital muscles. When adductor muscle spasm occurs also, Stanley (1981b) recommends that the doctor holds the woman's knees together firmly while she attempts to separate them; slowly she is allowed to succeed and during these manoeuvres she learns muscle relaxation and eventually allows access to the vagina. Concerning the relevant vaginal muscles, the female must learn which of them are involved and this may be done by voiding with the legs apart which excludes adductor activity. The flow is stopped during voiding which activates the specific muscles (Duddle & Brown, 1980) and if she can insert a finger into the vagina she will locate them. Contraction and relaxation of the pelvic floor should be repeated frequently every day.

The patient is encouraged also to insert her finger slowly into the vagina and after a time move it round; she will experience penetration and the movement helps to stretch the vagina and relax the muscles. In due course two fingers then vaginal dilators are inserted. The use of plastic gloves and lubrication are optional. Some women are unable to use their finger and prefer to employ a dilator; if so it is essential to ensure that their correct use is taught and that she can insert it satisfactorily and leave it in place for a short time. When the dilator is introduced with ease a larger one is tried. The patient should practice these techniques several times daily. The role of the partner is variable but frequently it is helpful for him to be taught how to insert his finger or a dilator.

Sometimes during therapy Stanley (1981a) incorporates a 'guided tour' of the female genitalia which involves the patient, doctor and preferably the partner. The woman adopts a half-sitting position with legs apart and a mirror placed so that she sees her vulva. She explores the lower genital tract which may include the cervix using a plastic speculum and light and the doctor explains the anatomy and physiology. Stanley's patients find it a valuable exercise, although sometimes embarrassing initially, as it often leads to a more open discussion of sexual matters.

A further helpful step is to encourage the use of tampons during menstruation as this provides another method of vaginal manipulation and often produces greater confidence in the use of the vagina. Vaginismus may be present for many years before help is sought and although initially the couple may function satisfactorily without intercourse, the constant failure to achieve penetration usually discourages contact. Therefore sexual counselling incorporating sensate focus is often required. Certain characteristics are frequently noted in these couples such as the presence of a good relationship, the female is of above-average attractiveness but she is the dominating partner who is unwilling to submit. If so the gentle male should be encouraged to be more forceful (Duddle, 1977).

When vaginal penetration has been established digitally and/or with dilators penile penetration should be tried. This is best achieved when stimulation has resulted in sufficient vaginal lubrication and swelling. The female superior position (Fig. 13.3) with the woman sitting astride the partner gives her full control and allows her to lower herself slowly onto the erect penis. No movement should occur until confidence is achieved thereafter gentle movements are started.

The results of treatment of vaginismus depend on many factors particularly the duration of the problem. Success rates of about 90 and 70 per cent have been reported by Ellison (1968) and Duddle (1977) in a series of 100 and 32 patients respectively. Finally, it is worth reiterating that vaginal dilatation under anaesthesia and perineotomy for this disorder are rarely indicated as they invariably aggravate the problem.

MALE DISORDERS

Erectile dysfunction
An organic cause is found in about 5 to 35 per cent of men with erectile dysfunction (Johnson, 1968; Spark et al 1980) therefore treatment should not start until this

possibility is excluded. Nevertheless counselling is usually necessary so that the male's maximum potential is achieved and to help him accept the disability (Duddle & Brown, 1980). The basic treatment of this disorder is sensate focus with an initial emphasis on the ban on intercourse and no goal-orientation, so that anxiety caused by the need for erection and intercourse is removed.

During non-genital touching the male is encouraged to relax and enjoy the sensations experienced and not to think about his performance i.e. 'spectate'. He may be surprised to find that erection occurs which may disappear when he is aware of it. Reassurance is necessary that erections come and go and this may be demonstrated during the next stage of genital touching when his partner stimulates him to erection, allows it to subside and stimulates him again until it reappears. This should be repeated several times. Finally, penetraton is encouraged using the female superior position (Fig. 13.3) and there should be no movement initially so that he can experience vaginal containment of the erect penis; thereafter gentle movements are started. Masters & Johnson (1970) found it helpful to emphasise that it is the female's responsibility to produce erection thereby reducing male anxiety.

The treatment of the primary disorder is generally more difficult as it may be due to a learning fault or psychological disturbance. The methods used for these include psychotherapy, training in social skills (Arkowitz, 1977) and desensitisation procedures (Duddle & Brown, 1980). Other treatments are available for erectile dysfunction. Many drugs have been tried such as androgenic hormones (Bancroft, 1977) which gave variable results and anti-depressants when there is coexisting depression, however, some of these interfere with erection and ejaculation. Mild tranquillisers have been shown in a controlled study to be as effective as conjoint (couple) therapy (Ansari, 1976). Some patients with an organic cause for example priapism, Peyronie's disease or following cystectomy may benefit from penile implants (Pryor, 1979); younger men who ejaculate normally but have no erection are particularly suitable. A variety of male appliances are available ranging from a rigid penile prosthesis attached to a waist belt to vibrators. Their purpose is to help female stimulation but they also ensure continuing sexual contact between the couple which is important (Rhodes, 1980). A popular device, the Blakoe ring, is available which is shaped like a flat Hodge pessary and fits round the base of the penis and scrotum. By means of its venous constricting effect and the small electric current set up between the skin and zinc and copper electrodes attached to it, erection is improved; good results with this device have been noted by Cooper (1974).

In general an improvement rate in erectile dysfunction of between one-half and two-thirds of patients may be expected (Matthews et al, 1976; Cooper, 1979) but the primary disorder is less amenable to treatment because of the psychological and other factors involved (Bancroft & Coles, 1976). When improvement occurs with the secondary dysfunction many men are disappointed that their previous levels of maximum erection are not achieved. This is due usually to ageing, therefore they should be encouraged to have realistic expectations (Cooper, 1979).

Ejaculatory disorders

Premature ejaculation
Many treatments have been tried for this disorder, for example distracting the man's

thoughts from the erotic excitement by thinking about work problems or counting backwards; also using a condom, alcohol or drugs to diminish sensation. None of these methods are particularly effective and usually if there is an improvement, say with a drug, it will last only as long as it is continued. The best treatment was developed by Semans (1956) and modified by Masters & Johnson (1970) as the 'squeeze technique' and Kaplan (1974) as the 'stop-start method'. The principle is for the man to recognise increasing excitement to the point at which ejaculation becomes inevitable, then stimulation is stopped just before 'ejaculatory inevitability' is reached.

This technique can be incorporated into sensate focus. The man lies on his back with his partner sitting facing him. She stimulates his genitals particularly the penis until he feels that climax is near. When he indicates this stimulation is stopped until the sensation has worn off, or alternatively the penis is squeezed firmly for 15 to 20 seconds by the female's fingers and thumb around the coronal ridge. Following either manoeuvre some erection will be lost but it will return with further stimulation and the process is repeated three or four times. Later this exercise is done using lubrication to simulate vaginal secretions. The final stage is for the woman, sitting astride her partner (Fig. 13.3), to place the erect penis in the vagina and at first to remain still so that the man experiences penetration; then gentle movement is added until he signifies that climax is near at which time the penis is removed from the vagina and the squeeze applied as before. Again the process is repeated several times on each occasion and the sessions should be repeated regularly until ejaculatory control is achieved.

For the male temporarily without a partner this method may be employed successfully using masturbation. The results are generally good and ejaculatory control is usually achieved within weeks of regular use.

Retarded ejaculation

The principle treatment is maximal penile stimulation by the female. Prognosis is improved if ejaculation already occurs during solitary masturbation. The female stimulates the penis to emission and gradually this is repeated closer to the vagina each time until, using the female superior position (Fig. 13.3), the penis is inserted into the vagina just before ejaculation occurs. Alternatively the male may have to masturbate himself in the presence of his partner and move closer to the vagina each time. Again sensate focus techniques may be used but if there is sexual conflict concerning soiling or damaging the woman, psychotherapy will be necessary (Duddle & Brown, 1980). In a small series of patients Masters & Johnson (1970) reported that the great majority were treated successfully.

CONCLUSION

This chapter has tried to demonstrate that sexual dysfunction is a common problem and that it has a wide variety of causes. Current demands on treatment facilities far outweigh the supply, therefore, interested clinicians should be encouraged to become involved in this field. Gynaecologists may be particularly suited for this work. Using the counselling techniques described much can be done for the couple with simple problems and more detailed treatment is available for complex disorders. Clinicians will find the work both interesting and rewarding and in general the results are good.

Acknowledgement
It is a pleasure to acknowledge the considerable help of Dr May Duddle, Consultant Psychiatrist in Manchester, who has developed much of the sexual counselling services in the North-West of England and trained many of those working in this field.

REFERENCES

Ansari J M A 1976 Impotence: prognosis. A controlled study. British Journal of Psychiatry 128: 194–198
Arkowitz H 1977 Measurement and modifications of minimal dating behaviour. In: Ersen M H, Eisler M, Miller P M (eds) Progress in behavioural modification. Academic Press, New York, ch 5, p 1–61
Bancroft J 1977 Hormones and sexual behaviour. Psychological Medicine 7: 553–556
Bancroft J, Bancroft J 1978 Man and woman. Self help with sexual problems. Pamphlet produced for Yorkshire Television series
Bancroft J, Coles L 1976 Three years' experience in a sexual problems clinic. British Medical Journal 1: 1575–1577
Beaumont G 1979 Sexual side-effects of psychotropic drugs. British Journal of Clinical practice (Symposium Supplement) 4: 45–47
Begg A, Dickerson M, Loudon N B 1976 Frequency of self-reported sexual problems in a family planning clinic. Journal of Family Planning Doctors 2: 41–48
Belliveau F, Richter L 1974 Understanding human sexual inadequacy. Coronet Books, London
Burnap D W, Golden J S 1967 Sexual Problems in Medical Practice. Journal of Medical Education 42: 673–680
Christensen H T, Gregg C F 1970 Changing sex norms in America and Scandinavia. Journal of Marriage and The Family 32: 616–627
Cooper A J 1974 A blind evaluation of a penile ring. A sex aid for impotent males. British Journal of Psychiatry 124: 402–406
Cooper A J 1979 A review of 215 cases seen in a sex clinic. British Journal of Sexual Medicine 6: 45: 38–42
Danesino V, Martella E 1976 Modern conceptions of corpora cavernosa function in the vagina and clitoris (Translated reprint from Archivo di Ostetricia & Ginecologia (Napoli) — quoted by Levin 1980)
Duddle C N 1975 The treatment of marital psychosexual disorders. British Journal of Psychiatry 127: 169–170
Duddle C M 1977 Etiological factors in the unconsummated marriage. Journal of Psychosomatic Research 21: 157–160
Duddle C M, Brown A D G 1980 Clinical Management of Sexual Dysfunction. Clinics in Obstetrics & Gynaecology 7: 2: 293–323
Ellison C 1968 Psychosomatic factors in unconsummated marriage. Journal of Psychosomatic Research 12: 61–65
Fagen J, Shepherd I C 1970 (eds) Gestalt therapy now. Harper & Row, London
Fox C A 1978 Recent Research in Human Coital Physiology. British Journal of Sexual Medicine 5: 41: 13–19
Fox C A, Meldrum S J, Watson B W 1973 Continuous measurement by radio-telemetry of vaginal pH during human coitus. Journal of Reproduction & Fertility 33: 69–75
Fox C A, Wolff H, Baker J A 1970 Measurement of intra-vaginal and intrauterine pressures during human coitus by radio-telemetry. Journal of Reproduction and Fertility 22: 243–251
Freud S 1905 Three essays on the theory of sexuality. Translation. (ed) Strachey J London: Hogarth Press and Institute of Psychoanalysis 1962
Gillan P 1979 Stimulation therapy in sexual dysfunction. British Journal of Sexual Medicine 6: 49: 13–14
Gillan P, Brindley G S 1979 Vaginal and pelvic floor responses to sexual stimulation. Psychophysiology 16: 471
Goodlin R C, Keller D W, Raffin M 1971 Orgasm during late pregnancy. Obstetrics & Gynaecology 38: 916
Goodlin R C, Schmidt W, Greevy D C 1972 Uterine tension and fetal heart rate during maternal orgasm. Journal of Obstetrics & Gynaecology 39: 125–127
Hallstrom T 1980 Sexuality in the climacteric. Clinics in Obstetrics & Gynaecology 4: 1: 227–239
Hawkins D F, Elder M G 1979 Human fertility control: theory and practice. Butterworth, London
Heiman J, Lopiccolo L, Lopiccolo J 1976 Becoming orgasmic: A sexual growth programme for women. Prentice-Hall, New Jersey
Hite S 1976 The Hite report. Talmy Franklin, London
Javert C T 1957 Spontaneous and habitual abortion. McGraw-Hill, New York

Johnson J 1968 Disorders of sexual potency in the male. Pergamon Press, Oxford
Kaplan H S 1974 The new sex therapy. Baillière Tindall, London
Kegel A H 1952 Sexual functions of the pubococcygeus muscle. Western Journal of Surgery in Obstetrics & Gynaecology 60: 521
Kinsey A C, Pomeroy W B, Martin C E, Gerhard P H 1953 Sexual behaviour in the human female. Saunders, Philadelphia
Kline-Graber G, Graber B 1975 A guide to sexual satisfaction — woman's orgasm Popular Library, New York p 21–54
Kumar R, Brant H A, Robson K M 1981 Childbearing and maternal sexuality: a prospective survey of 119 primiparae (in press)
Levin R J 1980 Physiology of Sexual Function in Women. Clinics in Obstetrics & Gynaecology 7: 2: 213–252
Levin R J, Wagner G 1977 Human vaginal fluid — ionic composition and modification by sexual arousal. Journal of Physiology 266: 62–63
Levin R J, Wagner G 1978 Mechanisms for vaginal ion movement in women. Journal of Physiology 284: 172–173
Levin R J, Wagner G 1980 Influence of atropine on sexual arousal and orgasm in women — a pilot study. In Medical Sexology (Proceedings of 3rd International Congress of Medical Sexology Rome) (ed) Forleo R, Pasini W pp 618–624 Littleton Massachusetts: PSG Publishing
Lopiccolo J, Lopiccolo L 1978 Handbook of sex therapy. Plenum Press, New York and London
Ludwig H, Metzer H 1976 The human female reproductive tract — a scanning electron microscopic atlas. Springer Verlag, Berlin p 14
Masters W H, Johnson V E 1966 Human sexual response. Little Brown, Boston
Masters W H, Johnson V E 1970 Human sexual inadequacy. Churchill Livingstone, Edinburgh
Matthews A, Bancroft J, Whitehead A, Hackman A, Julia D, Bancroft J, Gath D, Shaw P 1976 The behavioural treatment of sexual inadequacy: A comparative study. Behaviour Research and Therapy 14: 427–436
Naeye R L 1981 Coitus and antepartum haemorrhage. British Journal of Obstetrics & Gynaecology 88: 765–770
Newman G, Nichols C R 1960 Sexual activities and attitudes in older persons. Journal of American Medical Association 173: 33–35
Perkins R P 1979 Sexual behaviour and response in relation to complications of pregnancy. American Journal of Obstetrics & Gynaecology 134: 498–505
Perl J I, Milles G, Shimozato Y 1959 Vaginal fluid subsequent to panhysterectomy. American Journal of Obstetrics & Gynaecology 78: 285
Pfeiffer E, Verwoerot A, Davis G C 1972 Sexual behaviour in middle life. American Journal of Psychiatry 128: 1261–67
Pryor J P 1979 The surgery of erectile impotence. British Journal of Sexual Medicine 6: 50: 24–25
Rhodes P 1980 The use of aids in the management of disorder of sexual dysfunction. Clinics in Obstetrics & Gynaecology 7: 2: 421–432
Riley A J, Riley E J 1978 A controlled study to evaluate directed masturbation in the management of primary orgasmic failure in women. British Journal of Psychiatry 133: 404–409
Scott R S, Hsueh G S C 1979 A clinical study of the effects of galvonic muscle stimulation in urinary stress incontinence and sexual dysfunction. American Journal of Obstetrics & Gynaecology 135: 663
Semans J H 1956 Premature Ejaculation. A new approach. Southern Medical Journal 49: 353–7
Singer I 1973 The goals of human sexuality. Norton, New York
Solberg D A, Butler J, Wagner N 1973 Sexual behaviour in pregnancy. New England Journal of Medicine 288: 1098–1103
Spark R F, White R A, Connolly P B 1980 Impotence is not always psychogenic. Newer insights into Hypothalamic-Pituitary-Gonadal Dysfunction. Journal of the American Medical Association 243: 750–755
Stanley E 1981a Principles of managing sexual problems. British Medical Journal 282: 1199–1202
Stanley E 1981b Vaginismus. British Medical Journal 282: 1435–8
Stevens O J 1979 Awareness. Bantam Books, London
Wagner N N, Butler J C, Sanders J P 1976 Prematurity and orgasmic coitus during pregnancy: data on a small sample. Fertility and Sterility 27: 911–915
Wagner G, Levin R J 1978 Vaginal fluid. In: Hafez E S E, Evans T N (eds) Human vagina. North-Holland Publishing, Amsterdam, ch 8, p 121–137
Wagner G, Levin R J 1980 Effect of atropine and methyl atropine on human vaginal blood, sexual arousal and climax. Acta Pharmacologica et Toxiccologica 46: 321–325
Werner A 1975 Sexual dysfunction in college men and women. American Journal of Psychiatry 132: 164–168

SUGGESTED PAPERBACK READING LIST FOR COUPLES

Belliveau F, Richter L 1971 Understanding human sexual inadequacy. Hodder, London
Brown P, Faulder C 1978 Treat yourself to sex: a guide for good loving. Penguin, Harmondsworth
Delvin D 1975 Book of love: home doctor book of sex and marriage. New English Library, London
Piccolo L, et al 1977 Becoming orgasmic: a sexual growth programme for women. Prentice Hall, Hemel
  Hempstead

14. Cost-effectiveness of hormone therapy after the menopause

Wulf H. Utian

There are few areas in modern gynecology that excite as much controversy as the concept of long-term hormone replacement therapy to women in their postmenopausal years (Utian, 1980a). No method of treatment has been so widely applied to an otherwise normal population with so little background knowledge. An attempt at evaluation of the risk-benefit ratio of the long-term effects of pure estrogens or of estrogens with added progestogen highlights the fact that, compared to the great many carefully designed large-scale epidemiologic studies on the health consequences of oral contraceptive use, no comparable body of data is available for postmenopausal hormone replacement. Despite this lack, it is possible to subject the known risks and benefits and their potential costs, to some form of mathematical evaluation and analysis.

The purpose of this review is to outline the risks and benefits of postmenopausal hormone replacement therapy, to demonstrate how the risks, benefits and costs of such long-term therapy can be balanced by the application of general analytic methods, and thereby to provide acceptable guidelines for clinical practice. In all, the objective is to place current practice on a scientific rather than an emotive foundation (Utian, 1980a).

GENERAL ANALYTIC APPROACHES

Certain introductory comments on general analytic approaches are necessary. Various measures have been designed that can help guide decision making in medicine by systematic analysis. For example, several potential therapeutic modalities may need to be compared on a basis of population need, therapeutic risk and benefit, and overall cost. The answers so obtained could be of value to health care decision-makers in planning new facilities or in allotting limited available funds on a priority basis by providing a measure of health effectiveness and cost. Logically, the balancing of benefits of estrogen therapy against potential risks is a subject in need of such analysis. The answer we seek in this instance should help decide whether such therapy should be given or not.

To be of value, any form of analysis must be comprehensive and broadly applicable. This necessitates the availability of the best current information on both the efficacy of therapy and its costs, as well as the possible risks and their respective costs. Unfortunately, the available data base on the effectiveness of estrogen therapy and menopause is distressingly limited. The tendency among physicians and consumers to demand exact scientific proof is commendable and desirable but does not detract from the fact that until accurate information is obtained, current analysis and decision making must depend upon the best available current evidence. Nonetheless, any form of analysis should be structured to incorporate new data as it becomes available and even to suggest areas in need of future research (Weinstein & Stason, 1977).

An ideal measure of the effectiveness of a clinical practice needs to be outcome-oriented, with length and quality of life as the ultimate measures. Inevitably, when risks and benefits of a particular form of therapy are being evaluated, which in turn involve possible trade-offs between longevity and quality of life, subjective values have to be involved.

Another area that needs incorporation into any effective analysis is the balance between present and future health benefits and costs. Estrogen therapy, for example, can be considered as a preventative program in which the costs are immediate and ongoing, but the health benefits and risks may be in the future.

SPECIFIC ANALYTIC APPROACHES

Cost-benefit analysis (Bunker et al, 1977) and cost-effectiveness analysis (Weinstein & Stason, 1977) are two different analytic approaches that can be applied to the assessment of postmenopausal hormone therapy.

Cost-benefit analysis. Values all outcomes in economic (e.g. dollar) terms. This requires that human lives and quality of life be valued in dollars. Once the benefits and costs have been reduced to dollar values, the decision whether to administer estrogen, in theory at least, is simplified.

Cost-effectiveness analysis. In this instance priority is placed on alternate expenditures without requiring that the dollar value of life and health be assessed. Health effectiveness is measured in quality-adjusted life years (QALY) because it incorporates changes in survival and morbidity in a single measure that reflects tradeoffs between them. This will be further explained below. Health care costs are measured in dollars. The measure of cost-effectiveness then becomes a ratio of the cost in dollars to net health effectiveness measured in QALY. Thus, the lower the ratio, the better the result (Weinstein & Stason, 1977).

Net health care costs. There are various ways to measure the cost of medical care.

1. Direct (therapeutic) costs include payment for service by doctors, hospitals, laboratories, pharmacy, etc.
2. Use of indirect costs is a more comprehensive measure that takes into account the impact of illness, premature death, or disability on the economy. Being broader in concept, it is less easy to define.
3. Preventive costs involve the costs of a prophylaxis program which includes drugs, dispensing, education, physician time, etc. Savings on such a program can be calculated by deducting the actual preventive costs from the hypothetical costs of treating the disease in the absence of a prophylactic program. This difference could also be termed avoidable costs.

The following formula for calculation of health costs, modified from Weinstein & Stason (1977) takes all of the above factors, excluding indirect costs, into account:

$$HC = \Delta C_{RX} + \Delta C_{SE} - \Delta C_{BENEF} + \Delta C_{RX\Delta LE}$$

where HC = net health care costs (H.C.C.); ΔC_{RX} = all direct H.C.C. (drugs, physician, etc.); ΔC_{SE} = all H.C.C. due to side-effects of treatment; ΔC_{BENEF} = savings in H.C.C. due to disease prevention; and $\Delta C_{RX\Delta LE}$ = H.C.C. of diseases that would not have occurred if patients did not receive treatment.

Net health effectiveness. The measure of improvement or loss in quality of life is a controversial area. A weighting scheme or health status index (λS) (Bush et al, 1973; Weinstein & Stason, 1977) assigns a numerical weight (P) between zero and one to differentiate full health from varying degrees of disability or discomfort. The greater the number the worse the disability, i.e. 0.0 is virtually no disability and 1.0 would imply a patient condition tantamount to being dead, i.e. the probability (P) for death is 1.0. The health status index (λS) is then calculated as 1–P.

The number of years spent (YS) at this health status is multiplied by λS to yield the number of quality adjusted life years (QALY). This can be considered to be equivalent to the number of years spent in full health, the calculation is thus as follows:

$$\lambda S \times YS = \Delta Y_{BENEF} \text{ or } \Delta Y_{SE} \text{ in QALY}$$

where λS = H.S.I. or disability weight = 1–P, if P = probability of death; YS = years at health status; ΔY_{BENEF} = net health effectiveness; ΔY_{SE} = net health loss; and QALY = quality-adjusted life years.

The following example demonstrates the use of the Health Status Index to quantify the situation for a potential risk like uterine cancer:

Morbidity	P
A = Early cancer removed; no disability	0.05
B = Surgery plus radiotherapy; minimal disability	0.15
C = Vaginal stenosis and pain	0.35
D = Severe pain, recurrence	0.88
E = Advanced secondary disease	1.0

$$\lambda S = 1\text{–}P$$
and $\lambda S \times$ Years = ΔY_{CANCER} *in* QALY

The potential benefit for prevention of osteoporosis is:

Morbidity	P
A = Radiologic osteoporosis; no disability	0.1
B = Occasional discomfort on exertion	0.35
C = Fractured wrist	0.55
D = Femoral neck or vertebral compression fracture	0.85
E = Totally bedridden, disabled, intractable pain	1.0

$$\lambda S = 1\text{–}P$$
and $\lambda S \times$ Years = ΔY_{OSTEO} *in* QALY

The overall measure of improvement or loss in quality of life, or net health effectiveness, can be calculated from the following formula, also modified from Weinstein & Stason (1977) (Utian, 1978a).

$$HE = \Delta Y + \Delta Y_{BENEF} - \Delta Y_{SE}$$

where HE = net health effectiveness in QALY; ΔY = expected number of unadjusted life years; ΔY_{BENEF} = improvement in quality of life years due to reduction in morbidity or prevention thereof; and ΔY_{SE} = loss due to side effects of treatment.

The expected number of unadjusted life years (ΔY) can be derived from life tables. The measure of ΔY_{BENEF} and of ΔY_{SE} are calculated as previously described. The latter two measures are also calculated on an additive basis taking all the relative risks (for example, uterine cancer, surgery for gallstones, etc.) and benefits (for example, reduced bone fracture rate, feeling of well-being due to symptom relief, etc.) into account.

The overall *cost-effectiveness ratio* is thus calculated according to the following formula:

$$\frac{HC}{HE} = \frac{\Delta C_{RX} + \Delta C_{SE} - \Delta C_{BENEF} + \Delta C_{RX\Delta LE}}{\Delta Y + \Delta Y_{BENEF} - \Delta Y_{SE}}$$

A source of criticism of cost-effectiveness analysis is that data are not usually available to make these measures with certainty. Furthermore, the whole trade-off concept is difficult. Nonetheless, such trade-offs in therapeutic measures are made each day by doctors in clinical practice. All that health analysis does is to supply a quantification to make the measure explicit (Utian, 1978a; Weinstein & Stason, 1977).

COST-EFFECTIVENESS ANALYSIS APPLIED TO POSTMENOPAUSAL ESTROGEN THERAPY

Calculation of the cost-effectiveness of long-term estrogen therapy after the menopause is dependent upon numerous local factors in varying countries and communities and therefore needs independent analysis. The potential advantages and disadvantages will be dealt with below. Cost-effectiveness analysis takes present knowledge as a data base and allows future knowledge to be incorporated. Potential risks and benefits must be evaluated with this in mind.

Potential benefits

Numerous potential benefits have been claimed for postmenopausal replacement of the sex hormones, singly or in combination, in a vast medical literature that ranges from highly scientific to anecdotal (Utian, 1980a).

Relief of symptoms

The symptoms of menopause are summarized in Table 14.1 (from Utian, 1980a). Specific symptoms that are estrogen-related are more likely to respond to estrogen therapy. The specific early symptoms related to hot flushes and atrophic vaginitis have been shown to respond to short-term estrogen therapy as tested on single-blind estrogen-placebo crossover studies (Utian, 1972a; Utian, 1973), double blind studies (Campbell, 1976; Campbell & Whitehead, 1977), in innumerable clinical reports over the years (Dapunt, 1967; Kullander & Svanberg, 1975; Kupperman et al, 1959), and in most physicians' clinical experience.

It should come as no surprise that most nonspecific symptoms have been less successfully treated with estrogen. Moreover, late problems are unlikely to be

Table 14.1 Symptoms associated with menopause (from Utian, 1980a and reproduced courtesy of Appleton-Century-Crofts)

1. *Specific: True hormonal-related symptoms*
   Early: hot flushes; perspiration (night sweats).
   Later: relate to the metabolic change in the target organ affected; e.g., osteoporosis causing backache, vaginal atrophy causing dyspareunia, etc.
2. *Nonspecific: Psycho-socio-cultural symptoms*
   Determined by the woman's environment and the structure of her character; e.g., depression, irritability, insomnia, frigidity, headache, apprehension, etc.

responsive to estrogen replacement unless such therapy has been proven to cure the pathology as well. Backache due to osteoporosis, for example, is unlikely to respond to estrogens.

The mental tonic effect described by Utian (1972b) has been confirmed as an entity that is independent of vasomotor symptoms (Campbell, 1976; Campbell & Whitehead, 1977; Fedor-Freybergh, 1977). That is, post-menopausal women receiving exogenous estrogen therapy feel better in terms of mental awareness and ability to perform their daily duties, and thus have a generally improved feeling of well-being. This euphoric effect of general improvement in mental state probably accounts for the reduction in some nonspecific symptoms that are not directly related to estrogen deficiency.

The ability of exogenously administered estrogen to improve mental state may reflect a pharmacologic effect, rather than reversal of a post-menopausal phenomenon. Nevertheless, it is a distinct benefit and should be recognized as such.

The status of estrogens for the treatment of minor psychiatric symptoms (e.g. minor depression, irritability, insomnia) is less clear. Initially, an extraordinarily wide number of claims was made for beneficial effects of estrogens on psychological changes, but few have held up to scrutiny (Dennerstein & Burrows, 1978; Hawkinson, 1938; Ingvarrson, 1951). Many investigators were unable to differentiate estrogen effects on psychological symptoms from placebo responses (George et al, 1973; Thomson & Oswald, 1977; Utian, 1972a). Kantor et al (1968) and Michael et al (1970) reported estrogens to delay the 'psychological deterioration' that apparently occurs in untreated older women. Fedor–Freybergh (1977) confirmed the ability of estrogen to slow down the natural deterioration of some perceptual, attentional, and memory processes. Thomson & Oswald (1977) reported estrogens to increase rapid eye movement sleep, that is, to be of possible value in the postmenopausal patient complaining of insomnia.

The difficulty in reaching any significant conclusion as to the precise role for estrogens in relief of minor psychiatric symptoms could be blamed on a 'symptom-snowball' effect. The beneficial effect of estrogens on hot flushes reduces night sweats and this enhances the ability to sleep, which in turn, has a positive influence on mood, which increases the ability to concentrate, and so forth. There is a need for a randomized, controlled, prospective, double-blind study of the effects of estrogens in postmenopausal women without hot flushes for their effect on these minor symptoms (Campbell, 1976). In the interim, the mental tonic effect aside, the case for estrogens as a cure for minor psychiatric symptoms must be considered as possible, but unproven.

Weinstein (1980) in a major attempt to evaluate the cost-effectiveness analysis, incorporated 'hypothetical subjective evaluations of the effects of estrogens on the quality of life' into his analysis. He included relief from symptoms of menopause or sequelae of osteoporosis, hip fracture, and endometrial cancer. He allowed symptomatic improvement to provide the equivalent of 0.01 quality-adjusted year of life for each year on treatment. This figure represents his subjective assessment of the willingness of the patient to sacrifice 1 per cent of her life to get rid of the symptoms during those years. The author's experience with patients suffering severe perimenopausal symptoms would suggest this figure is extremely conservative.

No study exists at present in which an accurate cost-effectiveness analysis has been applied directly to symptom relief. Until such time as such statistics become available, subjective approximations such as those of Weinstein (1980) are the only figures available to be incorporated into the risk:benefit ratio.

Prevention of osteoporosis
The prevention of osteoporosis and its complications is one of the most cited indications for long-term estrogen therapy and has been reviewed in depth elsewhere (Utian, 1980a).

Osteoporosis appears to be an enormous problem. Despite a lack of well-defined prevalence, complication and disability rates for osteoporosis, the distinct relationship between this condition and bone fractures has become increasingly clear. For example, of all patients with hip fracture, more than 80 per cent have pre-existing osteoporosis. About 10 per cent of women may have symptomatic osteoporosis by age 55, and 20 per cent by the age of 68 (Bauer, 1970).

The major problem in investigation of the cause, development and response to treatment of osteoporosis has been the lack of a specific clinical tool to establish the diagnosis and to measure the change in bone density over any period of time. The application of modern techniques has provided a greater understanding of both the natural history of skeletal development, and of bone loss in relation to normal aging and specific pathological processes such as ovarian failure (Utian, 1980a).

A large amount of evidence indicates that normally functioning ovaries exert a protective effect on the skeleton. This protective effect is reduced and then lost during the perimenopause. Premature menopause or castration hastens this process. Removal of ovaries from premenopausal women is followed by significant calcium loss (Gallagher et al, 1972). When the indices of osteoporosis are related to the menopause, decreased vertebral density can be observed within five years.

In view of the relationship between ovarian function, menopause, osteoporosis and bone fracture rates, it is not surprising that estrogen therapy has been carefully scrutinized as a possible preventative or therapeutic measure for this problem. Such therapy has been shown to be effective at several levels in the prevention of bone metabolic changes that lead to osteoporosis. Estrogen replacement therapy in postmenopausal women induced positive calcium balance (Utian, 1972c). In turn, estrogen treatment started within two months of bilateral oophorectomy has been shown to prevent subsequent bone mineral loss (Aitken et al, 1973). This skeletal protective effect has been demonstrated to last as long as eight years. It should be emphasized that estrogen does not prevent all age-related bone loss, but does appear to abolish the sex difference.

While the evidence for a protective effect of estrogens against the development of osteoporosis is quite substantial, evidence that such hormone replacement therapy will alter fracture rates has been slower in forthcoming. Recent information based on the retrospective case-control study method has shown that women after the menopause who are on estrogen therapy are less likely to suffer osteoporosis-related bone fractures than similar women not on such treatment (Hutchinson et al, 1979; Weiss et al, 1980). It seems important that therapy needs to be administered over a prolonged period of time to be effective, and may even be more effective when administered within three years of the menopause.

The data of Hutchinson et al (1979) and Weiss et al (1980) suggest that women taking estrogens after age 50 are less than half as likely to sustain fractures of the wrist and hip than their untreated contemporaries. Presumably, this difference would only apply so long as therapy is continued. Gordon et al (1973) reported up to an eight-fold reduction of spinal compression fractures in a prospective cohort study in patients on doses of 1.25 mg per day of conjugated estrogens. Heaney (1976) has reported the mortality rate for hip fractures to be as high as 16 per cent.

Effect on skin
There is scant evidence that estrogen prevents skin atrophy but further study is necessary. For example, while the thickness of the epidermis and the number of mitoses decreases sharply after castration, it has been shown that pathological deterioration can be prevented or reduced with estrogen therapy (Punnonen, 1972). At this point in time, it is not possible to determine a health-effectiveness value for this skin effect.

Benefits claimed but unproven
Many other potential benefits of long-term estrogen replacement have been claimed, but are unproven. A few are worthy of discussion.

Prevention of aging. Claims have been made for estrogen in the prevention of aging. In this context 'aging' is a nebulous term that needs definition and quantification. If reduced bone loss or deceleration of skin atrophy are components of prevention of aging, then the claim may be true. Otherwise there is as yet no satisfactory study that differentiates estrogen effect from the concurrent processes in a general aging population over a sufficient period of time and in a large enough study group. Until some preliminary evidence is forthcoming, the case must be considered unproven. Estrogen, moreover, could only be one small factor out of many that relate to the aging process.

Prevention of coronary heart disease. The apparent protective effect of the ovary in development of atherosclerosis and coronary heart disease has led to claims that long-term estrogen therapy may reduce the incidence of coronary heart disease. Such claims have not held true. The subject has been extensively reviewed elsewhere (Utian, 1980a).

Improvement in libido. Unsubstantiated claims have also been made for the use of estrogen in improving libido after menopause. Decreased libido due to vaginal atrophy (that is, the patient who 'wants' but 'can't') will respond to local effects of estrogen on the vaginal epithelium (Utian, 1970). Estrogen replacement, in the absence of local vaginal problems, has been shown to be of no benefit in the treatment of decreased or absent libido (Utian, 1975; Dennerstein et al, 1977).

Potential risks

The possible risks of estrogen therapy, in general, have been as poorly defined as the potential benefits due to the many problems involved in analyzing risk. It is extremely difficult to assess the risk attributable to one factor like estrogen without considering the synergistic effects of other health risk factors such as smoking, obesity, and hypertension, and possible other coincidental factors which are not as easily identified. For example, contraceptive pill users who are non-smokers appear to be at lower risk of heart disease mortality than pill users who do smoke cigarettes (Jain, 1977). Does the same apply to pure estrogen? Moreover, these synergistic influences vary in different countries and within different socioeconomic groups in a given country.

Despite the above limitations, certain risks of long-term estrogen usage have become obvious and merit consideration.

Postmenopausal bleeding and unnecessary surgery

This is a real disadvantage of postmenopausal estrogen therapy. The incidence will vary depending on prescribing practices, drug selection, and dosage, and on patient response (Gambrell et al, 1978). Older women strongly associate bleeding after menopause with cancer, and they should be spared this unnecessary cause for anxiety. Differentiation is occasionally made between 'on-pill' bleeding and 'between-pill' bleeding. In either event, endometrial biopsy and even dilation and curettage is usually indicated, particularly as a regular bleeding response to estrogen is no guarantee of a healthy endometrium (Sturdee et al, 1978).

The increased incidence of postmenopausal bleeding may directly affect the incidence of diagnostic curettage and hysterectomy. For instance, the rate of hysterectomy in the United States is said to have increased from 602/100 000 in 1970 to 727/100 000 in 1975 (Editorial, 1977; Kistner, 1976). What is not known is the influence, if any, of estrogen therapy on this increase.

Uterine cancer

A series of reports since 1975 have linked postmenopausal estrogen usage with the possibility of an increased risk of uterine cancer (Antunes et al, 1979; Gray et al, 1977; Horwitz & Feinstein, 1978; Jick et al, 1979; McDonald et al, 1977; Mack et al, 1976; Smith et al, 1975; Weiss et al, 1976; Ziel & Finkle, 1975).

The annual risk of development of endometrial cancer in untreated women after the menopause with an intact uterus is usually accepted as being about one in every thousand. The general consensus of the studies linking long-term estrogen therapy to endometrial cancer is that the annual cancer risk will be increased to between four and eight cases per thousand.

In particular, the following factors seem to enhance the relationship between estrogen and cancer:

1. An increase in duration of therapy to more than three years doubles the risk ratio from 4.6 to 9.2 (Gray et al, 1977; Ziel & Finkle, 1976).

2. The type of drug may be of importance, nonsteroidal estrogens and estrone preparations possibly being of greater risk. In fairness, however, these were also the most available and frequently used estrogens, and this aspect needs further clarification.
3. The risk increases with higher dosage of estrogen.
4. Continuous unopposed estrogen administration is a greater risk factor than cycled therapy in the risk production (Whitehead, 1978). Two studies call this statement into question, and at this time the matter remains unresolved (Hammond et al, 1979; Jick et al, 1979).

Two important issues need to be raised. First, the question as to whether estrogen is a carcinogen or a cocarcinogen is not the pertinent one. The maximal definable risk is the pertinent issue. The question is not whether estrogen causes cancer, within present knowledge, but what is the worst possible risk that may be entailed if estrogen does cause cancer. The answer, as stated above, appears to lie between an extra four to eight cases per year per 1000 women treated. Second, if such an increased relationship does exist, and the evidence now appears strong, then what factors could explain this increased risk and are such factors avoidable? Again, the consensus of the above studies appears to indicate that the risk is maximized in unselected women placed on continuous high dosage of estrogen over a long period of time.

Certain individuals do appear to be at increased risk for endometrial cancer (Gusberg, 1976; Klopper & Farr, 1978). Moreover, a continuous high-estrogen status is nonphysiologic (Gurpide, 1976). It is possible that lower doses of selected estrogen given cyclically, with added progestogen in some instances (Gambrell, 1978; Hammond et al, 1979; Kistner 1976; Sturdee et al, 1978), to a patient without known cancer-risk factors and who is adequately and regularly observed, may result in an incidence of carcinoma similar to that of nontreated patients. There is theoretical reason to expect this but little proof, and the final answer will have to await the reports of various avenues of research currently in progress.

The case-fatality rate for endometrial cancer has been estimated at 10 per cent, reflecting the fact that most cases reported under such circumstances have proven to be of early stage (Hulka et al, 1980).

Obviously, women with previous hysterectomy are not candidates for uterine cancer. The calculation of cost-effectiveness must thus allow for the prevalence of hysterectomy in the total group to be treated. This could account for up to 30 per cent of the total group (Hulka et al, 1978).

Breast cancer

The relationship between estrogen therapy and the risk for development of breast cancer is less clear. A possible marginal increase in breast carcinoma in estrogen-treated patients has been reported (Hoover et al, 1976) but has not been confirmed (Burch et al, 1974; Boston Collaborative Drug Surveillance Program, 1974). At worst, the relative risk appears to be increased by a factor of 1.3 at 12 years of estrogen therapy and by a factor of two after 15 years of usage (Hoover et al, 1976). The risk appears to be related to the continuous long-term use of relatively high dosages of estrogens, as with estrogens and endometrial cancer. There is, as yet, no evidence as to whether cyclical low-dose estrogen with added progestogen will affect the development of breast cancer. Experience from use of the oral contraceptive is reassuring in this respect. None of the published retrospective studies or prospective studies have indicated any overall relationship between oral contraceptive use and breast cancer.

Mammography has been of considerable value in evaluating the breast. However, estrogen therapy after menopause can produce changes in the breast demonstrable as cystic or dysplastic by mammography (Peck & Lowman, 1978). These changes regress on cessation of therapy and it has therefore been suggested that such therapy be discontinued before mammography so that clinical and radiologic evaluation can be enhanced.

Deep vein thrombosis and thromboembolism

Unlike the information on oral contraceptive usage, there are few statistics for deep venous thrombosis and thromboembolism on estrogen therapy when given alone.

The question of thromboembolic risk is extremely important. The concept of long-term estrogen replacement following menopause implies that such drug usage will reduce certain risk factors such as the development of osteoporosis. The value would be negated were one risk factor to be replaced by another; the same argument, holds true for endometrial cancer. Moreover, it would appear that the patients who receive postmenopausal estrogens would be at higher risk for development of thromboembolism, often being obese, hypertensive, cigarette smokers, and mostly over the age of 50.

There is preliminary evidence to suggest that the risk of thromboembolism may be increased in postmenopausal estrogen users compared to nonusers. The risk appears to be increased in users of synthetic unconjugated steroids (ethinyl-estradiol and mestranol) (Gow & MacGillivray, 1971) as compared to users of conjugated equine estrogen (Bolton et al, 1975; Notelovitz & Greig, 1975), estradiol valerate, or estriol succinate (Toy et al, 1978). The latter finding does seem to be a specific drug-related response, rather than a dose-related effect, in that all the estrogens thus far incriminated in clinical reports as potential thrombogenics are unnatural compounds with an alkylated side chain which renders their metabolism and inactivation slow and inefficient. It is possible that the use of natural estrogens such as estradiol, estrone or estriol would avoid the problem of thrombosis.

The significance of the reported effects of different estrogens on various coagulation-related factors in clinical terms is far from clear. The early promise that naturally occurring estrogens may be safer than synthetic estrogens is inconclusive but encouraging. Until the situation is clarified, estrogen usage should be avoided in patients with pre-existing risk factors for thromboembolism, particularly a previous history of deep venous thrombosis or severe varicosities, obesity, hypertension, diabetes, and heavy smoking. It is likely that postmenopausal estrogen replacement will carry a clinical risk of thromboembolism greater than that of the contraceptive pill in view of the type of population to receive such therapy. Large epidemiologic, clinical, and laboratory based studies are urgently needed. One reassuring factor has been the failure to find a statistically significant association between current regular use of estrogen and nonfatal acute myocardial infarction or stroke (Rosenberg et al, 1976).

Increase in blood pressure

Estrogens are not generally associated with any significant elevation of diastolic blood pressure in postmenopausal women (Utian, 1978b). Nevertheless, some postmenopausal women have an idiosyncratic response to conjugated estrogens with blood pressure elevations (Notelovitz, 1975; Utian, 1978b). In view of the potential adverse effects of such a blood pressure increase, all women on long-term estrogen treatment should have blood pressure readings taken every six months as part of their routine medical follow-up examination.

Gallstones

The incidence of gallstones, or certainly that of gallstones requiring surgical treatment, has been reported to be increased in women taking estrogens after menopause (Boston Collaborative Drug Surveillance Program, 1974). In real figures, the incidence rate of gallbladder disease requiring surgical treatment increases from 87/100 000 per year in healthy women aged 45 to 49 not on estrogens to 218/100 000 for estrogen users. This is a relative risk of 2.5 times that of a control group. The case-fatality rate for cholecystectomy is estimated at 0.28 per cent for patients between the age of 50 and 69 (Weinstein, 1980).

Changes in glucose tolerance

Most carbohydrate metabolism studies on estrogens and progestogens have been applied to oral contraceptive populations and very few in relation to use after menopause. In general, the effect of exogenous estrogens on glucose tolerance of postmenopausal women has been reassuring. Few significant changes have been found in either the fasting glucose values, glucose tolerance curves, or on plasma insulin levels. However, some idiosyncratic responses may occur (Notelovitz, 1976; Spellacy et al, 1972; Thom et al, 1976).

Notelovitz (1976) felt that conjugated estrogens could impair glucose tolerance in a small percentage of patients. Thom et al (1976) however found that conjugated equine estrogen or estradiol valerate did not impair glucose tolerance. Goldzieher and co-workers (1978) in an extremely well-controlled study, were unable to show any adverse effect of ethinyl estradiol or mestranol on carbohydrate metabolism or any effect of added progestogen compounds on estrogen-treated women. Nonetheless, Spellacy et al (1972) believe that estrogen-progestogen combinations may have a synergistic effect and impair glucose tolerance, and, indeed, Thom et al (1976) did show a significant deterioration of carboyhdrate tolerance in patients on combinations of ethinyl-estradiol or mestranol with progestogens.

Spellacy et al (1972) reported a significant increase in bodyweight in patients on estrogen therapy. This finding was not confirmed by Utian (1978b) nor by McKay et al (1978) who found a decrease in weight on estrogen therapy. Goldzieher et al, 1978 have emphasized that glucose intolerance and diabetes mellitus are not the same thing, and it is inappropriate to infer that any steroid-induced changes carry with them the long-term hazards associated with diabetes mellitus.

It would seem at present that correct estrogen usage does not generally result in significant or prolonged alterations in glucose tolerance. However, risk factors such as a family history of diabetes, suggestive obstetric history of potential diabetes, and obesity should be carefully evaluated before prescribing estrogens. Diabetes does not of itself stand as an absolute contraindication to estrogen treatment. It is recommended that a two-hour post-glucose blood level be measured once a year in all patients, diabetic or not, on long-term estrogen therapy. The latter then should be the only direct cost incurred in this respect.

Costs — direct and indirect

In a world beset with problems of inflation, disparity of health programs, and variable health needs, it would be more than presumptuous to attempt to advise on the desirability of a general estrogen prophylaxis program and to estimate costs for such a program for any specific region. Costs can be calculated according to the formula already presented utilizing local statistics. The following information is of general interest.

Direct treatment costs

Aitken (1976) and Dewhurst (1976) independently estimated that the total annual drug bill for Britain would be about £90 000 000 (approximately $183 000 000) if conjugated estrogens were routinely prescribed for prophylaxis. Dewhurst calculated that the bill for medical services would add a further £65 000 000 ($132 000 000) per year. Greenwald et al (1977) estimated that 14 per cent of American women over the age of 45 were taking estrogens in 1975, predominantly conjugated estrogen at a cost of $82 777 000. Aitken estimated that general use of conjugated equine estrogens in Britain could cost about £88 500 000 ($180 000 000) whereas cheap synthetics would cost about £2 600 000 ($5 300 000).

Controversy exists in drug selection and different estrogens do appear to exert different effects. In addition to usage of local statics, cost-effectiveness analysis should be applied to the use of all the presently available types of estrogen.

On an individual basis, therapeutic costs depend not only on drug costs, but also the number of physician visits and special tests performed. Minimal annual costs in the United States calculated for cyclic conjugated estrogen (0.625 mg) treatment would be:

Pill costs	$100
Physician follow-up visits — (2) —	$ 50
Endometrial biopsy	$100

The patient can therefore expect an annual cost of $150 without endometrial biopsy, $250 with biopsy and additional costs for any other specific tests, for example, lipid analysis or blood glucose level.

Potential side-effect costs

D & C for postmenopausal bleeding. Weinstein (1980) has estimated that 0.3 per cent of patients will require D & C during the first two years of estrogen treatment at a cost of $500 per operation and a case-fatality rate of 0.1 per cent.

Uterine cancer. Average treatment costs per case in the United States have been calculated to be $3200 (11.7 days of hospitalization at $200 per day, plus surgeon's fee of $700, plus incremental cost of radiotherapy) (Weinstein, 1980).

Breast cancer. The treatment cost per case has been estimated by Weinstein, 1980 to be $3500 (11.7 hospital days at $200/day plus surgeon's fee $700, plus allowance for radiotherapy and prosthesis). Annual mammography as a screening procedure would add to direct costs.

Cholecystectomy. The cost per case would be about $3500 (14.4 hospital days at $200/day plus surgeon's fee of $600) (Weinstein, 1980).

Potential savings

Osteoporosis. Weinstein (1980) estimated the cost of treatment per hip fracture to be about $6000 in the United States (24 hospital days at $200/day, plus surgeon's fee $700, plus nursing and rehabilitation costs). Treatment of wrist fracture was estimated to cost $250 if handled on an outpatient basis.

Aitken (1976) calculated that the annual cost of treating femoral neck and Colles' fractures in a stable population of 200 000 people (in which population there would be about 38 000 women over 45) would be about £40 000 ($81 500), or looked at in wider context, about £10 000 000 ($21 000 000) for the whole of Britain per year. This would allow £1 ($2.00) per head per annum before the cost of prophylaxis exceeded the likely cost of treating complications of osteoporosis as they arose. Unfortunately, the British figures do not take into account the Health Status Index, that is, the cost to the patient of being in pain or disabled or unable to live an independent existence. Recalculation of the figures with true cost-effectiveness analysis would therefore be of greater value. In Britain, nonetheless, the cost of prevention of osteoporosis clearly far exceeds the cost of treatment of the developed problem.

BALANCING THE RISKS AND BENEFITS

It is obvious that the tradeoff between risks and benefits, or risk:benefit ratio, is finely balanced. This leads to difficulty in deciding whether estrogen should be administered or not. The logical response is to apply what may be termed the '*minimax concept*' (Utian, 1978a); that is, aim to minimize the risks and maximize the benefits. This necessitates giving due care to factors such as detailed clinical evaluation so that patients with risk factors do not receive therapy, specific selection of drug, therapeutic regime, added progestogen, detailed follow-up, and so forth.

Application of specific analytic methods to long-term estrogen therapy is of value in that it forces physicians and health planners to be explicit about the beliefs and values that underlie their decisions. Where points of view differ, the relative trade-offs can be compared more directly.

The balance of risks and benefits is dependent upon a number of unanswered questions. At the present time the decision to prescribe long-term estrogen therapy must rest upon a choice between relying on a proper analysis despite the present imperfections, or on no analysis at all. To quote Weinstein & Stason (1977): 'The former, in these times of increasingly complex decisions, difficult tradeoffs, and limited resources, is by far the preferred choice'.

Until further results are forthcoming, the following attitudes toward practice could be adopted:

1. Short-term estrogen therapy for specific menopausal symptoms (hot flushes and atrophic vaginitis) is fully acceptable.
2. Long-term hormone therapy is justified in young women undergoing premature menopause, provided the due precautions are observed. This applies particularly to women undergoing early surgical loss of uterus and ovaries. Clearly the absence of risk of uterine cancer and the definitive risk of osteoporosis warrants a recommendation for long-term hormone replacement.
3. Long-term therapy cannot yet be recommended for all women after menopause. It is not, however, justifiable to withhold such treatment from a normal informed patient who requests it on an individual basis, provided there are no contraindications and the patient agrees to regular checkups.
4. Certain rules for estrogen usage and patient follow-up exist and must be observed. In particular, the drug should be administered cyclically or intermittently, and in the lowest effective dose and the patient must be well informed (Utian, 1978c, 1980b).

The menopause and estrogen therapy are emotional subjects, not only to women but to men and to doctors. It is mandatory to keep an open mind on the subject, as new evidence is bound to accumulate at an accelerating pace in the near future. In the interim, the advantages should be maximized and the disadvantages minimized for each potential patient.

Acknowledgements
The author expresses his appreciation to the following publishers for allowing abstracts from or reference to their respective publications:

S. Karger A G, Basel (Utian, W H, 1978, Frontiers Hormone Research, 5: 26–39).

New England Journal of Medicine (Weinstein M C, and Stason W B, 1977, 296: 716; Weinstein M C, 1980, 303: 308–316).

Appleton-Century-Crofts, New York (Utian, W H, 1980. Menopause in Modern Perspective, Appleton-Century-Crofts, New York).

REFERENCES

Aitken J M 1976 Bone metabolism in post-menopausal women. In: Beard R (ed) The menopause. MTP Press, Lancaster, p 95–142

Aitken J M, Hart D M, Lindsay R 1973 Oestrogen replacement therapy for prevention of osteoporosis after oophorectomy. British Medical Journal 3: 515–518

Antunes C M F, Stolley P D, Rosenshein N B et al 1979 Endometrial cancer and estrogen use: report of a large case-control study. New England Journal of Medicine 300: 9–13

Bauer G C H 1970 Epidemiology of fractures. In: Barzel US (ed) Osteoporosis. Grune & Stratton, New York, p 153–163

Bolton C H, Ellwood M, Hartog M et al 1975 Comparison of the effects of ethinyl estradiol and conjugated equine estrogens in oophorectomized women. Clinical Endocrinology 4: 131–138

Boston Collaborative Drug Surveillance Program 1974 Surgically confirmed gallbladder disease, venous thromboembolism and breast tumors in relation to postmenopausal estrogen therapy. New England Journal of Medicine 290: 15–19

Bunker J P, Barnes B A, Mosteller F 1977 Costs, risks and benefits of surgery. Oxford University Press, New York

Burch J C, Byrd B F, Vaughn W K 1974 The effect of long-term estrogen on hysterectomized women. American Journal of Obstetrics and Gynecology 118: 778–782

Bush J W, Chen M M, Patrick D L 1973 Health status index in cost-effectiveness analysis of PKU program. In: Berg R L (ed) Health status indices. Hospital Research and Educational Trust, Chicago

Campbell S 1976 Double blind psychometric studies on the effects of natural estrogens on post-menopausal women. In: Campbell S (ed) The management of the menopause in post-menopausal years. University Park Press, Baltimore, MD, p 149–158

Campbell S, Whitehead M 1977 Oestrogen therapy and the menopause syndrome. In: Greenblatt R B, Studd J W W (eds) Clinics in obstetrics and gynecology, 4: No 1. Saunders, Philadelphia, p 31–47

Dapunt O 1967 The treatment of climacteric symptoms with oestradiol valerate, Medizinische Klinik 62: 1356–1361

Dennerstein L, Wood C, Burrows G D 1977 Sexual response following hysterectomy and oophorectomy. Obstetrics and Gynecology 48: 92–96

Dennerstein L, Burrows G D 1978 A review of studies of the psychological symptoms found at the menopause. Maturitas 1: 55–64

Dewhurst C J 1976 Financial implications of hormone replacement therapy. In: Campbell S (ed) The management of the menopause and postmenopausal years. University Park Press, Baltimore, MD, p 429–430

Editorial: 1977 Rate of hysterectomy increases. Obstetrical and Gynecological News 12: 2

Fedor-Freybergh P 1977 The influence of oestrogens on the wellbeing and mental performance in climacteric and postmenopausal women. Acta Obstetrica et Gynecologica Scandinavica Supplement 64: 1–91

Gallagher J C, Young M M, Nordin B E 1972 Effects of artificial menopause on plasma and urine calcium and phosphate. Clinical Endocrinology 1: 57–64

Gambrell R D 1978 The prevention of endometrial cancer in postmenopausal women with progestogens. Maturitas 1: 107–112

Gambrell R D, Castaneda T A, Ricci C A 1978 Management of postmenopausal bleeding to prevent endometrial cancer. Maturitas 1: 99–106

George G C W, Utian W H, Beumont P J V, Beardwood C J 1973 Effect of exogenous oestrogens on minor psychiatric symptoms in postmenopausal women. South African Medical Journal 47: 2387–2388

Goldzieher J W, Chenault C B, de la Pena A, Dozier T S, Kraemer D C 1978 Comparative studies of the ethinyl estrogens used in oral contraceptives. VI. Effects with and without progestational agents on carboyhydrate metabolism in humans, baboons, and beagles. Fertility and Sterility 30: 146–153

Gordan G S, Picchi J, Roof B S 1973 Antifracture efficacy of long-term estrogens for osteoporosis. Transactions Association of American Physicians 86: 326–332

Gray L A Sr, Christopherson W M, Hoover R N 1977 Estrogens and endometrial carcinoma. Obstetrics and Gynecology 49: 385–389

Greenwald P, Caputo T A, Wolfgang P E 1977 Endometrial cancer after menopausal use of estrogens. Obstetrics and Gynecology 50: 239–243

Gurpide E 1976 Hormones and gynecologic cancer. Cancer 38 (1): 503–508

Gusberg S B 1976 The individual at high risk for endometrial carcinoma. American Journal of Obstetrics and Gynecology 126: 535–542

Hammond C B, Jelovsek F R, Lee K L et al 1979 Effects of long-term estrogen replacement therapy. II Neoplasia, American Journal of Obstetrics and Gynecology 133: 537–547

Hawkinson L F 1938 The menopausal syndrome. One thousand consecutive patients treated with estrogen. Journal of the American Medical Association III: 390–393

Heany R P 1976 Estrogens and postmenopausal osteoporosis. Clinical Obstetrics and Gynecology 19: 791–803

Hoover R, Gray L A Sr, Cole P, MacMahon B 1976 Menopausal estrogens and breast cancer. New England Journal of Medicine 295: 401–405

Horwitz R I, Feinstein A R 1978 Alternative analytic methods for case control studies of estrogens and endometrial cancer. New England Journal of Medicine 299: 1089–1094

Hulka B S, Hogue C J R, Greenberg R G 1978 Methodologic issues in epidemiologic studies of endometrial cancer and exogenous estrogens. American Journal of Epidemiology 107: 267–276

Hulka B S, Fowler W C, Kaufman D G et al 1980 Estrogen and endometrial cancer. American Journal of Obstetrics and Gynecology 137: 92–101

Hutchinson T A, Polansky S M, Feinstein A R 1979 Postmenopausal oestrogens protect against fractures of hip and distal radius: A case-control study. Lancet 2: 705–709

Ingvarsson G 1951 Hormone treated cases of menopausal psychosis. Acta Psychiatrica et Neurologica Scandanavia 26: 155–175

Jain A K, 1977 Mortality risk associated with the use of oral contraceptives. Studies in Family Planning 8: 50–54

Jick H, Watkins R N, Hunter J R et al 1979 Replacement estrogens and endometrial cancer. New England Journal of Medicine 300: 218–222

Kantor H I, Michael C M, Shore H, Ludvigson H W 1968 Administration of estrogens to older women, a psychometric evaluation. American Journal of Obstetrics and Gynecology 101: 658–661

Kistner R W 1976 Estrogen and endometrial cancer. Obstetrics and Gynecology 48: 479–482
Klopper A, Farr J 1978 The epidemiology of endometrial cancer. Frontiers in Hormonal Research
    5: 89–100
Kullander S, Svanberg L, 1975 On climacteric symptoms and their treatment with a new non-steroidal
    estrogen. International Journal of Gynaecology and Obstetrics 13: 277–281
Kupperman H S, Wetchler B B, Blatt M H G 1959 Contemporary therapy of the menopausal syndrome.
    Journal of the American Medical Association 171: 1627–1637
MacGillivray I, Gow S 1971 Metabolic, hormonal and vascular changes after synthetic oestrogen therapy in
    oophorectomized women. British Medical Journal 2: 73–77
Mack T M, Pike M C, Henderson B E et al 1976 Estrogens and endometrial cancer in a retirement
    community. New England Journal of Medicine 294: 1262–1267
Michael C M, Kantor H I, Shore H 1970 Further psychometric evaluation of older women — the effect of
    estrogen administration. Journal of Gerontology 25: 337–341
McDonald T W, Annegers J F, O'Fallon W M, Dockerty M B, Malkasian G D Jr, Kurland L T 1977
    Exogenous estrogen and endometrial carcinoma: case-control and incidence study. The American
    Journal of Obstetrics and Gynecology 127: 572–580
McKay Hart D, Lindsay R, Purdie D 1978 Vascular complications of long-term oestrogen therapy.
    Frontiers in Hormonal Research 5: 174–191
Notelovitz M 1975 Effect of natural oestrogens on blood pressure and weight in postmenopausal women.
    South African Medical Journal 49: 2251–2257
Notelovitz M, Greig H B W 1975 The effect of natural oestrogens on coagulation. South African Medical
    Journal 49: 101–105
Notelovitz M 1976 The effect of long-term oestrogen replacement therapy on glucose and lipid metabolism
    in postmenopausal women. South African Medical Journal 50: 2001–2003
Peck D R, Lowman R M 1978 Estrogen and postmenopausal breast. Mammographic considerations.
    Journal of the American Medical Association 240: 1733–1735
Punnonen R 1972 Effect of castration and peroral estrogen therapy on the skin. Acta Obstetrica et
    Gynecologica Scandinavica Supplement 21: 44
Rosenberg L, Armstrong B, Jick H 1976 Myocardial infarction and estrogen therapy in postmenopausal
    women. New England Journal of Medicine 294: 1256–1259
Smith D C, Prentice R, Thompson D J, Hermann W L 1975 Association of exogenous estrogen and
    endometrial carcinoma. New England Journal of Medicine 293: 1164–1167
Spellacy W N, Buhi W C, Birk S A 1972 The effect of estrogens on carbohydrate metabolism: glucose,
    insulin, and growth hormone studies on one hundred and seventy one women ingesting premarin,
    mestranol, and ethinyl estradiol for six months. American Journal of Obstetrics and Gynecology
    114: 378–392
Sturdee D W, Wade-Evans T, Paterson M E L, Thom M, Studd J W W 1978 Relations between bleeding
    pattern, endometrial histology, and oestrogen treatment in normal women. British Medical Journal
    1: 1575–1577
Thom M, Chakravarti S, Oram D H, Studd J W W 1976 Effect of hormone replacement therapy on glucose
    tolerance in postmenopausal women. British Journal of Obstetrics and Gynecology 84: 776–783
Thomson J, Oswald I 1977 Effect of Oestrogen on the sleep, mood, and anxiety of menopausal women.
    British Medical Journal 2: 1317–1319
Toy J L, Davies J A, Hancock K W, McNicol G P 1978 The comparative effects of a synthetic and a natural
    oestrogen on the haemostatic mechanism in patients with primary amenorrhea. British Journal of
    Obstetrics and Gynaecology 85: 359–362
Utian W H 1970 Use of vaginal smear in assessment of oestrogenic status of oophorectomized females.
    South African Journal of Obstetrics and Gynecology 8(2): 69–72
Utian W H 1972a The true clinical features of postmenopause and oophorectomy and their response to
    oestrogen therapy. South African Medical Journal 46: 732–737
Utian W H 1972b The mental tonic effect of oestrogens administered to oophorectomized females. South
    African Medical Journal 46: 1079–1082
Utian W H 1972c Effects of oophorectomy and subsequent oestrogen therapy on plasma calcium and
    phosphorous. South African Journal of Obstetrics and Gynaecology 10: 8–13
Utian W H 1973 Comparative trial of P1496, a new non-steroidal estrogen analogue. British Medical
    Journal 1: 579–581
Utian W H 1975 Effect of hysterectomy, oophorectomy and estrogen therapy on libido. International
    Journal of Gynaecology and Obstetrics 13: 97–100
Utian W H 1978a Application of cost-effectiveness analysis to postmenopausal estrogen therapy. Frontiers
    in Hormonal Research 5: 26–39
Utian W H 1978b Effect of postmenopausal estrogen therapy on diastolic blood-pressure and bodyweight.
    Maturitas 1: 3–8

Utian W H 1978c The menopause manual: A woman's guide to the menopause. MTP Press, Lancaster
Utian W H 1980a Menopause in modern perspective. Appleton-Century-Crofts, New York
Utian W H 1980b Your middle years: A doctor's guide for today's woman. Appleton-Century-Crofts, New York
Weinstein M C 1980 Estrogen use in postmenopausal women — costs, risks, and benefits. New England Journal of Medicine 303: 308–316
Weinstein M C, Stason W B 1977 Foundations of cost-effectiveness analysis for health and medical practices. New England Journal of Medicine 296: 716–721
Weiss N S, Szekely D R, Austin D F 1976 Increasing incidence of endometrial cancer in the United States. New England Journal of Medicine 294: 1259–1262
Weiss N S, Ure C L, Ballard J H, Williams A R, Daling J R 1980 Decreased risk of fractures of the hip and lower forearm with postmenopausal use of estrogen. New England Journal of Medicine 303: 1195–1198
Whitehead M I 1978 The effects of oestrogens and progestogens on the postmenopausal endometrium. Maturitas 1: 87–98
Ziel H K, Finkle W D 1975 Increased risk of endometrial carcinoma among users of conjugated estrogens. New England Journal of Medicine 293: 1167–1170
Ziel H K, Finkle W D 1976 Association of estrone with the development of endometrial carcinoma. American Journal of Obstetrics and Gynecology 124: 735–740

15. Advances in the treatment of carcinoma of the cervix and corpus uteri

Per Kolstad

INTRODUCTION

No dramatic changes have taken place in the treatment of carcinoma of the cervix and corpus uteri during the last two decades. Indeed, two of the early pioneers of gynaecological oncology, Margareth Cleaves and Wertheim, published their first reports on the results of the use of intracavitary radium treatment and radical surgery for carcinoma of the cervix at the beginning of this century. These methods remain the corner stones in the management of malignant disease of the uterus. The improvements in the prognosis of both cervix and corpus cancer seen the last two decades are first and foremost dependent upon an earlier stage distribution of the clinical material. Furthermore, the histopathological classification has become more precise with a subgrouping of the different tumours which undoubtedly influence both the choice of treatment and the end results.

Surgeons can today perform extensive radical surgery, e.g. exenteration procedures. This is not only because the surgeons are better trained, but also because they cooperate with well trained specialist teams. The anaesthetists provide optimal surgical conditions with a relaxed and well oxygenated patient, and accurately monitor the balance between fluid and blood loss and input during and after radical pelvic surgery. Within radiobiology, knowledge about the radiosensitivity and radioresistance of different histopathological tumours, the importance of the oxygenation and the effect that radiosensitisers can play in selected patients, occupies an important role in the treatment of cervical cancer. Both experimental and clinical studies indicate that a higher cure rate may be achieved if an optimal oxygen tension can be delivered to the cancer cells, e.g. by the use of atmospheric or hyperbaric oxygen breathing or by overcoming hypoxia by the use of radiosensitisers. Use of heavy particles, as neutrons, protons and pi-mesons, is also intensively studied today, but such sophisticated and expensive treatment schedules are not available for general use. The same holds true for hyperthermic radiotherapy. Within the field of hormone treatment of cancer, carcinoma of the corpus is an excellent model for studies both of preoperative, postoperative and adjuvant treatment with gestagens and/or anti-oestrogens, and also for studies of the role of hormone treatment in patients with advanced stages of the disease.

New chemotherapeutic drugs are placed at our disposal almost every month. It is difficult to evaluate their place in the treatment of gynaecological cancer. These drugs present a challenge to the clinician who must explore both the short- and the long-term effects in early, advanced, and recurrent disease. Gynaecological oncologists should, however, be cautious about changing their treatment methods too frequently because reports on new combination chemotherapeutic regimes seem to show better treatment results. In our cancer centre in Oslo, the Norwegian Radium Hospital (NRH), we have tried a variety of regimes, especially in invasive carcinoma of the cervix and ovarian cancer. In the last decade between 300 and 400 new cases of invasive carcinoma of the cervix, 200 to 300 cases of ovarian cancer and 180 to 200 cases of corpus cancer have been referred each year. Almost all recurrences return to our unit for evaluation to decide if additional treatment including chemotherapy may be helpful. Our many attempts with different combination regimes to help these unfortunate patients cannot so far be claimed to be very successful. My personal opinion is that the so-called 'complete' or 'partial' response rates, which are the most frequently used parameters in the evaluation of the results achieved, do not give a true picture of the patients' situation. Most gynaecological oncologists know that even where a toxic combination therapy regime may give a higher 'complete' response rate, it may not be the best treatment in the single case. What about the long-term survival, and more important, the quality of life of those women who may live two, four, six or perhaps even 12 months longer than those who receive less toxic regimes? More and more oncologists emphasise this point. When a so-called 'complete' cure cannot be achieved, the goal must be palliation, which means both physical and psychological comfort. In this context, the hospice concept for terminally ill patients is now generally accepted (McGowan, 1978).

Information about different treatment regimes can be obtained by protocols which are used by cooperating clinics. However, compiling data from clinics which have a small number of cancer patients can be misleading. There will always be selection factors in such series. It is much better if gynaecological cancer is centralised to a few large units with experienced full-time oncologists who are able to agree upon carefully designed treatment protocols. The best way of answering a clinical question is usually to randomise the patients into two or three groups. The series should not be split up in too many groups. It is better to ask one, or perhaps two questions at a time.

Some smaller units have presented remarkably good results. However the problem of selection must be taken into account. The procedures of staging and the different consultants' surgical and/or radiological skill certainly will influence the fate of the patients. If some stage I cases are allotted to stage II, and some stage II cases are allotted to stage III, the end results will be better stage by stage. Upstaging or downstaging makes it difficult to compare results from different oncological centres. Another important factor is the completeness of the follow-up system. When data are presented, which do not take into account that from 5 to 10 or even as many as 20 per cent of the patients have moved to other regions or to other countries where they cannot be traced, the statistical data are not reliable. Among the non-traced patients a high percentage may have died from their disease.

It is also a prerequisite that the records which form the data base for the statistical analysis are designed to allow retrieval of the pertinent information, e.g. as in a computerised system. However, the computer will not provide the final answer to the question of the value of the different treatment methods and, as the old saying goes, 'garbage in, garbage out': we must ensure that the medical records contain only relevant and important data.

Currently a large number of articles are published about treatment methods and results and assessments often difficult. Nevertheless, some advances in the treatment of carcinoma of the cervix and corpus uteri seem to repeat themselves from clinic to clinic. Some of the information which has appeared during the last decade will be reviewed.

CARCINOMA OF THE CERVIX

Epidemiology

Although this chapter is concerned mainly with treatment methods and results, some comments about epidemiology of cervical cancer are pertinent. There are still differences of opinion about the value of screening for cervical carcinoma. Nevertheless, data has accumulated which shows that in areas where cytological screening has been carried out for a sufficient period of time, which means at least 10 to 15 years, both the incidence and mortality of invasive carcinoma of the cervix has been reduced (Fidler et al, 1970; Hakama & Räsänen-Virtanen, 1976; MacGregor, 1976). Furthermore, also in regions where the use of cytologic smears has not been part of a systematic screening programme, but nevertheless commonly used in general practice, the stage distribution of cases detected has improved. The main problem today is to reach those women who are at the highest risk of developing invasive cancer. Such high risk groups, which usually belong to the lower socio-economic classes are more apt to avoid screening centres, and furthermore, they are late in consulting a doctor when they get symptoms. If a computerised invitation programme could reach and encourage all women within the age groups which ought to have a regular gynaecological examination each year including the taking of smears (women between 20 to 25 and 55 to 60 years of age), a significant reduction in the mortality of cancer of the cervix could possibly be obtained. Within these age groups all studies have shown that the yield from screening is so high that it is worthwhile to use part of our medical and economical resources to conduct such screening programmes. This seems to be an established truth in the United States, in Canada and in several other countries both in Europe and other parts of the world.

Histopathology

The international histological classification of malignant tumours of the cervix uteri is shown in Table 15.1. This classification has been agreed upon by the World Health Organisation Group of Histopathologists, the International Federation of Gynecology

Table 15.1 Histological classification of malignant tumours of the cervix uteri

Epithelial tumours
1. Squamous cell carcinoma (epidermoid carcinoma)
   - (a) Keratinising
   - (b) Large-cell non-keratinising
   - (c) Small-cell non-keratinising
2. Adenocarcinoma, endocervical type
3. Endometrioid adenocarcinoma
4. Clear cell (mesonephroid) adenocarcinoma
5. Adenoid cystic carcinoma
6. Adenosquamous carcinoma
7. Undifferentiated carcinoma

Non-epithelial tumours
1. Leiomyosarcoma
2. Embryonal rhabdomyosarcoma (sarcoma botryoides)
3. Müllerian mixed tumour

and Obstetrics and the American Joint Committee. In this review I will not discuss non-epithelial tumours, sarcomas, mixed tumours or secondary tumours.

In agreement with other histopathologists, we have not been able to confirm that grading systems as those suggested by Martzloff (1923), Broders (1926), Wentz & Reagan (1959) are of value for deciding upon treatment. There are, however, some tumours that should be excluded from our statistics on treatment results. An example of this is the so-called apudomas. The ultimate diagnosis of these rare endocrine secreting tumours can be done by electron-microscopic studies. Local control can be achieved by irradiation or surgery, but they behave clinically as the oat-cell tumours of the lung with early distant metastases.

It seems also reasonable that clear cell adenocarcinomas, the so-called adenoid cystic carcinomas (which usually are found in older women) and the adenosquamous carcinomas should not be included in the statistics about treatment results in carcinoma of the cervix. All adenomatoid lesions, endocervical, endometrioid and the above mentioned apudomas should be reported separately.

Stage distribution

As long ago as 1929 Heyman, Lacassagne & Woltz agreed upon a clinical staging of carcinoma of the cervix. Their pioneer work is still the basis for our present management of women with cervical cancer.

The distribution by stages will of course influence the choice of therapy. Stage grouping of carcinoma of the cervix, which is internationally agreed upon, can be studied in detail in the 17th Annual report on the results of treatment of gynecological cancer (1979). In Table 15.2 this staging system is presented.

Table 15.2   Stage grouping of carcinoma of the cervix

Pre-invasive carcinoma	
Stage O	Carcinoma in situ, intra-epithelial carcinoma
	Cases of Stage O should not be included in any therapeutic statistics for invasive carcinoma.
Invasive carcinoma	
Stage I	Carcinoma strictly confined to the cervix (extension to the corpus should be disregarded).
Stage Ia	Microinvasive carcinoma (early stromal invasion).
Stage Ib	All other cases of stage I. Occult cancer should be marked 'occ'.
Stage II	The carcinoma extends beyond the cervix, but has not extended on to the pelvic wall. The carcinoma involves the vagina, but not the lower third.
Stage IIa	No obvious parametrial involvement.
Stage IIb	Obvious parametrial involvement.
Stage III	The carcinoma has extended on to the pelvic wall. On rectal examination there is no cancer-free space between the tumour and the pelvic wall. The tumour involves the lower third of the vagina. All cases with a hydro-nephrosis or non-functioning kidney should be included, unless they are known to be due to other cause.
Stage IIIa	No extension on to the pelvic wall.
Stage IIIb	Extension on to the pelvic wall and/or hydro-nephrosis or non-functioning kidney.
Stage IV	The carcinoma has extended beyond the true pelvis or has clinically involved the mucosa of the bladder or rectum. A bullous oedema as such does not permit a case to be allotted to Stage IV.
Stage IVa	Spread of the growth to adjacent organs.
Stage IVb	Spread to distant organs.

Stage O

Because of the wide-spread use of exfoliative cytology and in the later decades also colposcopy, more and more young females are detected with precursors to invasive carcinoma of the cervix. Papanicolaou published his first paper on the detection of cancer cells in smears from the vagina in 1928, and Hinselman described his method of colposcopy in 1925. The real value of these two pioneers' observations was not recognised until several decades later. Papanicolaou was proposed as candidate for the Nobel Prize. There is no doubt that he would have deserved this high award.

The method of detecting cervical cancer by cytology was refined and spread in the United States, while the method of colposcopy was taken up by gynaecologists in German-speaking countries, in Eastern Europe, in France, in Spanish-speaking countries in South America, and in Australia. Today, most gynaecologists dealing with preinvasive lesions of the cervix agree that cytology and colposcopy are complementary methods that will make it possible to decide upon a precise and as a rule conservative treatment for preinvasive cervical lesions which mostly affect women in the childbearing years of their life.

In English-speaking countries a so-called 'suspect' or 'positive' smear was 10 to 20 years ago followed either by conisation or hysterectomy. If dysplasia or carcinoma in situ was found in the cone specimen, hysterectomy was recommended. This means that most females with a 'suspect smear' lost their uterus irrespective of their age. It has been clearly documented that the combined use of cytology and colposcopy enable much more conservative therapy. Many of the preinvasive lesions in young women are today treated by thermocautery, or cryosurgery, and recently by Laser-evaporation. However, all patients who have had a precursor to invasive cervical cancer are at risk to recurrences or the development of new lesions either in the cervix, vagina or the vulval region. Life-long follow-up is essential (Kolstad & Klem, 1976).

Stage Ia
The concept of early invasive cancer of the cervix, 'microcarcinoma', is controversial. Other terms used are 'occult', 'pre-clinical', and 'small'. In the literature, we find that some oncologists who are of the opinion that invasion 1 mm below the basement membrane should be classified as stage Ia lesions, and all other cases should be classified to the stage Ib. It is difficult to understand why gynaecological oncologists disagree so much about the definition of stage Ia carcinoma of the cervix. The acceptable limit of extension into the stroma varies from 1 to 7 mm. Furthermore, some histopathologists measure the invasion into the stroma from the basement membrane, others measure the invasion from the surface of the epithelium on the ecto- or the endocervix, and some measure the invasion into the stroma from the lowermost gland in the area.

The International Federation of Gynecology and Obstetrics has up to date not been able to agree upon a precise definition of stage Ia cancer of the cervix, 'microinvasive carcinoma'. In the 17th Annual report on the results of treatment of gynecologic cancer (1979) stage Ia lesions are defined as follows:

'Stage Ia represents those cases of epithelial abnormalities in which histological evidence of early stromal invasion is unambiguous. The diagnosis should be based on microscopical examination of tissue removed by biopsy, conisation, portio amputation or the removed uterus.' This definition is vague and the biopsy diagnosis cannot be accepted. Furthermore, the definition does not take into account the depth and extent of the disease. Therefore, at the International Congress of FIGO in Tokyo in 1979 a subcommittee was appointed to try to solve some of the definition problems

(R. Scully, M.D., E. Burghardt, M.D., and the author of this article). The committee has found that there are three methods to define microinvasive carcinoma of the cervix. The most sophisticated definition proposed by Professor Burghardt and his colleagues in Austria and Germany includes a volume measurement. The Harvard group is of the opinion that 2 to 3 mm of invasion into the stroma measured from the basement membrane is the limit for classifying the lesion as microinvasive carcinoma. All other cases should be allotted to stage Ib. A compromise would be that the lesion should always be measured on a cone specimen in two dimensions. Growth into the stroma of 4 to 5 mm measured from the surface epithelium or 2 to 3 mm from the basement membrane, and at the same time not more than up to 10 mm in the longitudinal direction measured on the ecto- or endocervix should be classified as 'microcarcinoma' or stage Ia.

Another difficult area is the importance of invasion into lymphatic vessels or blood vessels. The opinions among both clinicians and histopathologists on this question vary so much that I would recommend that invasion into endothelial lined spaces should not be included in the definition of stage Ia. The clinician with experience in this problem has to take such an observation into account when deciding upon treatment. We all have to work with our own histopathologists.

The World Health Organisation has pointed out that in some cases the very earliest signs of invasion into the stroma are buds of cells connected with the surface epithelium which penetrate not more than 1 mm into the underlying stroma. These cases are called carcinoma in situ which questionable (minimal) stromal invasion (Poulsen et al, 1975) and can safely be treated for example by conisation. Larger lesions must be measured in two dimensions and in such cases conisation may be used as the ultimate treatment as long as there are no signs of invasion into lymph vessels. If tumour cells are found in endothelial lined spaces, in our experience, the patients should be treated either by simple hysterectomy with pelvic lymphadenectomy or intracavitary radiotherapy followed by external radiation to the pelvic lymph nodes (Iversen et al, 1979).

Stage Ib

The decision about treatment in carcinoma of the cervix stage Ib is dependent on several factors: histopathology, size of tumour, location in the ectocervix or endocervix, the age of the patient, and complicating diseases. Arguments about the radiosensitivity of the adenocarcinomas are still going on. They possibly are slightly more radioresistant than the squamous cell carcinomas.

The majority of the stage Ib lesions are of the squamous cell type. Grading of these tumours was first performed by Martzloff in 1923 and Broders in 1926. However, clinicians have not been able to prove that any grading system can be used in practice to decide upon type of treatment. This also holds true for the system suggested by Wentz & Reagan (1959). They divide the squamous cell lesions of the cervix into small cell carcinomas, large cell non-keratinising and large cell keratinising carcinomas. Some studies seem to show that the small cell carcinomas have a poorer prognosis, but other observations do not confirm that this is true (Beecham et al, 1978). This discrepancy may be due to the fact that the endocrine secreting apudomas in most series have been listed as 'poorly differentiated', 'undifferentiated' or 'small cell carcinomas'.

Today, it seems that more and more centres individualise treatment in stage Ib lesions, especially in the younger age groups. In small lesions which by clinical examination and colposcopy are shown to be located to the ectocervix, radical surgery with removal of the uterus, the cervix, the parametria, the upper part of the vagina, and the lymph nodes, but with preservation of the ovaries, is in many centres the treatment of choice. Larger tumours, and especially those which are located in the endocervix with a barrel-shaped cervix, are not so easily operated upon. By using preoperative intracavitary treatment with radium, caesium or cobalt sources, radical surgery with lymphadenectomy can more safely be done, with less infections in the postoperative period (Rampone et al, 1973). In the older age groups, many clinicians prefer radiotherapy combining intracavitary treatment and external highvoltage radiotherapy.

In the 17th annual report on the results of treatment in carcinoma of the cervix and other gynaecological cancers the larger centres with wide experience either in surgery or in radiotherapy present approximately the same treatment results.

There are differences of opinion about the value of lymphadenectomy. It should be realised, however, that so-called 'lymphadenectomy' may include everything from sampling of a few nodes, which Wertheim performed, up to complete removal of all nodes in the pelvis draining the cervix and the corpus uteri. Preferably, the completeness of the procedure should be controlled by intra-operative lymphographic films (Kolbenstvedt & Kolstad, 1976). If this is not performed, usually a large number of nodes will be left behind. By meticulous dissection and a meticulous histopathological study of the removed nodes, it has been found that in stage Ib lesions there are approximately 25 per cent of node involvement, and even in the common iliac region the figure is as high as 20 per cent (Kolbenstvedt & Kolstad, 1976). Many authors believe that lymphadenectomy will not increase the survival rate. In our own series we have found that the salvage rate in stage Ib lesions has gone up from approximately 75 per cent to 85 to 90 per cent by using intra-operative control of the completeness of the removal of the lymph nodes. By giving high voltage irradiation to the patients with positive nodes, between 50 and 60 per cent survive five years. It is important to stress, however, that we cannot really compare results from country to country or from clinic to clinic. In stage I carcinoma of the cervix involvement of lymph nodes in the pelvis has been found in between 8 to 9 per cent up to 25 per cent of the cases (Gad, 1976; Kneale, 1970; Kolbenstvedt & Kolstad, 1976; Nieminen et al, 1977). These discrepancies may in part be due to many cases of stage Ia lesions (microcarcinomas) being included in the series with the lowest percentage of node involvement, and also to a systematic upstaging of cases.

Both radical surgery, modern radiotherapy and combined treatment may give approximately the same end results in stage I carcinoma of the cervix. However, more and more young females are detected with stage Ia and small stage Ib carcinomas. Surgical treatment may in these cases be the treatment of choice. Hospitalisation will be short, and the cost of treatment less expensive. Furthermore, preservation of the ovaries is also an important point. Spread to the ovaries from cervical cancer in the early stages is extremely rare. The ovaries should in young women be transposed outside a possible postoperative radiation field if metastases are found to the pelvic lymph nodes.

It should also be emphasised that the 17th annual report on the treatment of gynaecological cancer (1979) indicates that small stage IIa lesions should be treated by combined radiotherapy and surgery rather than by surgery alone or radiotherapy alone. A multivariant analysis performed by Dr Folke Pettersson seems to show that combined treatment methods should be recommended in the future.

Stages II, III and IV
Surgical treatment of the more advanced cases, stages IIb, III and IV, seems only to have a place in recurrent disease. Primary treatment with surgery in the larger stage IIb lesions and in stages III and IV is not to be recommended. Combined intracavitary and high voltage external radiation should be preferred. The best schedule is to give external irradiation to shrink the tumour before intracavitary radium, cobalt or caesium sources are applied.

In earlier years, external irradiation was given by ordinary 200 to 300 kV machines with a four field technique. The distribution of irradiation to the lateral pelvic wall and to the parametrium was poor. After the introduction of cobalt sources the results seemed to improve. Betatron machines and linear accelerators were found to be more flexible and give better end results than the cobalt machines.

At present, the best and most flexible machines probably are the linear accelerators. At an energy above 4 to 7 MeV, they deliver an ideal dose to the parametria and the lateral pelvic wall. Data presented by Bush (1979) clearly show that linear accelerators and betatron machines are superior to cobalt machines in gynaecological cancer.

The importance of oxygenation, radiosensitisers and heavy particles is at present being tested in many centres. It has been proved beyond doubt that hypoxic cells are two to three times less radiosensitive than well oxygenated cells (Gray, 1961). This fact has led to a series of trials all over the world. In our institution atmospheric oxygen breathing was used during a clinical trial, and a small difference was found between the group receiving oxygen as compared to the controls (Bergsjö & Kolstad, 1968). There are trials reported on hyperbaric oxygen radiotherapy which seem to prove that some patients will benefit from such therapy (Bates & Churchill-Davidson, 1975). However, the method is time-consuming, and there are also some hazards involved in using high oxygen pressure. Therefore, radiosensitisers have become more popular in attempts to increase the results of radiotherapy in large stage IIb, III and IV lesions. Piver et al (1974) have used hydroxurea in connection with radiotherapy and claim that the results were improved. Other sensitisers which are at present being investigated are Metronidazole and Misonidazole. It is too early to evaluate if Misonidazole and radiotherapy are an acceptable combination for overcoming the radioresistance of poorly oxygenated cancer cells in carcinoma of the cervix. The same holds true with attempts at using heavy particles (neutrons, pi-mesons) and hyperthermia during radiotherapy. However, some promising results have been reported, although the numbers are small and the follow-up relatively short.

Chemotherapy
Most oncologists do not believe that carcinoma of the cervix is sensitive to chemotherapeutic agents. In the literature we can find that most of the drugs which we have at our disposal today, have been tried either as single drug or in combination therapy.

In preinvasive lesions in the vulval region, the vagina and the cervix, topical application of 5 per cent 5-fluoro-uracil has been used with success in young women (Ballon et al, 1979). Bleomycin cream as suppositories have also been shown to be effective against carcinoma in situ of the vagina.

In invasive cervical carcinoma both alkylating agents, antimetabolites, vinca alkaloids and antibiotics have been used in recurrent and advanced cases. There is no doubt that some of these drugs can give palliation for some months, especially pain relief. Thiotepa, cyclophosphamide and 5-fluoro-uracil have been used for this purpose.

Bleomycin was early on thought to be the drug of choice since good results could be achieved in squamous carcinomas of the head and neck, and also in vulval carcinomas. However, the trials to date have been disappointing. A regimen with Bleomycin and Methotrexate was some years ago reported to give a relatively high response rate (Conroy et al, 1976). This combination chemotherapy has, however, with increasing experience, also been a disappointment. The same holds true for Adriamycin. A realistic picture of the current situation concerning chemotherapy in carcinoma of the cervix is shown by the fact that during the last congress of the International Federation of Gynecology and Obstetrics in 1979 in Tokyo nearly 1000 papers were delivered and only five papers were concerned with some form of chemotherapy in cervical cancer (Sakamoto et al, 1980).

Combining chemotherapy and radiation has also been studied. As mentioned above, Piver et al (1974) reported that hydroxurea improved the control and length of survival in cancer of the cervix. This drug was used because of experimental evidence suggesting that it had a synergistic effect with radiation. Another trial combining radiation and 5-fluoro-uracil has shown no additional benefit. Nevertheless, the use of chemotherapeutic agents in the treatment of cancer of the cervix needs to be explored further. It does seem, however, that we cannot obtain better treatment results by adding chemotherapy to conventional surgical or radiation therapy. On the contrary, it might be that chemotherapy may reduce the immunological surveillance of the host. We still have to set up our trials with chemotherapy only in those cases that cannot be adequately treated either by surgery or radiotherapy. In our unit we have seen responses with reduction of lung metastases following the use of both alkylating agents, antimetabolites, antibiotics or combination of several of these drugs. In the last years we have also tried cis-platinum with some subjective and objective effect, but unfortunately this has been short-lasting.

The value of carcinoembryonic antigen studies in the evaluation and follow-up of cancer of the cervix

Several investigators have demonstrated that there is a direct correlation between tumour volume and plasma values of carcinoembryonic antigen (CEA) in carcinoma of the cervix (Khoo & Mackay, 1974; Van Nagel et al, 1975). However, it has not been demonstrated that a high pretreatment value of CEA is related to a poor prognosis. Van Nagel et al (1975) stated that pretherapy plasma values were of no value in predicting which patients would develop recurrence. Their material included a large percentage of advanced cases. In a recent study by Kjörstad & Örjasaeter (1981) a good correlation between the plasma values and prognosis in stages I and II was found. Furthermore, the same authors (Kjörstad & Örjasaeter, 1977) showed that in adenocarcinoma of the cervix stage I there was a direct correlation between metastases to the lymph nodes and an elevated CEA in plasma. No patient with localised disease had a value over 4.0 n/ml. It was found that adenocarcinomas of the cervix and corpus had different biological properties, and that in adenocarcinoma of the cervix determination of CEA is a reliable indicator of the extent of the disease.

The failing prognostic value of CEA in the advanced stages of squamous cell carcinoma is difficult to explain. It is obvious that CEA can only reflect tumour burden in patients with CEA releasing tumours. Therefore, in advanced stages of the disease low values are equivocal, meaning in many cases a lack of CEA releasing capacity. Sequential post-therapy determination of CEA may be especially helpful in the detection of patients with recurrent disease in stages I and II. Many of the patients in whom the diagnosis of recurrence in based solely on the presence of an elevated CEA, will be without symptoms. In most cases, it is extremely difficult to determine the site of recurrence, and so far, such studies have not been of much practical value in the treatment of recurrences. This is especially so since chemotherapy has a very small place in the treatment of squamous cell carcinoma of the cervix.

CARCINOMA OF THE CORPUS UTERI

Epidemiology

In many western countries endometrial carcinoma has become the most common gynaecological malignancy, but the mortality from this disease is much less than that for ovarian and cervical malignancies. It is difficult to assess this possible increase in endometrial carcinoma because for many years in statistical reports a large number of cases have been recorded as 'uterus unspecified'. The increase may also be due to the fact that a larger proportion of the population is now post-menopausal, and endometrial carcinoma is well known to be more frequent after 50 to 60 years of age. Nevertheless, some cancer registries show data which seem to indicate that the age-specific incidence rate of carcinoma of the endometrium is significantly higher in some age groups compared to 20 years ago (Gusberg, 1980; The Cancer Registry of Norway, 1972; Walker, 1980).

The aetiology of endometrial carcinoma is unknown, but there are certain factors which are associated with predisposition to this malignancy. The patients are usually post-menopausal, obese, with a low infertility index, and a relatively high percentage have pre-diabetes or diabetes. During their younger years, and especially before menopause, a history of irregular menstruation with anovulatory bleedings can be obtained. Hypertension is also more common among women with endometrial cancer as compared to the normal population.

These observations suggest that there is an abnormality in the hypothalamic-pituitary ovarian hormonal axis. It has also been shown that androstendione can act as a precursor of oestrone, and this conversion most probably takes place in fat tissue. Other factors that indicate a hormonal factor in endometrial cancer is that relatively young women with Stein-Leventhal syndrome, which is associated with menstrual irregularities, infertility, obesity, and hirsutism have a relatively high frequency of endometrial carcinoma. The same holds true for those patients with oestrogen-producing tumours, especially thecomas and granulosa-theca cell tumours of the ovaries.

Histopathology

Carcinoma of the corpus develops from the endometrial glands. In this chapter the malignant tumours developing from the fibrous and mesenchymal stroma or the myometrial part of the corpus uteri will not be discussed.

The adenocarcinomas are usually divided into three grades:

1. Highly differentiated adenocarcinomas (G1)
2. Moderately differentiated adenocarcinomas (G2)
3. Poorly differentiated carcinomas or mainly solid carcinomas (G3).

It is important to keep in mind that the G3 tumours are much more malignant than the G1 and G2 tumours.

For many years a special group of tumours, the so-called 'adeno-acanthomas', in some studies were found to have a good, in other studies a poor prognosis. Today most histopathologists agree that adeno-acanthomas only represent adenocarcinomas with some areas of squamous metaplasia. If there are no signs of atypicality of the metaplastic epithelium, the prognosis is only dependent upon the differentiation of the adenomatous part of the lesion.

However, other types of tumours certainly carry a poorer prognosis, the so-called 'adenosquamous carcinomas' and the mesonephroid or clear cell carcinomas of the corpus uteri (Scully, 1980). The last mentioned tumours are frequently misinterpreted as true adenocarcinomas, because they do not always show the typical clear cells, but mostly so-called 'hob-nail' cells. Areas with 'hob-nail' structures may be difficult to recognise during routine histopathological work. If the adenosquamous carcinomas and the clear cell (hob-nail) carcinomas could be separated from the true adenocarcinomas, it would help to guide therapy and prognosis.

Stage distribution

The group from Radiumhemmet, Stockholm, Sweden, especially Heyman and Kottmeier have made major contributions to our knowledge about the fate of the patients with different stages of carcinoma of the corpus. The FIGO staging of carcinoma of the corpus which is at present accepted by most authorities around the world, is shown in Table 15.3. Unfortunately, even well known authorities within gynaecological oncology tend to modify this staging system. This makes it difficult to compare treatment results on an international basis. Since radiotherapy alone with,

Table 15.3 Stage grouping of carcinoma of the corpus

Stage O	Carcinoma in situ. Histological findings suspicious of malignancy. Cases of Stage O should not be included in any therapeutic statistics.
Stage I	The carcinoma is confined to the corpus including the isthmus.
Stage Ia	The length of the uterine cavity is 8 cm or less.
Stage Ib	The length of the uterine cavity is more than 8 cm.
Stage II	The carcinoma has involved the corpus and the cervix, but has not extended outside the uterus.
Stage III	The carcinoma has extended outside the uterus, but not outside the true pelvis.
Stage IV	The carcinoma has extended outside the true pelvis or has obviously involved the mucosa of the bladder or rectum. A bullous oedema as such does not permit a case to be allotted to Stage IV.
Stage IVa	Spread of the growth to adjacent organs as urinary bladder, rectum, sigmoid, or small bowel.
Stage IVb	Spread to distant organs.

for example, packing of the uterus followed by external irradiation may be compared with combined treatment or surgery only, it is essential to use a clinical staging system. Findings of spread to the ovaries or other structures in the pelvis will often make the oncologist change his staging when reporting treatment results.

The most controversial question in the clinical staging of carcinoma of the corpus is how to prove that there is extension to the cervix, or in the later stages, that there is extension to other pelvic organs. Fractional curettage may show tumour cells in the specimen received from the cervix before dilating the internal os (stage II), but these fragments may only be contamination from the tumour in the uterus (Onsrud et al, 1981).

Furthermore, it is often difficult to perform clinical staging of these patients even under anaesthesia. They are frequently obese, and the details of the anatomical structures in the pelvis are not easy to evaluate. Fortunately, the majority belong to stage I, which means that the tumour by ordinary clinical examination including fractional curettage is located only to the endometrium, infiltrating more or less into the myometrium of the body of the uterus.

Treatment

Stage O

There is no doubt that so-called 'adenomatous atypical hyperplasia' of the endometrium is a precursor to invasive carcinoma of the corpus. Unfortunately, different histopathologists still do not agree upon the classification of the very early stage of endometrial carcinoma. It is difficult to decide if a lesion is to be classified as benign adenomatous hyperplasia, adenomatous atypical hyperplasia, 'carcinoma in situ', or a well differentiated carcinoma, when the histopathologist is only examining curettings from the endometrial cavity. As in carcinoma of the cervix, the histological decision upon the differentiation between an in situ lesion or a lesion which should be classified as invasive carcinoma must usually be made on an operation specimen, which means that we have to remove the uterus. Such a decision is not difficult in women who have had the children they want, but in some cases in the age group below 40 years of age a wish to become pregnant may influence our decision about therapy. Results have been presented that show that treatment with progestagens may eradicate early endometrial lesions (Kistner, 1970; Kjörstad, 1978). It must also be added that the prognosis for those with invasive stage I carcinoma grade I below 40 years of age is extremely good even if treatment is not carried out immediately.

Treatment with high doses of progestagens over six to 12 months will in the majority of cases of atypical adenomatous hyperplasia lead to a normalisation of the histopathological appearance of the endometrium. It must, however, be emphasised that in long-term follow-up of such cases, the preinvasive lesion usually recurs.

Stage I

The diagnosis of stage I carcinoma of the corpus is made by clinical examination, fractional curettage, X-ray examination of the thorax and the skeleton and intravenous pyelograms. In some clinics hysterography and/or hysteroscopy either with the use of carbon dioxide or hiscon, or so-called contact hysteroscopy, are used to find out if the lesion is extending into the endocervix.

Cervical scraping is a controversial method. It is easy to get contamination of cancer cells from the endometrium even if one is extremely careful in not dilating the internal os before starting the scraping of the cervix. In our experience, the occurrence of so-called 'free floating tumour cells' in the endocervical curettings do not confirm a diagnosis of a stage II lesion (Onsrud et al, 1981). Such free floating tumour cells should not alter the decision on therapy as they do not influence the survival rate of these patients compared with unequivocal stage I lesions.

Many oncologists throughout the world are still of the opinion that every patient irrespective of the grade of the tumour, the size of the uterine cavity, or complicating factors such as obesity or diabetes, should receive preoperative irradiation either with intracavitary sources of radium, caesium or cobalt, or by external irradiation. It is, however, becoming more and more usual to perform immediate hysterectomy in all stage I lesions of the corpus. The treatment results after primary surgery compared with those who receive combined radiotherapy and surgery do not show any difference, although randomised clinical studies are lacking. This holds true even for the G3 tumours and for those with a cavity more than 8 cm.

It seems to be well documented that the patients should receive some form of irradiation to the vaginal vault postoperatively. By vaginal applicators which deliver a moderate dose of radiation affecting only the surface epithelium of the vagina, the recurrence rate at this site can be reduced from 10 to 12 per cent to 2 to 4 per cent. The complication rate of vaginal irradiation is minimal.

A much more controversial question is whether patients should receive any treatment to the lymph nodes in the pelvis and the paraaortic region. For decades it has been postulated that corpus cancer has a tendency to spread to the paraaortic glands in the renal hilus. This cannot be confirmed by carefully conducted studies, which have tried to find out if recurrences in this region are common in corpus carcinoma (Conroy et al, 1976). Studies on removal of the lymph nodes have revealed metastases from corpus cancer stage I in between 8 to 14 per cent of the cases. Most commonly spread is found in those with G3 tumours (Boronow, 1976; Morrow et al, 1973).

Since pelvic lymphadenectomy in old often obese patients is difficult, particularly if so-called 'complete dissection' of all the lymph nodes is attempted, it was decided to perform a controlled clinical trial with irradiation to the lateral pelvic walls after primary operation for carcinoma of the corpus (Aalders et al, 1980). In 540 cases, which were randomised to an irradiation group or to a control group, no effect on the five-year or 10-year survival rates was found. However, it was found that by giving external irradiation to the pelvis, a better local control of the tumour was achieved. On the other hand, the patients who received external irradiation had more distant metastases. Those patients who had not had any external irradiation and during follow-up were found to have local recurrences in the pelvis, could be treated by external irradiation with or without gestagens.

Cases with tumour cells in endothelial lined spaces in the myometrium had a greater tendency to spread to the pelvic lymph nodes. Therefore, we now prefer primary surgery followed by external irradiation to those cases with poorly differentiated (G3) tumours penetrating more than half way through the myometrium. Postoperative high voltage irradiation is also given to cases with growth almost throughout the myometrium irrespective of the differentiation, and to those with tumour cells in endothelial lined spaces.

Stage II

Stage II disease is defined as endometrial carcinoma with extension to the endocervix, but with no clinical evidence of tumour beyond the uterus. Extension to the endocervix traditionally has been verified by fractional curettage. In some clinics the extension to the endocervix is evaluated by hysteroscopy. There is no doubt that the stage II lesions have a poorer prognosis than the stage I lesions and that the percentage of metastases to the pelvic wall is higher in these cases. Most clinics therefore prefer combination therapy in stage II carcinoma of the corpus, e.g. with preoperative intracavitary radium or caesium sources followed by surgery and thereafter external irradiation. Radical hysterectomy with lymphadenectomy has also been recommended (Stallworthy, 1971).

It should be emphasised, however, that the diagnosis of spread to the endocervix is often difficult. In many cases one may find tumour cells floating free in the curettings from the cervical canal. If these cases receive some sort of irradiation preoperatively, one will usually not be able to decide if the tumour has penetrated into the fibromuscular part of the cervix. Cases with free floating tumour cells have a prognosis which is comparable to stage I lesions, while in cases with gross tumour invasion, the prognosis is poor. In our randomised clinical trial (Onsrud et al, 1981) we also found that additional external irradiation to the pelvic wall did not make any difference to the treatment results in these two groups. The series was, however, small and so far no definite conclusions can be made. Currently we prefer to perform primary surgery in most cases of stage II carcinoma of the corpus. If there are gross (macroscopic) signs of invasion or if we find curettings from a cavity in the endocervix, we perform radical hysterectomy, otherwise simple hysterectomy. We have not planned lymphadenectomy in these old, obese patients, but we prefer to give external high voltage irradiation, 5000 rads (50 Gy), to the pelvic lymph nodes. The future will show if this is a safe way of treating these patients.

Stage III

If the tumour has involved the parametrium or the ovaries but is still within the pelvis, the prognosis decreases further. Fortunately, there are few patients who show up with stage III disease. If the clinical examination indicates involvement of one or both ovaries, primary operation should be performed because one can never be sure that the lesion is primary in the endometrium or in the ovaries. All these cases should receive external irradiation either to a pelvic field or to a combined pelvic and para-aortic field according to the findings during laparotomy. In addition, long-term treatment with progestogens for one to two years may possibly increase the salvage rate.

Stage IV

Very seldom one may find that endometrial cancer, which extends to the endocervix, also involves the rectal or bladder mucosa, which indicates a stage IV lesion. Distant metastases also means that the case belongs to stage IV. It is difficult to give advice about the treatment schedule in such cases. However, it seems that all cases should receive progestogens for the rest of their life. Remarkable regressions of metastases have been seen during such treatment. If possible, a combination of intracavitary and external irradiation to the pelvis may also give a palliation and local control of the tumour. If progestogens do not seem to work after two to three months, additional chemotherapy with, for example 5-fluorouracil may increase the response rate. Adriamycin has also been used in such cases. Fortunately, there are few cases which present themselves in stage IV. The overall survival rate in this stage is only 5 to 10 per cent.

Recurrent disease

Although most patients have a stage I lesion when they are first seen, metastases will be found in the pelvis, along the para-aortic region and in bone and lung. To date, recurrences from carcinoma of the corpus have been treated with high doses of progestogens, either 17-hydroxyprogesterone acetate or medroxyprogesterone. In most series the response rate with hormone treatment has been between 25 and 30 per cent. The highest response rates will be found in those with lung metastases. It is not unusual to find that lung metastases disappear completely after two to three months of hormone therapy. In some cases one may achieve permanent cure. It should be emphasised, however, that when a good response has been achieved and, for example, lung metastases have disappeared, one should not stop treatment because it is the experience of most authors that the metastases start growing as soon as the progestogen is stopped.

There is now an increasing interest in progesterone and oestrogen receptor studies which seem to help in predicting the response to hormone treatment of advanced or recurrent endometrial carcinoma. Erlich et al (1980), Iacobelli et al (1980), Kauppila et al (1980) all conclude that there is a good correlation between receptor activity and the response to progestogen therapy.

Chemotherapy in corpus cancer has not been well evaluated, mainly because of the good response to progestogens. However, drugs as 5-fluorouracil or melphalan may add to the response rate if hormone therapy fails (Piver et al, 1980).

REFERENCES

Aalders J, Abeler V, Kolstad P, Onsrud M 1980 Post-operative external irradiation and prognostic parameters in stage I endometrial carcinoma. Obstetrics and Gynecology 56: 419–427

Annual report on the results of treatment in gynecological cancer 1979 vol 17, Radiumhemmet, Stockholm, Sweden

Ballon C B, Roberts J A, Lagasse 1979. Obstetrics and Gynecology 54: 163–166

Bates T D, Churchill-Davidsen I 1975 Hyperbaric oxygen combined with irradiation in the treatment of advanced carcinoma of the cervix (Ch. 4 In: Brush M G, Taylor R W (eds) 1975 Gynecological malignancy. Baillière Tindall, London

Beecham J B, Halvorsen T, Kolbenstvedt A 1978 Gynecologic Oncology 6: 95–105

Bergsjö P, Kolstad P 1968 Clinical trial with atmospheric oxygen breathing during radiotherapy of cancer of the cervix. Scandinavian Journal of Clinical Laboratory Investigation 22, Suppl 106: 167–171

Boronow R C 1976 Endometrial cancer. Not a benign disease. Obstetrics and Gynecology 47: 630–634

Broders A C 1926 Carcinoma grading and practical application. Archives of Pathology 2: 376–381

Bush R S 1979 Malignancies of the ovary, uterus and cervix. Arnold, London, ch 13

Conroy J F, Lewis G C, Brady L W, Brocsky I, Kahn S B, Ross, D, Nuss R 1976 Cancer 37: 660–664

Erlich C E, Cleary R, Young P 1980 Which endometrial cancers respond to progestin therapy? Contemporary Obstetrics and Gynecology 15: 139–140

Fidler H K, Boyes D A, Nichols T M, Worth A J 1970 Cervical cytology in the control of cancer of the cervix. Modern Medicine of Canada 25: 9–15

Gad C 1976 Treatment and survival in 631 patients with invasive carcinoma of the cervix. British Journal of Obstetrics and Gynaecology 83: 560–566

Gray L H 1961 Radiobiological basis of oxygen as a modifying factor in radiation therapy. American Journal of Roentgenology 85: 803–815

Gusberg S B 1980 The changing nature of endometrial cancer. New England Journal of Medicine
302: 729–731

Hakama M, Räsänen-Vitanen V 1976 Effect of a mass screening program on the risk of cervical cancer.
American Journal of Epidemiology 103: 512–517

Iacobelli S, Longo P, Scombia G, Natoli V, Sacco R 1980 Progesterone receptors and hormone sensitivity
of human endometrial carcinoma. In: Iacobelli S, Di Marco A (eds) Progress in cancer research and
therapy, Rowen Press, New York, vol 15, p 97–106

Iversen T, Abeler V, Kjörstad K E 1974 Factors influencing the treatment of patients with stage Ia
carcinoma of the cervix. British Journal of Obstetrics and Gynaecology 86: 593–597

Kauppila A, Jarme O, Kujansuu E, Vihko R 1980 Treatment of advanced endometrial adenocarcinoma
with a combined cytologic therapy. Predictive value of cytosol estrogen and progestin receptor levels.
Cancer 46: 2162–2167

Khoo S K, Mackay E V 1974 Carcinoembryonic antigen by radioimmunoassay in the detection of
recurrence during long-term follow-up of female genital cancers. Cancer 34: 542–548

Kistner R W 1970 Effects of progestational agents on hyperplasia and carcinoma in situ of the
endometrium: 10 year follow-up. International Journal of Gynecology and Obstetrics 8: 561–572

Kjörstad K E, Örjasaeter H 1977 Studies on carcinoembryonic antigen levels in patients with
adenocarcinoma of the uterus. Cancer 40: 2953–2956

Kjörstad K E, Örjasaeter J 1982 Cancer (in press)

Kjörstad K E, Welander C, Halvorsen T, Grude T, Onsrud M 1978 Progestogens as primary treatment in
premalignant changes of the endometrium. In: Brush M G, King R J B, Taylor R W (eds) Endometrial
cancer. Baillière Tindall, London, ch 21

Kneale B 1970 Pelvic lymph node metastases in carcinoma of the cervix. Australia and New Zealand
Journal of Obstetrics and Gynaecology 10: 167–171

Kolbenstvedt A, Kolstad P 1976 The difficulties of complete lymph node dissection in radical hysterectomy
for carcinoma of the cervix. Gynecological Oncology 4: 244–254

Kolstad P, Klem V 1976 Long-term follow-up of 1121 cases of carcinoma in situ. Obstetrics and
Gynecology 48: 125–129

Krupp P J, Bohm J W 1978 Obstetrics and Gynecology 51: 702–705

Macgregor J E 1976 Evaluation of mass screening programmes for cervical cancer. Tumori 62: 287–295

Martzloff K H 1923 Relative malignancy of cancer of the cervix uteri as indicated by the predominant
cancer cell type. Bulletin of the Johns Hopkins Hospital 34: 141–149, 184–195

McGowan W 1978 The dying gynecologic cancer patient and society. Gynecologic Oncology.
Appleton-Century-Croft, New York, ch 25, p 416

Morrow C P, DiSaia P J, Townsend D E 1973 Current management of endometrial carcinoma. Obstetrics
and Gynecology 42: 399–403

van Nagel J R, Meeker W R, Parker J C 1975 Carcino-embryonic antigen in patients with gynecologic
malignancy. Cancer 35: 1372–1376

Nieminen U, Hiilesmaa V K, Timonen S 1977 Results of treatment of carcinoma of the cervix 1964–1969.
A report of 768 cases. Annales chirurgiae et gynaecologiae 66: 234–239

Onsrud M, Aalders J, Abeler V, Taylor P 1981 Gynecologic Oncology (in press)

Papanicalaou G N, Traut H F 1943 Diagnosis of uterine cancer by the vaginal smear, Commonwealth
Fund, New York

Piver M S, Barlow J J, Vangtama V, Webster J 1974 Hydroxurea and radiation therapy in advanced
cervical cancer. American Journal of Obstetrics and Gynecology 120: 969–972

Piver M S, Lele S, Barlow J J 1980 Melphalan, 5-fluorouracil and medroxyprogesterone acetate in
metastatic endometrial carcinoma. Proceedings of the American Association of Cancer Research 21: 425

Poulsen H E, Taylor C W, Sobin L H (eds) 1975 Histological typing of female tract tumours. World Health
Organization, Geneva

Rampone J F, Klem V, Kolstad P 1973 Combined treatment of stage Ib carcinoma of the cervix. Obstetrics
and Gynecology 41: 163–167

Sakamoto S, Tojo S, Nokayama T (eds) 1980 Gynecology and obstetrics. Excerpta Medica, Amsterdam

Scully R E 1980 Cancer of the uterine corpus — pathologic types. International Journal of Radiology,
Oncology, Biology and Physics 6: 361–364

Stallworthy J A 1971 Surgery of endometrial cancer in the Bonney tradition. Annals of the Royal College of
Surgeons 48: 293–305

The Cancer Registry of Norway. Trends in cancer incidence in Norway 1955–67. Universitetsforlaget,
Oslo, 1972

Walker J H 1980 The epidemic of endometrial cancer. American Journal of Public Health 70: 264–267

Wentz W B, Reagan J W 1959 Survival in cervical cancer with respect to cell type. Cancer 12: 384–388

Woodruff J D 1965 Treatment of recurrent carcinoma in situ of the lower genital tract. Chir Obstet Gynec
8: 757–760

Index

Abnormalities, of fetal heart rate, 28–33
    baseline fetal bradycardia, 29
    fetal heart rate patterns, 30–33
    tachycaria, 28–29
    variability of baseline rate, 30
Abortion, risk from amniocentesis, 52–53
Acute group B streptococcal sepsis (GBS), 140–143
    antenatal prevention, 142
    neonatal signs and diagnosis, 142
    prevention in the neonate, 143
Affection, bonding of *see* mother-infant interaction
Air leaks, in respiratory distress syndrome, 140
Amenorrhoea, lactational, 196
Amniocentesis, 47–67
    complications of,
        fetal, 51–53
        maternal, 51
    indications for,
        amniography, 66–67
        genetic disease and congenital abnormality *see*
            Genetic amniocentesis
        maturity studies, 64–66
        polyhydramnios, 66
        rhesus incompatibility, 61–64
    technique of,
        early pregnancy, 49–50
        late pregnancy, 50
Amniography, 66–67
Amniotic fluid,
    clinical physiology, 47–49
    sampling *see* Amniocentesis
Antenatal cardiotocography *see* Cardiotocography
Asia, trends in perinatal mortality in, 203–205
Asphyxia, antepartum, 22–23
Aspirator, for oocyte retrieval, 268, 269

Basal body temperature, in detection of ovulation,
    221–226
Blood gas monitoring, in labour, 37–39
    in respiratory distress syndrome, 138–139
Bonding, infant, *see* Mother-infant interaction
Bradycardia, fetal, 29
Breast cancer, 315–316
Breast feeding,
    and fertility *see* Lactation
    and immunology, 175
Breast milk,
    antibacterial aspects of, 122
    changes in composition, 122
    hormones and prostaglandins in, 123
    human milk banks, 129

Breast milk (*cont.*)
    pre-term, 129–130
Breech delivery, 133
Bromocriptine, for dysovulatory infertility, 254
Bronchopulmonary dysplasia (BPD), 140

Caesarean section, and respiratory distress
        syndrome, 133
Caine drug effect, 32–33
Cancer,
    breast, 315–316
    cervical *see* Cervical cancer
    endometrical *see* Endometrial cancer
    uterine, 314–315
Carcinoembryonic antigen (CEA), in cervical
        cancer, 333–334
Cardiography, 18–23, 25–27
    frequency of recording, 22
    interpretation of, 20–21
    oxytocin stress test (OCT), 18
    unstressed, 19
    see also Fetal heart rate
Catheter, for embryonic transfer, 276–277
Cervical cancer, 325–339
    carcinoembryonic antigen in, 333–334
    chemotherapy, 332–333
    epidemiology, 327
    histopathology, 327–328
    stage distribution, 328–332
Cervical mucus,
    periovulatory changes,
        chemical constituents, 230–231
        physical, 226–230
Cervix,
    cancer of *see* Cervical cancer
    morphological changes, 231
Childbirth, fertility after *see* Fertility
Clinical diabetes mellitus, in pregnancy, 100–110
    assessment of fetal wellbeing, 105
    classification, 100–101
    complications of, 103–105
    control of, 102–103
    general problems, 101
    infants of diabetic mothers, 107–110
        malformations, 108
        perinatal morbidity, 108–110
    labour and, 107
    management, 101–102
    mode of delivery, 106–107
    timing of delivery, 105–106
    see also Diabetes mellitus

Clomiphene (Clomid), 248–250
  and corticosteroids, 249
  and HCG, 250
  and oestrogen, 249–250
Collagen diseases, in pregnancy, 82–83
Continuous tissue pH, 35–37
Continuous tissue PO2(TCPO2), 37–39
Contraception,
  during lactation, 196–197
  supplementary food during breast feeding and,
    189–191
Corpus uteri,
  cancer of see Endometrial cancer
Cost-benefit analysis, 308
Cost effectiveness analysis, 308
  applied to post menopausal hormone therapy see
    Post menopausal hormone therapy

Daily fetal movement count (DFMC), see Fetal
    movement recording
Danazol (Danocrine), 255
Decelerations, in fetal heart rate, 30–33
Deep vein thrombosis, 316
Delivery,
  blood lactate levels during, 39
  in diabetic mothers, 105–107
  maternal position at, 41
Detection of ovulation,
  hormone assays see Hormone assays
  intermenstrual pain, 233–234
  periovulatory effects,
    basal body temperature, 221–226
    cervical morphology, 231
    cervical mucus, 226–231
    endometrial histology, 232
    vaginal cytology, 232
  premenstrual symptoms, 234
  saliva, 233
  ultrasonography, 234–235
Developing world, perinatal mortality see Perinatal
    mortality
Diabetes mellitus,
  and pregnancy, 83, 95–110
    clinical see Clinical diabetes mellitus
    gestational see Gestational diabetes mellitus
    history, 95–97
    physiology, 97
Dietary needs, of pre-term infants, 124–127
  caloric intake, 126–127
  carbohydrate, 125–126
  fat, 25
  minerals, 126
  protein, 124–125
  vitamins, 26
Doppler ultrasound cardiography, 27
Dysovulatory infertility, 241–256
  initial assessment of the couple, 246–247
  menstrual cycle and, 241–246
  treatment, 247–255
    bromocriptine, 254
    clomiphine see Clomiphene
    danazol, 255

Dysovulatory infertility, treatment (cont.)
    gonadotrophin releasing hormone (GnRH), 255
    human gonadotrophins see Gonadotrophins
    oestrogen and progesterone, 251
    placebo effect, 251
    summary and conclusions, 255–256

Ejaculation,
  premature, 292
  retarded, 292
Electrocardiography, fetal, 25–27
Embryo transfer (ET), 259–280
  catheters, 276–277
  developmental stage of embryo, 273–274
  difficulties, 278
  number of embryos transferred, 274–276
  post ET care, 280
  route of transfer, 276
  successful, 278–280
  technique of transcervical transfer, 277–278
  see also In vitro fertilisation
Endometrial cancer, 325–339
  epidemiology, 334
  histopathology, 335
  recurrent disease, 339
  stage distribution, 335–336
  treatment, 336–339
Endometrium,
  cancer of see Endometrial cancer
  histology, 232
Erectile dysfunction,
  characteristics, 291–292
  premature ejaculation, 292
  retarded ejaculation, 292
  treatment, 302–303
Estrogen therapy, postmenopausal, 310–320
  benefits,
    effect on skin, 313
    prevention of osteoporosis, 312–313
    relief of symptoms, 310–312
    unproven, 313–314
  costs, 318–319
  risks,
    breast cancer, 315–316
    changes in glucose tolerance, 317
    deep vein thrombosis, 316
    gallstones, 317
    increase in blood pressure, 317
    postmenopausal bleeing, 314
    uterine cancer, 314–315
Ethology, 161–162

Feeding, pre-term infants,
  adaptation to extrauterine feeding, 123–124
  amino acids, 121
  breast milk see Breast milk
  dietary needs see Dietary needs, of pre-term
    infant
  methods of, 127–130
    milk, 128–130
    total parenteral nutrition (TPN), 127–128
  physiological response to, 123

Fertilisation,
    culture *see* Fertilisation culture
    in vitro *see* In vitro fertilisation
Fertilisation culture, 268–273
    insemination, 272–273
    oocyte identification, 270–272
    quality control procedures, 268–270
Fertility,
    after childbirth *see* Lactational infertility
    assessment, 262
    detection of ovulation *see* Detection of ovulation
Fetal heart rate,
    abnormalities of *see* Abnormalities of fetal heart
        rate electrocardiography, 25–27
        Doppler ultrasound, 27
        external, 26
        phonocardiography, 26–27
    interpretation of patterns, 28–33
Fetal monitoring, in labour, 25–42
    computers for, 41–42
    electrocardiography *see* Fetal heart rate
    fetal blood sampling, 33–34
    fetal heart rate *see* Fetal heart rate
    radiotelemetry, 41
    recent developments, 34–39
    selection of patients for, 39–40
    tocography, 27–28
Fetal movement recording, 13–18
    daily fetal movement count (DFMC),
        clinical application, 16
        clinical interpretation, 16–18
    future developments, 18
Follicle stimulating hormone (FSH),
    in lactation, 193
    in regulation of ovulation, 215–217

Gallstones, 317
Genetic amniocentesis, 53–61
    chromosomal abnormalities, 57–61
    neural tube defects, 55–57
    X-linked recessive disorders, 61
Genetic-obstetric clinic, 54–55
Genital secretions, 284–285
Gestational age, estimation of, 64–66
Gestational diabetes mellitus, 97–100
    diagnosis of, 98–99
    infant mortality and, 100
    management of, 99–100
Glomerulonephritis, in pregnancy, 80–82
Glucose tolerance, 317–318
Gonadotrophin releasing hormone (GnRH), 255
Gonadotrophins,
    during lactation, 193
    human, for dysovulatory infertility, 251–253
        chorionic (HCG), 250–252
        menopausal (HMG), 251–252
        pituitary (HPG), 251–252
        treatment with, 252–253

High risk pregnancy, monitoring of, 3–23
    antenatal cardiotocography *see* Cardiotocography
    clinical techniques, 3–9

High risk pregnancy, monitoring of (*cont.*)
    dynamic tests of fetal wellbeing, *see* Fetal
        movement recording
    hormone assays, 12
    ultrasonography *see* Ultrasonography
    uterine growth, 9–10
Hormone assays,
    and ovulation,
        luteinising hormone, 219–220
        oestrogens, 220–221
        pregnanediol, 217–219
        progesterone, 217–219
    in high risk pregnancy, 12
Hormone therapy, postmenopausal *see*
        Postmenopausal hormone therapy
Human milk banks, 129
Human placental lactogen (HPL), 12
Hypertonus, 33
Hypothalamus, sensitivity in lactation, 193–194

Idiopathic infertility, 260
Impotence *see* Erectile dysfunction
India, perinatal mortality in, 203–204
Indonesia, perinatal mortality in, 204
Infertility,
    detection of ovulation for *see* Detection of
        ovulation
    dysovulatory *see* Dysovulatory infertility
    idiopathic, 260
    lactational *see* Lactational infertility
    tubal, 259–260
Insemination, and fertilisation culture, 272–273
Intensive care, neonatal, 118–121
Intermenstrual pain, 233–234
Intrapartum fetal monitoring *see* Fetal monitoring
Intraventricular haemorrhage, 146–148
In vitro fertilisation (IVF), 259–280
    embryo transfer *see* Embryo transfer
    fertilisation culture *see* Fertilisation culture
    pretreatment investigation, 264–265
    retrieval of mature oocytes, 266–268
    selection of patients, 262–264
    treatment cycle, 265–266
Isoimmunisation, 51

Japan, perinatal mortality in, 205

Karyopyknotic index (KPI), 232
Kidney, in pregnancy,
    anatomical changes, 71
    blood pressure regulation, 73–74
    functional changes, 71–73
Korea, perinatal mortality, 204

Labour,
    ambulation in, 40–41
    blood lactate levels during, 39
    control of diabetes in, 107
    fetal monitoring in *see* Fetal monitoring
    premature, 52–53
Lactate, blood levels in labour and delivery, 39
Lactation,
    contraception during, 196–197

Lactation (*cont.*)
effect on fertility, 181–187
gonadotrophins during, 193
hypothalamic sensitivity during, 193
ovarian sensitivity during, 194–196
ovulation during, 183–184
urinary steroid secretion during, 184–186
Lactational amenorrhoea, 196
Lactational infertility, 181–197
assessment of, 183
see also Lactation and Ovulation
Laparoscopy,
in assessment of pelvic status, 262–263
in retrieval of mature oocytes, 267
Low birthweight,
care of infants *see* Low birthweight infant
mortality from in developing world, 205–206
Low birthweight infant, care of, 115–148
effectiveness of intensive care, 118–121
feeding *see* Feeding pre-term infants
intraventricular haemorrhage, 146–148
mortality from in the developing world, 205–206
necrotising enterocolitis in *see* Necrotising
enterocolitis
post-natal wards, 116–118
respiratory distress syndrome *see* Respiratory
distress syndrome
streptococcal sepsis *see* Acute group B
streptococcal sepsis
Luteinising hormone (LH),
assay for, 219–220
during lactation, 193
in regulation of ovulation, 215–217, 219–220

Malaysia, perinatal mortality in, 205
Menopause, therapy *see* Postmenopausal hormone
therapy
Menstrual cycle,
abnormalities of, 241–242
evaluation of, 242–246
fertile, 241–242
hormone levels during, 215–217
Menstruation, effect of breast feeding on, 186–187
Mittelschmerz *see* Intermenstrual pain
Mortality,
neonatal, 53, 118–120
perinatal *see* Perinatal mortality
Mother-infant interaction, 161–178
bonding of affection, 162–163, 168–170
effects of drugs, 172–173
encouragement of, 173–174
general policy, 175–177
historical perspectives, 164–165
low birthweight and, 173
neonatal sensory system *see* Neonatal sensory
system
socio-economic influences, 174
vulnerable mother and, 170–172

Necrotising enterocolitis, 143–146
aetiology, 143–145
diagnosis, 145

Necrotising enterocolitis (*cont.*)
prevention, 145
treatment, 145–146
Neonatal mortality,
and amniocentesis, 53
effect of neonatal intensive care, 118–121
Neonatal sensory system, 166–168
attentive behaviour, 166
hearing, 168
individuality and adaptability, 168
interpreting need states, 166–167
smell, 168
vision, 167
Neonatal unit,
admission to, 116–117
effect on mortality, 118–121
see also Low birthweight infant
Net health care costs, 308–309
Net health effectiveness, 309–310
Non-stress test (NST), 18, 19

Oestradiol, in regulation of ovulation, 215–217
Oestriol, assay in pregnancy, 12
Oestrogens,
assay for ovulation, 220–221
in dysovulatory infertility, 249–250, 251
in postmenopausal therapy *see* Estrogen therapy
Oocyte,
identification, 270–272
retrieval for in vitro fertilisation, 266–268
Orgasm,
blended, 286
effect in pregnancy, 293
uterine, 286
vulval, 286
Orgasmic dysfunction,
primary, 289
secondary, 289
treatment, 299–300
Osteoporosis, 312–313, 319
Ovary,
access to for oocyte retrieval, 267
sensitivity during lactation, 194–196
Ovulation,
and breast feeding, 187–192
malnutrition, 191–192
supplementary food, 189
and lactation, 183–184, 192–197
and malnutrition, 191–192
detection of *see* Detection of ovulation
dysfunction of *see* Dysovulatory infertility
hormonal regulation, 215–217
relationship to first menstruation after birth,
186–187
Oxytocin stress test (OCT), 18

Patent ductus arteriosus (PDA), 139–140
Perinatal morbidity,
in diabetes mellitus, 108–110
renal disease and, 78
Perinatal mortality,
and renal disease, 78

Perinatal mortality (*cont.*)
  in diabetes, 100
  in the developing world, 201–211
    Asia, 203–205
      low birthweight and, 205–206
      model of perinatal care *see* Singapore
Periovulatory hormone effects *see* Detection of
    ovulation
Phillipines, perinatal mortality in 205
Phonocardiography, 26
Phospholipid spot area ratio (LSAR), 64–66
Polycystic kidney disease, 83
Polyhydramnios, 66
Postmenopausal bleeding, 314
Postmenopausal hormone therapy, cost
      effectiveness, 307–320
    analytical approaches, 307–310
    balancing risks and benefits, 319–320
    costs, 328–319
    oestrogen therapy *see* Estrogen therapy
Postnatal wards, 116–118
Pre-eclampsia,
    in diabetes mellitus, 104
    incidence with pre-existing renal disease, 77–78
Pregnancy,
    diabetes mellitus in *see* Diabetes mellitus
    effect on blood pressure, 76
    effect on the kidney, 71–74
    high risk *see* High risk pregnancy
    renal disease in *see* Renal disease
    sexuality in, 292–294
Pregnanadiol, assay for ovulation, 217–219
Prenatal assessment, 5–7
Progesterone,
    assay for ovulation, 217–219
    in dysovulatory infertility, 251
Prolactin, and lactational amenorrhoea, 196

Radiotelemetry, 41
Renal biopsy, in pregnancy, 86–87
Renal disease, in pregnancy, 71–91
    acute renal failure. 90–91
    management, 85–87
    nephrotic syndrome, 84–85
    pathophysiology of, 74–75
    problems, 76–78
    renal function during pregnancy, 75
    specific diseases, 80–84
Renal transplantation, and pregnancy, 87–90
    allograft rejection, 89
    counselling, 89–90
    management, 87–88, 89
    neonatal problems, 89
Respiratory distress syndrome (RDS), 130–140
    acid-base homeostasis, 137
    blood pressure and volume, 137
    complications, 139–140
    delivering premature infants, 133
    drug therapy, 137–138
    feeding and, 135
    fluid and electrolyte balance, 135–136
    management of, 133–134

Respiratory distress syndrome (*cont.*)
    monitoring infants with, 138–139
    surfactant physiology, 131–133
    ventilatory assistance, 137
Rhesus incompatibility, amniocentesis and, 61–
      64
Risk card, in pregnancy, 3–5

Saliva, periovulatory changes, 233
Semen, analysis, 262, 265
Sensate focus, 297–299
Sexual anatomy and physiology, 283–287
    effect of ageing, 287
    genital secretions, 284–285
    orgasm, 286–287
    pelvic vascularity and musculature, 283–
      284
Sexual counselling, 295–296
Sexual disorders, 283–304
    classification, 287
    diagnosis, 294–295
    female,
      causes, 290–291
      general, 289
      orgasmic dysfunction *see* Orgasmic
        dysfunction
      vaginismus *see* Vaginismus
    male,
      erectile dysfunction *see* Erectile dysfunction
    sexual counselling, 295–296
    treatment, 296–303
    see also Sexual dysfunction
Sexual dysfunction, 283–304
    incidence, 287–288
    sexuality in pregnancy, 292–294
    treatment, 296–303
    see also Sexual disorders
Sexual response, 285–286
Singapore, model of perinatal care, 207–211
    causes of perinatal death, 207–209
    domicilary after care services, 207
Spermatozoa, abnormality, 260–262
Sri Lanka, perinatal mortality in, 204
Surfactant, infant lung,
    composition, 131
    synthesis and release, 131–133

Tachycardia, fetal, 28–29
Thailand, perinatal mortality in, 204
Thromboembolism, 316
Tocography,
    external, 27–28
    internal, 28
Total parenteral nutrition (TPN), 127–128
Transcervical transfer, 277–278
Tubal infertility, 259–260
Tubulointerstitial disease, 83

Ultrasonography,
    assymetrical growth retardation, 11–12
    in detection of ovulation, 234–235
    poor intrauterine fetal growth, 11

Ultrasonography (*cont.*)
routine scanning, 10–11
symmetrical growth retardation, 11
Urolithiasis, 83–84
Uterine cancer, 314–315

Vagina, cytology of, 232
Vaginismus,
characteristics, 289–290
treatment, 300–301